Problems in the Behavioural Sciences

GENERAL EDITOR: Jeffrey Gray

EDITORIAL BOARD: Michael Gelder, Richard Gregory, Robert Hinde, Christopher Longuet-Higgins

Human organic memory disorders

Problems in the Behavioural Sciences

Human organic memory disorders

Andrew R. Mayes
Manchester University

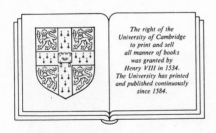

The right of the
University of Cambridge
to print and sell
all manner of books
was granted by
Henry VIII in 1534.
The University has printed
and published continuously
since 1584.

CAMBRIDGE UNIVERSITY PRESS

Cambridge
New York   New Rochelle   Melbourne   Sydney

Published by the Press Syndicate of the University of Cambridge
The Pitt Building, Trumpington Street, Cambridge CB2 1RP
32 East 57th Street, New York, NY 10022, USA
10 Stamford Road, Oakleigh, Melbourne 3166, Australia

First published 1988

Printed in the United States of America

Library of Congress Cataloging-in-Publication Data

Mayes, A. R. (Andrew Richard)
Human organic memory disorders.

(Problems in the behavioural sciences)
Bibliography: p.

1. Memory, Disorders of.   2.Memory.   I. Title.
II. Series.   [DNLM: 1. Memory – physiology.   2. Memory
Disorders.   WM 173.7 M468h]
RC394.M46M39   1988   616.85′232   87–30103

British Library Cataloguing in Publication Data

Mayes, Andrew

Human organic memory disorders.

1. Memory, Disorders of   2. Neurophysiology
I. Title
616.85′23   BF376

ISBN 0 521 34418 2 hard covers
ISBN 0 521 34879 X paperback

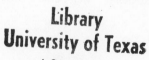

Contents

Acknowledgements

This book began as a joint effort with Peter Meudell, who very generously allowed me to use the material he had gathered on memory assessment, auditory–verbal short-term memory deficits, and semantic memory deficits. My views on these and other topics have benefited from many discussions with him and with Alan Pickering. I am particularly indebted to Jeffrey Gray for the great care and acumen with which he read the various drafts of the manuscript that finally led to this book. His comments helped shape my thinking and focus my conclusions in a more explicit and satisfactory form. I would also like to thank Peter Harforth for all his hard work with the preparation of the figures and Fran Morris for typing the references.

1   Healthy and pathological memory: the underlying mechanisms

Section One: The aims of this book

What were you doing immediately before you picked up this book? This question should cause you little difficulty, but there are people who would find it very hard to answer. For these people, known as organic amnesics, life must be experienced as if they were continually waking from a dream. Brain damage has made them very poor at remembering recently experienced events and at learning new information. It also makes them poor at remembering things that were learnt up to many years prior to the brain trauma. Despite such memory impairments, organic amnesics may have normal or superior intelligence. Not all memory deficits caused by brain damage are like organic amnesia, however. Other patients with lesions different from those responsible for organic amnesia show a very rapid loss of spoken information whilst possessing good longer term remembering of most things. For example, such a person might be unable to repeat back more than two spoken digits even with no delay but be able to give the gist of a newspaper article recounted by someone else on the previous day (something well beyond the powers of an organic amnesic). This kind of short-term memory failure is associated with the language disorder known as conduction aphasia and is clearly distinct from the memory deficits seen in organic amnesia, although both are caused by brain damage.

Brain damage is not, however, an essential prerequisite for memory pathology. More popular, at least in novels and films, are lapses of remembering caused by some unbearable emotional strain – the so-called functional amnesias, in which forgetting is thought to be motivated by an unconscious wish not to recall unpleasant memories. In other words, the memories are too painful for the victim to recall. A recent example is provided by the film *The Return of the Soldier*, based on a novel by Rebecca West. In the story, the hero returns from the trenches, apparently intact, except that he can no longer remember anything about his life at home, including the fact that he is married and that his son died in childhood. All that he can remember are the halcyon days of many years before when he was courting his first love. In the dénouement, the shock of being told about his son restores the lost memories. Cases like this are rare but probably authentic. Furthermore, not only do they not require brain damage, but such damage rarely causes so severe a memory loss of this kind. The nearest approximation is seen in senile dementia, but dements have many intellectual deficits not found in functional amnesics.

These examples of organic and functional memory deficits indicate that mem-

1

ory breaks down in a number of ways. The main aim of this book is to examine the variety of memory deficits that are caused by brain damage in order to gain insight into how the various kinds of memory are mediated by the brains of intact people. In order to do this, it is important, however, to be able to distinguish between organic and functional causes of poor memory. This is not easy to do, partly because such poor memory often has both organic and functional causes. For example, it is not uncommon to find that murderers cannot recall the circumstances of their crimes. These amnesias are sometimes found in individuals who were drunk when they killed their victims, so it is difficult to determine to what extent their forgetfulness is caused by alcohol-induced brain dysfunction at the time of the crime and to what extent by the need to repress painful memories on later occasions. The question of how we can distinguish between functional and organic memory failures is discussed briefly in chapter 2, which is about the assessment of memory problems.

In human beings, brain damage is an adventitious matter, which usually affects several brain regions that control different functions. Thus patients may simultaneously show several kinds of memory failure as well as other cognitive problems. If they do, it becomes hard to know whether the cognitive and memory failures are related and, indeed, whether there is truly one memory deficit or several, dissociable ones that happen to be occurring together. The analysis attempted in this book seeks to identify and characterize those memory disorders that are not made up of further, more selective memory deficits. In other words, it seeks to construct a kind of 'periodic table' of memory disorders and to analyse what underlies each elementary disorder. This goal can be achieved only by gradual approximations. Its fulfilment depends on the accurate description of the functions that have been lost and on the precise location of the brain lesion that causes such losses. It is difficult to be sure that a memory deficit is an elementary one. The ultimate test is whether smaller lesions in the same area where lesions cause the putatively elementary deficit produce merely a less severe problem of the same kind or whether they ever produce a more selective memory deficit. For example, organic amnesia can be caused by lesions in a brain region known as the medial temporal lobes, and involves poor ability to learn new information and poor memory for information acquired pre-traumatically. If it is an elementary memory disorder, it will be impossible to find cases where smaller lesions of the medial temporal lobes ever cause a problem either with new learning in isolation or with pre-traumatic memories in isolation. Such null hypotheses are notoriously hard to establish, but greater confidence in their truth is achieved if patients can be shown to have very circumscribed lesions and if theories of memory derived from studies of intact people suggest that only one memory process has been lost. These checks are, however, fallible because even small brain lesions may compromise several functional systems and because the study of intact people does not provide powerful evidence for the development of memory theories. Such theories are therefore likely to be inadequate and insufficiently articulated. Realistically, then, this book will aim to identify those memory deficits that are most selective and to specify what brain damage causes them.

If it is known what brain damage causes elementary kinds of memory deficit, where a single function is lost, then it becomes possible to consider how the healthy brain performs that function in intact people. It is too simple to assume without further evidence that the damaged region itself performs the lost function because the activity of apparently intact and normal brain regions may be disturbed by the lesion. Provisional identification of the damaged region as the one that normally performs the lost function may, however, be supported by studies that record electrophysiological and metabolic activity in the brains of intact people whilst they are learning and remembering. For example, recordings of electrophysiological activity made by electrodes placed in the medial temporal lobes of patients during memory tasks are consistent with the idea that this region helps mediate those memory processes disturbed in organic amnesics. Further confidence in the critical role of damaged structures may be gained through a knowledge of their inputs, outputs, and physiology. This knowledge may also provide significant constraints about how the lost function is performed and may ultimately lead to the development of a theory about how neural structures mediate the relevant function. Such theoretical advances are likely to depend heavily on animal studies. These studies not only allow the modelling of human organic amnesia and detailed physiological analysis of the structures damaged in this syndrome, but also may help determine whether there are more specific memory pathologies that have not been found in isolation in brain-damaged people. In this book, discussion of animal models of human memory pathologies and of the physiology and biochemistry of damaged regions will be directed mainly at organic amnesia, but physiological knowledge will be related to the other organic memory deficits where it is relevant.

Organic memory disorders are caused by particular brain regions working poorly either because they have been destroyed (lesioned) or because a biochemical abnormality makes them malfunction. Such disorders are surprisingly common. Apart from selective disorders, such as organic amnesia and the short-term memory deficit, mentioned in the first paragraph, an incomplete list of well-known conditions that are associated with poor memory of various kinds would include normal ageing and pathological ageing, particularly as in Alzheimer's dementia, Parkinson's disease, Huntington's chorea, multiple sclerosis, depression, and schizophrenia. In addition, more exotic kinds of brain damage have been linked with poor memory. For example, severing the fibres that link the two hemispheres of the human brain, an operation that has been performed on certain epileptic patients to relieve their seizures, has been claimed to cause some difficulty with the learning of new information. A subsidiary aim of this book is to discuss such memory disorders briefly to determine whether they are best construed as compounds of the elementary memory deficits that will be tentatively identified or whether they may involve novel kinds of memory impairment, the identification of which will require more research. The book is not concerned specifically with remediation, although this will be discussed when it fits naturally with a discussion of biochemical or other matters.

In summary, this book will outline the ways in which brain damage in humans causes memory to break down by constructing a 'periodic table' of memory disorders. The nature of the lost psychological functions underlying these elementary memory deficits will be characterized as fully as possible, and an attempt will be made to identify the lesions that cause them. The nature of the inputs, outputs, and physiology of the damaged regions will be discussed, and, where possible, animal models of particular deficits will be considered, in order to develop hypotheses about how the brain mediates the disturbed memory processes. In pursuing these aims, some attention will be paid to less well-specified organic memory problems, such as those associated with ageing and multiple sclerosis, to see whether they can be understood as compounds of the elementary memory disorders.

Although research on human memory pathologies began about 100 years ago, it has mushroomed only in the past 20 years, during which time it has been guided by theoretical ideas drawn from studies of intact people. For this reason, an outline of these ideas is given in the next section. It has already been indicated, however, that research on the memory of intact people may not be a powerful source of ideas about basic memory processes. Neuropsychologists who study organic memory deficits would therefore be unwise to follow too slavishly ideas drawn from this area. The information they discover may indeed be inexplicable in terms of current memory theories and may lead to the emergence of new ideas about memory. But if this is to happen, patients must be studied by researchers who are not blinkered by current theoretical preconceptions – open-mindedness is essential. The section on theoretical ideas drawn from studies of healthy people is followed by one on the ideas about memory that have emerged from physiological studies of memory in animals. The final section sketches the main memory deficits considered to be elementary in this book and introduces the brain regions, damage to which causes these deficits.

Section Two: Theories derived from the study of normal people

Introduction

Research on memory in normal people has been shaped by three theoretical distinctions. The first and oldest hypothesis, made by Plato and Aristotle, divides memory into three stages: registration, storage, and retrieval. In its inchoate form, this theory provides no new information about how human and animal memory works, as any memory system must logically be divisible into these three stages. Modern interest in it lies in the way the stages should be characterized. The nature of these characterizations determines the acceptability of the other two theories. According to the first of these, memory for rapidly forgotten information is mediated in a basically different way from memory for slowly forgotten information. Somewhat different versions of this theory have been used to explain short- and long-term memory in humans and physiological data with simpler kinds of memory in animals. The third kind of theoretical distinction differentiates among several kinds of long-term memory.

The potential application of these hypotheses to the interpretation of memory pathologies is obvious. As later chapters will show, memory breakdowns have been ascribed to selective failure of registration, storage, or retrieval; to selective failure of short- or long-term memory; and to selective failures of various kinds of long-term memory. To enable the reader to assess these explanations better, the three major kinds of theoretical distinction will be discussed more fully and the types of evidence relevant to them will be considered.

The division of human memory into the stages of registration, storage, and retrieval in itself says nothing about such memory. What matters is the specification of the characteristics of each stage. To do this, the Greeks relied on analogies that compared human memory to the storage of books in a library or of birds in an aviary. In these analogies, what is registered corresponds to a particular book or bird, storage corresponds to keeping the book in the library or the bird in the aviary, and retrieval corresponds to finding the book or bird later. These analogies say next to nothing about the kinds of information processing involved in registration and retrieval or about the way in which information is organized in storage. They also differ from organic memory in one fundamental respect. In human and animal memory, what is registered is not the thing itself but some representation of it. This commonplace distinction between an object and its representation is not apparent in the library and aviary analogies of memory.

What has been learnt about memory's three stages through a century of research into normal human memory?

Encoding and retrieval

One generalization that has emerged to become fashionable in the past decade is the view, developed from the work of Craik and Lockhart (1972), that things are remembered better if they are registered so as to be meaningful to the learner. This view has been supported by many experiments in which subjects are instructed to process verbal or non-verbal stimuli either in terms of meaning or in terms of physical features. For example, a subject might be told either to say which semantic category a word belongs to or to say whether it is written in upper- or lower-case letters. The subjects usually remember the meaningfully processed material better, even if they were not informed during presentation that their memories would be tested later. Originally, Craik and Lockhart argued that meaningfully processed material was better remembered because it was processed more deeply, and more deeply processed information was forgotten more slowly. Neither of these notions has stood up very well over the past decade. 'Depth' was a concept that rested on the assumption that semantic or meaningful information was extracted at a later stage in the sequence of information processing than were physical features, such as shape or colour. It has been found, however, that subjects can sometimes report semantic details of presented material more quickly than they can report some physical features (for a discussion, see Lloyd, Mayes, Manstead, Meudell, & Wagner, 1984). This has been taken as indicating that semantic features can be registered fairly early in the processing sequence. Similarly, it has been reported that information about semantic features can be forgotten as fast as information about physical features (Nelson & Vining, 1978). More popular now is the view that meaningfully registered or encoded information is remembered better for two reasons: It is encoded so as to be distinct from other information in memory, and the encoded information is better linked to other information in memory. The effect of these encoding advantages is to render such memories easier to find and identify.

The concept of 'distinctiveness' may be intuitively appealing, but it lacks precision. One way to clarify its use is by conceiving of the registration of events in terms of the encoding of a list of features. The distinctiveness of the encoding would then be determined by the number of features uniquely related to the event. This distinctiveness depends on the conditions of retrieval as well as those of learning (see Bransford, 1979). Encoding that is 'transfer-appropriate' leads to the best memory. For example, if subjects are asked about a word's size at retrieval, they will remember best if they encoded the word's physical attributes rather than its meaning. In other words, memory is best when there is correspondence between features encoded and those that are later used as cues during retrieval.

Distinctive and transfer-appropriate kinds of registration not only lead to good recall and recognition, but also are regarded as effortful forms of encoding. They are so regarded because the encoding of meaningful features typically involves processing additional information not immediately apparent in an experienced event. If these kinds of encoding are effortful, then they should be disrupted when subjects perform other cognitive activities at the same time, and effortful encoding should disrupt other cognitive activities. All effortful processes compete with one another in this way and are probably intended behaviours in that, for example, the encoder can indicate what he is aiming to encode. Hasher and Zacks (1979) have contrasted effortful encoding of this kind with automatic encoding of information. In their view, automatic encoding uses minimal attentional capacity and occurs without intentional direction so that other cognitive activities undertaken at the same time are minimally disturbed. Also, automatic encoding is only minimally disrupted by the simultaneous performance of other cognitive operations. Hasher and Zacks have argued that spatiotemporal features of events are automatically encoded and that this ability is fully developed in young children. More polemically, they have claimed that spatiotemporal features can be encoded only automatically and are not more effectively encoded if effort is applied. In contrast, they have also argued that people learn to encode some semantic features of words automatically. Kellogg (1980) has even shown that faces can be remembered at an above-chance level when little attention is paid to them during learning, which suggests that some facial features can be encoded automatically. No one denies, however, that face memory is much better when effortful registration can occur undisrupted by simultaneous performance of irrelevant cognitive operations. Both effortfully and automatically encoded features are necessary for good memory. It is interesting, therefore, that deficits in long-term memory have been attributed both to selective failures in automatic encoding and to selective failures in effortful encoding. The plausible underlying assumption is that different brain regions mediate the two forms of registration. The assumption is made more plausible by the sharp distinction drawn by Hasher and Zacks between the processes responsible for automatic and effortful encoding.

Appropriate encoding is necessary, but not sufficient, for good subsequent remembering. This is because what is encoded is not necessarily well stored or stored at all. For good subsequent remembering to occur, further storage processes must take place. It is unreliable to decide what information has been encoded by examining the contents of memory after a delay because some of the encoded information may not have been properly stored. If this point is not grasped, there is a danger of blurring the processes of storage with those of registration. The correct way to decide what has been registered is to find out what knowledge the learner can indicate he has at the time of learning so that a minimal memory load is imposed. The subject can indicate this knowledge either explicitly by an appropriate verbal or non-verbal response, such as pointing to an encoded sensory attribute, or implicitly when his behaviour indirectly reflects a recent experience. Implicit encoding can occur without explicit encoding, but explicit encoding always indicates implicit encoding. For example, if a person is shown a picture with a duck hidden in it, then she is usually unable to report seeing the duck. She may, however, be more likely to give 'duck' as a response when asked to give the name of the first farm animal that comes to mind, thus demonstrating that implicit encoding has occurred. If the duck had been identified initially, however, both forms of encoding would have occurred.

One of the discoveries of modern research is that implicitly encoded information has some impact on memory, albeit of a different kind from that found when the information has been explicitly encoded. The rememberer cannot describe the contents of what has been implicitly registered, but can indicate memory by indirect means. For example, Kunst-Wilson and Zajonc (1979) showed subjects irregular polygons for 0.001 sec each, too brief for conscious perception. Although conscious recognition of these shapes did not exceed a chance level, the subjects showed an aesthetic preference for the polygons they had been shown relative to similar novel polygons. Why is the explicit registration of events necessary for their later recognition, but not for the creation of more indirectly indicated memories? The answer is not yet available, but probably relates to the way in which the information is registered. In the example of the picture with the duck hidden in it, what is the difference between registering the duck's features explicitly or implicitly? The older view is that what is registered is the same, but for unknown reasons, the registered information is explicitly accessible in the former case only. A more recent proposal (Marcel, 1983) is that explicitly registered information is integrated, whereas implicitly registered information is fragmented. This proposal implies that the representation of an implicitly registered complex consists of a number of unintegrated fragments. Explicit registration means that these fragments are 'glued' together in an integrated whole. The idea can be tested because the components of an integrated representation should act as more effective cues for the rest of the representation than components of a fragmented representation. This idea is still primitive, but it may help explain organic amnesia because patients with this disorder, although still conscious, may store fragmented representations, just as if they were encoding implicitly.

In registration, information is processed so that a representation usually, but not necessarily, can be made of some external event. This representation may then be stored with varying degrees of efficiency. Unfortunately, modern research has had little useful to say about different modes of representation that may be used by the brain. It is not even clear what is meant by asking how information is represented. Thus it is not clear whether the same information about an external event can be represented in several different ways or whether different modes of representation mean that different aspects of the event and things related to it are being represented. For example, it is a matter of argument whether representing an event verbally uses a basically different code from the one used in representing it in terms of imagery. If the codes differ, the verbal one may be digital and the imagery one may be analogue, although no one has yet advanced a convincing test of this possibility. One reason for this failure is that representations cannot be directly examined because we can see their effects only after decoding. At present, psychology lacks a theory of how representations are encoded and decoded. Nevertheless, it seems likely that differences in mode of informational representation exist and, if they do, may well be associated with distinct registration, storage, and retrieval processes. If brain lesion A disturbs one kind of memory but not another, and lesion B has the reverse effect, this could be a weak indication that these two kinds of memory use distinct representational codes. Further evidence for this view would be available if the two brain regions were organized anatomically in very different ways.

How information is represented at registration and how it is represented in storage are closely related issues, and probably even less is known about the latter. Questions concerning the properties of storage are very poorly addressed by the study of intact human memory. Indeed, a recent review of human memory completely ignored storage processes and focused entirely on registration and retrieval systems (Horton & Mills, 1984). This is unfortunate for the neuropsychology of memory because some brain lesions may cause storage deficits. For example, it has been suggested that certain organic disorders of language arise partly because the patient has lost stored information about words. If so, current knowledge derived from studying intact people will not help in the more detailed characterization of such disorders. It would be useful to have knowledge about storage at two levels. The first level is the microscopic one and concerns those physiological changes within and between neurons that underlie memory. Fortunately, research on animal models has led to a partial elucidation of these processes, as will be described in the next section. The second level is the macroscopic one and concerns the way in which information is organized in the brain during storage. Second-level questions are far harder to answer than first-level questions, but can be divided into subquestions, some of which are easier to broach. Thus it is easier to determine where information is stored in the brain and whether different kinds of information are stored in different places. Furthermore, answers to these questions may be needed to resolve the trickier issue of how information is represented in storage. Preliminary attempts to answer the easier questions are discussed in the next section.

It is likely that the acquisition of complex information about events or general knowledge involves the registration and storage of many distinct features that are linked together in a Gestaltic unit. For example, remembering that one talked to two people on a certain London street yesterday involves storing information about the people's features, what was said, what the street was like, and so on, and all these things must be integrated so that they can be retrieved as a single event. Remembering occurs later when, during retrieval, some features of the originally encoded memory reactivate some of or all the other features. A very influential hypothesis about retrieval is the encoding specificity principle (see Tulving, 1984), which states that retrieval cues are effective only in so far as they have been encoded during original learning. When features constituting part of an original memory are re-encoded, there is (or may be) an automatic reactivation of the rest of the memory that does not further involve voluntary search processes. The more cues encoded at retrieval and the more distinctively they characterize the relevant memory, the better will be the remembering. Evidence shows that changes of background context, mode of presentation of information, and mood or physiological state between acquisition and retrieval lead to worse remembering (see Horton & Mills, 1984). This indicates that even those features unrelated to an event's interpretation form part of that event's representation in memory.

In contrast to Tulving, Jones (1979) has distinguished between cues that depend on intrinsic knowledge (encoded during original learning) and cues that depend on extrinsic knowledge (not so encoded). He argues that whereas intrinsic-knowledge cues are associated with rapid, automatic, and unconscious retrieval, extrinsic-knowledge cues are associated with a slower, more conscious, effortful, and inferential retrieval – sometimes called recollection. Recollection tends to occur when memories cannot readily be accessed. It seems to involve the use of extrinsic knowledge to find cues that will be sufficient to activate the automatic retrieval process. For example, in order to remember what one was doing on one's last birthday, it may be necessary to fill in a considerable amount of background before arriving at cues that will be sufficient to trigger the key information. The interplay of automatic and effortful processes in retrieval resembles that found at registration. The resemblance may be more than coincidence, for it is implicit in much recent theorizing that there is considerable overlap between the processes of registration and retrieval. Effortful registration and retrieval both involve planning activities, so if the capacity to plan is compromised, one would expect both effort-ful encoding and recollection to be affected. For example, as will be discussed later, lesions to the frontal lobes of the brain may impair memory at least partly for this reason. Furthermore, overlap is also likely because distinctive encodings require the retrieval of semantic information, whereas retrieval requires the en-coding of appropriate cues. But there is less reason to believe that the processes involved in more automatic kinds of registration and retrieval are the same.

Recognition and recall

There has been much discussion of and controversy about the processes required for recognition and recall of memories. An early view was that recall involved two processes: a process of generating candidate memories, and a process of iden-tifying the generated items as false or true memories. Recognition was thought to be usually superior to recall because it involved only the identification pro-cess, leap-frogging the generation process. If correct, this generate–recognize hypothesis might explain why recall is more affected than recognition in several organic memory disorders. The hypothesis is, however, almost certainly wrong (for discussions, see Horton & Mills, 1984; Tulving, 1984). Neither automatic nor effortful retrieval involves the systematic generation of candidate memories; accessing is more direct than the hypothesis suggests.

Even so, there is some evidence that recognition and recall depend on different kinds of information. For example, Fisher (1979) has shown that only recall is affected by the strength of the links between memory cues and the thing to be remembered, and only recognition is affected by the strength of the links between the thing to be remembered and background memory cues. Such cues are defined in contrast to the information on which attention is primarily focused. It has been argued by Baddeley (1982) that changes in background context, mood, or physio-logical state during the time between learning and retrieval, which probably do not alter the interpretation of target items, impair recall but have no effect on recognition. These features have been referred to as extrinsic context because it is plausible to argue that they do not influence the interpretation of the target information. Baddeley's claim about the absence of effects on recognition due to changes in extrinsic context seems to contradict Fisher's demonstration that recognition depends on the strength of the links between the thing to be remem-bered and background memory cues. The claim is open to challenge, however. For example, changes in mode of item presentation do impair recognition (for example, see Morton, Hammersley, & Bekerian, 1985), even though they are unlikely to alter interpretation of target material. It has also been found that changes in intrinsic context (which affects interpretation of target material) impair both recognition and recall.

Both recognition and recall depend on the ability of particular cues to activate other aspects of a complex memory. Recall seems to involve cues that help to link items to others acquired in the same context and cues that involve extrinsic context that may lead to the target items themselves. In contrast, with recognition, the main cue is the target item itself; to be accepted as a memory, this item must be re-encoded in the same way as it was during learning. If the encoding is sufficiently similar, then other aspects of the memory will be activated (perhaps those concerned with the mode of item presentation or the item's intrinsic context) and recognition will occur.

Mandler (1980) has argued, however, that there are two distinct recognition processes: familiarity and retrieval of an event's or item's context. The first operates with recognition of recently perceived items, and the second with recognition of older and weaker memories. His account of the mechanism underlying recognition of recently perceived items has been extended by Jacoby (in press), who argues that with such items, recognition is a product of the more rapid processing that they receive. Subjects attribute their greater processing speed to the items' familiarity. If correct, familiarity should not be affected by the absence of extrinsic contextual information available during learning, but merely require a probably automatic judgement that a recognized item has been processed faster than it would have been if unfamiliar. When memory becomes poorer, however, recognition requires the retrieval of a target's contextual background. In support of this view, Mandler has shown that recognition after a delay is influenced by the same organizational factors that link one event to another and that are known to affect recall. Recognition of recently perceived targets is not affected in this way. If Mandler's account of delayed recognition is correct, one would expect that it should be impaired by changes in background context. The explanation of how recognition is achieved after brief delays does face serious difficulties, however, because the notion that increased rapidity of processing recently perceived items makes them seem familiar is problematic. Thus it is unclear how subjects become aware of such increased processing rates, and, even if awareness is possible, there is evidence that increases in processing rate can occur for an item without its recognition (see chapter 6). Therefore, it could be that recognition always requires the retrieval of links between targets and their background or extrinsic context. Organic amnesics are poor at recognizing even recently perceived targets and may therefore be unable to access the targets' background context. It might be argued, however, that increased item-processing speed depends on retrieving extrinsic context, and so recognition would involve retrieval of such contextual features, faster item processing, and a judgement that faster processing has occurred (see the last section of chapter 6 for further discussion). If this possibility obtains, then poor recognition could result from a failure to retrieve extrinsic context cues, an impaired ability to base familiarity judgements on faster processing speeds, or other unspecified failures.

Storage and forgetting

Quite how recognition and recall differ from each other remains unclear. It is likely, however, that some processes are common to both, whereas other processes may be specific to recall or to recognition. If so, it is possible that some brain lesions will impair both, whereas others may disturb either recall or recognition in a relatively selective way. Although much still needs to be resolved, studies of intact people's memories have unearthed enough interesting phenomena to constrain thinking about registration and retrieval so as to provide a guide for neuropsychological theories of memory deficits. As already indicated, the same cannot be said about storage. Without reference to the physiological bases of storage, it is almost impossible to identify storage factors unequivocally as causes of memory effects in intact people. Two examples of this difficulty may have particular relevance to the interpretation of some memory pathologies. The first concerns the question of whether differences in memory are determined solely by variations in registration and retrieval or whether they are also caused by variations in storage efficiency. The second concerns the problem of what causes forgetting as the time from learning increases.

The difficulty in resolving the first question is illustrated by considering why applying increased attentional effort to target material usually improves subsequent memory. It is hard to imagine how an increase in effort can be obtained without affecting registration. Although some have claimed that they were able to manipulate effort in order to affect memory without influencing registration, this claim has proved polemical and not easy to substantiate (Tyler, Hertel, McCallum, & Ellis, 1979). Whether attentional effort modulates initial storage processes as well as registration therefore remains uncertain. In general, theories of normal memory offer no guidance to neuropsychologists about the kinds of processing deficits that will impair storage.

Uncertainty about the causes of forgetting over time does not persist because of a lack of experimentation. The problem is one of the most explored in memory research with intact people. All theories are of two main kinds. Forgetting is said either to result from decay of the store as time passes or to be caused by increased difficulty with retrieval as new memories are laid down. (Some have also argued that previously acquired memories exert a growing effect as time passes.) The second hypothesis is called the interference theory of forgetting. Because decay cannot be examined directly, research has focused on interference processes. Interference certainly causes forgetting, apparently by degrading retrieval cues for target material by attaching the cues to other memories as well. The extent to which it is responsible for normal forgetting over time is another matter. Even so, it is plausible to argue that as the amount of interference increases, so does forgetting. If so, brain damage that increases susceptibility to interference might also increase forgetting rate. The relationship of decay and interference to the shape and steepness of the forgetting function is, however, a mystery. Whereas Ebbinghaus and others have found that the rate of forgetting decreases steadily as the retention interval increases, it has been recently shown by Bahrick (1984) that for very overlearnt material, forgetting occurs in this way for only the first 3 to 6 years, and then for the next 30 years there may be no forgetting. Explanation of these functions may be possible only when storage can be more directly indexed. At present, it is controversial whether brain damage can cause pathologically fast forgetting or whether it merely lowers initial levels of remembering, leaving the rate of forgetting normal. It is also unknown whether brain damage can affect the shape of the forgetting function. If such effects occur largely because of storage deficits, then once again, knowledge derived from studying intact people will offer little guidance in interpreting the deficits. Guidance will come in the end from physiological studies of animals.

What, then, has been learnt about the three stages of memory by examining normal human performance? There is evidence that both registration and retrieval of complex information depend on automatic processes that require minimal intentional direction and on effortful processes that do require intentional direction and also use attentional resources. The same processes may well be involved in registration and retrieval, although each of the two memory stages probably also depends on other processes that are specific to it. Good memory very likely requires the operation of automatic and effortful processes at registration. The former may encode mainly contextual features at the periphery of awareness, whereas the latter is most effective if information is encoded distinctively and so as to be linked to other information already in memory. Retrieval is affected by the availability of contextual cues, and because recognition and recall are differently affected, they may depend on partially distinct retrieval processes. Despite these advances, little has been learnt about the extent to which storage variations are responsible for memory differences and, relatedly, about the way in which complex information is represented in the brain. Unfortunately, this ignorance is important when it comes to assessing the other two theoretical distinctions influential in contemporary thinking: that between short- and long-term memory, and that among different kinds of long-term memory. This point will be further discussed in the final section of this chapter, but for the moment it suffices to indicate that basic distinctions among kinds of memory probably reflect differences in modes of storage and representation, rather than simply differences in registration and retrieval processes.

Short-term memory

Originally, the idea of a short-term store was used to explain why so much information is rapidly forgotten. For example, Atkinson and Shiffrin (1971) proposed the existence of a store holding a limited amount of verbal information, encoded in terms of acoustic or articulatory features, for a short period of time. They believed that the fate of incoming information is a function of structural constraints, provided by the limited-capacity short-term store, and of control processes, which decide how information is registered and later retrieved. Information reaches long-term memory only after first passing through the short-term store. Other kinds of short-term store for non-verbal information have been postulated, but less often. Evidence regarded as favouring the existence of the short-term store typically showed that memory for rapidly forgotten verbal material is affected by factors different from the ones that influence more slowly forgotten information. Wickelgren (1974) has argued, however, that such dissociations are equally compatible with there being a single memory trace and storage strength depending on input conditions. In his view, fast forgetting occurs when storage is weak or there are similar competing items in memory, but not because information is in short-term storage.

Dissociable effects of variables on rapidly and slowly forgotten information therefore provide a necessary, but not a sufficient, condition for postulating a distinct short-term store. For example, being highly aroused or excited is believed often to impair short-term recall, but to improve longer term recall (see Eysenck, 1977). This effect could show that high arousal improves storage in a single system and also temporarily disrupts retrieval. The alternative, that the arousal strengthens long-term storage whilst weakening short-term storage, is no more plausible. Indeed, it is less plausible if one accepts Atkinson and Shiffrin's (1971) view that information is serially processed from the short-term store into the long-term one; disturbing the former should decrease the amount of information reaching the latter. The components of a single system of registration, storage, and retrieval might interact to give the superficial appearance that there were two storage systems. This has been argued by Wickelgren (1974), who has shown that the forgetting curves for short- and long-term retention are distinct, but then proposed that this is because of the greater amount of interference operating in short-term-recall tasks.

Short- and long-term recall are certainly affected by different factors. How these differences should be interpreted, however, is difficult to resolve, although most researchers still probably believe in distinct stores. Even so, the idea that there are distinct stores requires further elaboration and is only weakly supported by studies of intact people's memories. Such studies reveal little about the processes of storage. Without additional support (perhaps from neuropsychology), it might be safer to refer simply to short-term memory ability or abilities that are dissociable from long-term memory abilities. Convincing proof of the existence of a short-term store or stores will require convergent support from evidence derived from physiological research as well as studies of normal people.

Atkinson and Shiffrin's (1971) conception of short-term memory has been modified in two major ways in the past decade (Baddeley & Hitch, 1974). First, more than one kind of short-term store is now explicitly posited. As well as a store that holds verbal inputs (the phonological store), theorists have argued for another store that holds motor outputs (particularly those concerned with articulation) and for stores that hold sensory information (particularly visuospatial information in the 'visuospatial scratchpad') in a relatively 'raw' form (Baddeley & Hitch, 1974). Recently, Broadbent (1984) has further proposed that an abstract short-term memory system exists. Both he and Baddeley and Hitch believe that informational exchanges among these stores and between them and long-term memory are mediated by a general-purpose central executive. In Broadbent's view, the executive recodes information so that it can be transferred from one store to another, whereas Baddeley and Hitch also allow the executive a planning or organizational role. The second modification in thinking about short-term memory is that there is an increased interest in the functions of the system. It has been argued that its subsystems act as a working memory necessary for normal performance in tasks involving reasoning, comprehension, speech, and mental arithmetic, as well as the transfer of information into a long-term store. Working memory is then hypothesized to comprise several subsystems, each with its own specific functions. In principle, lesions should be capable of selectively impairing these subsystems, and, if so, their postulated functions should also be impaired. Whether the analysis of such lesion effects has helped distinguish between the view that separate short-term stores exist and the view that there are merely short-term-memory abilities operating within a single system for storing different kinds of complex memory will be discussed in chapter 3.

Long-term memory

Research on intact people has investigated primarily memory for complex things, such as knowledge about the world or language or about day-to-day autobiographical information. Within this domain, some workers have wished to distinguish between different kinds of long-term memory. As with the arguments for a separate short-term memory system, attempts to differentiate several long-term systems have been based on the search for dissociations between the possibly distinct systems. The implicit assumption underlying such attempts is that the occurrence of dissociations indicates the existence of two systems of registration, storage, and retrieval. Further, two systems of this kind are far more likely to exist if the information they store is represented in a different form. The path between dissociations and there being basically distinct kinds of long-term memory is, however, long and tortuous. For this reason, theorists are drawing increasingly on evidence from the effects of brain damage, which they believe to be convergent in its implications with that gathered from intact subjects.

Several distinctions have been proposed. First, many believe that the systems mediating remembering of verbal and visual information are separate and different. The stores involved are regarded as distinct from those required for short-term recall of these kinds of information. There has also been much, as yet inconclusive, discussion about whether visual and verbal materials are represented in radically different ways by the brain. It is known, however, that for visual and verbal materials memories are largely unrelated abilities, and there is much less interference among items held in the hypothetically distinct systems than there is among items held in the same system (see Broadbent, 1984). If visual and verbal long-term memory systems are indeed separate, future work may further subdivide them into several visual and verbal systems.

Second, Tulving (1984) has recently elaborated on a distinction, originally advanced a decade ago, between episodic and semantic memory. Episodic memory is the system concerned with remembering personally experienced autobiographical information, whereas semantic memory is the system concerned with remembering world and language knowledge without any necessary reference to the conditions of acquisition. In a recent review, Tulving (1984) lists 28 differences between episodic and semantic memory, although critics of the distinction do not regard these differences as sufficient reason for postulating two memory systems. The problem is that there is no theory of the two kinds of memory that enables one to interpret the observed differences. Without such a theory, it is difficult to apply Tulving's 'logic of dissociations', according to which if a variable differently affects episodic and semantic memory, then this shows they are distinct systems. Unfortunately, without a theory, there is no way of deciding whether the processing difference is trivial or of major significance. A memory taxonomy should be based on a theory that distinguishes between trivial processing differences and ones of central significance. Because no available theory does this, taxonomists interpret the logic of dissociations according to their intuitions.

A third kind of long-term memory distinction usually groups episodic and semantic memory together as kinds of declarative memory, the contents of which can be made directly accessible to consciousness. Such memories can be brought to mind as verbal propositions or as images, and may be of both personal episodes and impersonal facts. In contrast, procedural memory can be expressed only indirectly through skilled actions and perhaps conditioned responses or other behaviours that allow one to infer that the performer possesses certain kinds of knowledge. It is attributable to memory modifications that occur to processing operations. This kind of memory therefore includes knowledge necessary for displaying motor skills (such as riding a bicycle), perceptual skills (such as the ability to read mirror-reversed words), and certain 'intuitive' cognitive skills (such as the ability to make sound judgements from complex data without being able to say how one did so). It also includes what is usually referred to as 'priming', which occurs when an item is processed differently as a result of having been perceived at a point in the recent or fairly recent past. The change can often be described as one of increased efficiency of processing and has been shown to occur independently of the ability to recognize or recall the item in question (see Jacoby and Witherspoon, 1982). For example, when subjects are shown certain words and these words are subsequently displayed briefly in a list containing non-words and words, the subjects are quicker and more accurate at identifying them as words as distinct from non-words. Priming seems to be less affected by elaborative semantic encoding at input and to be forgotten at a different rate from declarative memories (for example, see Shimamura, 1986).

The status of these three distinctions is a matter of controversy. If the distinctions are valid, then exemplars of one putative kind of long-term memory must share more features and differ in fewer significant ways than putatively different kinds of memory. Also, if valid, the distinctions apply at different levels of generality, suggesting a hierarchical taxonomy (Table 1.1). At the highest level, declarative memories are distinguished from procedural ones. Declarative memory is then divided into semantic and episodic memory, and procedural memory is divided into memory for skills and for priming. Finally, semantic memory may be subdivided into verbal memory and various kinds of sensory memory, and episodic memory may be subdivided either in a similar way or in its own specific fashion (for example, into memory for target information and memory for background context). Correspondingly, skill memory may fractionate, and there may be different kinds of priming. No one denies that there is some flow of information among these hypothetically distinct memory systems. This flow and other planned processing activities could be mediated by the same central executive mentioned in connection with the working memory hypothesis.

The hierarchically arranged long-term memory distinctions, just discussed, broadly apply to complex memory. People and animals also show classical and instrumental conditioning, habituation, and simple kinds of sensory learning. Whether these constitute radically different types of memory, operating in isolation from the more complex types, or whether they can be satisfactorily construed as subvarieties of procedural memory has been inadequately explored, but will be briefly considered in the next section in connection with the memory taxonomy of Oakley (1983). His taxonomy is explicitly based on physiological observations of animal memory and human neuropsychological data, and draws very little from studies of intact people. There is a growing trend to follow his example. The hypotheses of short- and long-term memory adumbrated above, as well as those concerning registration and retrieval processes in complex memory, predict that brain damage should, in principle, cause selective deficits in the postulated processes and systems. For example, one might expect selective deficits in declarative and procedural memory, in aspects of semantic and episodic memory, and in verbal and visual memory. Although selective deficits like these are found, careful analysis may show that they only weakly support the postulated distinctions.

In summary of this section, it must be said that studies of intact people have thrown very little light on the processes of storage and the different possible ways of representing information. The studies have suggested, however, that the way items are encoded and retrieved plays a central role in determining how well they are remembered, that short- and long-term memory may be distinct, and that several forms of long-term memory have very different properties. It is tempting to predict that memory disorders will cleave along similar lines; for example,

Table 1.1. *A hierarchical taxonomic scheme for memory*

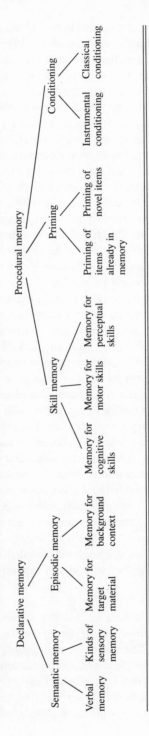

This is one way that a hierarchical taxonomy of the kinds of memory might work, although it is not intended to be comprehensive. Because the taxonomy is hierarchical, all forms of declarative memory must share characteristics not possessed by any form of procedural memory, although subvarieties of declarative memory will differ in subtle ways. For example, verbal and sensory memory must share characteristics of which episodic memory is devoid. The suggested distinction between semantic and episodic memory is not, in fact, accepted in this book.

there will be memory failures caused by poor encoding and retrieval, short-term memory deficits, and deficits of different kinds of long-term memory. The pattern of breakdown found tests these ideas and, when unpredicted, suggests that new ideas must be introduced. In the next section, a discussion of physiological research will examine what we have learnt about storage processes, for they may well be disturbed in memory disorders.

Section Three: Theories derived from physiological studies of memory in animals

The modular organization of memory systems

Most physiological research on memory has been performed on animals. It can be conveniently divided into attempts to elucidate the microscopic changes that underlie storage at the neuronal and subneuronal levels and the larger scale organizational changes that enable complex information to be encoded in the store. The second, macroscopic goal is probably beyond current techniques, so much work has been directed at solving the essential preliminary problem of discovering where different kinds of information are stored in the brain. In discussing this more modest macroscopic goal, Thompson (1986) refers to the essential memory-trace circuit, which includes all the neuronal circuitry from input to output that is necessary and sufficient for generating a particular learnt behaviour. Within this circuit lies the essential memory trace, which comprises the plastic neuronal processes necessary and sufficient for storing the memory relevant to the learnt behaviour and which changes the organization of the essential memory-trace circuit. Thus, for example, he argues that the cerebellum forms part of the essential memory-trace circuit for some kinds of conditioning and that the memory trace lies within the cerebellum as well as perhaps elsewhere. Macroscopic and microscopic levels also interact as, for example, the neuronal changes necessary for storage are modulated by processes organized at a macroscopic level. To some extent, the work to be described in this section is the mirror image of that reviewed in the last because it focuses on storage processes and reveals little about registration and retrieval.

At the macroscopic level, the first thing clearly to emerge is that hypothetically different kinds of memory do indeed appear to be stored in separate brain regions. Oakley's (1983) memory taxonomy (Table 1.2), when it is not simply speculative, is based largely on lesion evidence that addresses the problem of where various kinds of memory are located. His scheme is hierarchical, and he distinguishes initially between those kinds of early learning that must occur within a critical period of development and those that can occur throughout most of life. The distinction is plausible, but currently is somewhat speculative. There is, however, some evidence that imprinting (a form of early learning) in chicks is blocked by lesions of the hyperstriatum that have no effect on a superficially similar type of

Table 1.2. *A simplified version of Oakley's taxonomic scheme for memory*

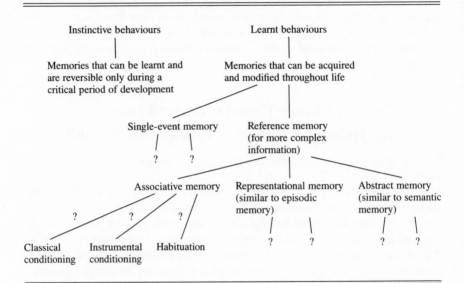

visual-discrimination learning that is not confined to a critical period (see Horn, 1985). It may be, however, that such hyperstriatal lesions are actually compromising two forms of avian learning that can occur throughout most of life. Thus imprinting may involve visual recognition, and visual discrimination learning could be a kind of procedural learning. As early learning probably plays an important role in human development, it is interesting to consider whether it can be selectively compromised by lesions in infancy or before. Selective effects of this kind would be expected on Oakley's view. At the next level down in his scheme, Oakley distinguishes single-event memory from reference memory, which is for more complex information. The postulation of a separate event memory, which Oakley regards as a sensory trace of an experienced event of a kind that might occur in eidetic imagery, is still very speculative. Reference memory is, however, further subdivided, and its components correspond to kinds of memory already mentioned. They are associative memory (including habituation as well as classical and instrumental conditioning), representational memory (which is very like episodic memory), and abstract memory (which is very like semantic memory).

It is never explicitly stated by Oakley that each of the five hypothetical kinds of memory must possess its distinctive modes of registration, storage, and retrieval. What he does stress is that each is mediated by different brain regions. There is, for example, increasing evidence that some kinds of conditioning and habituation can occur relatively normally after forebrain removal and even in isolated spinal cords (see Oakley, 1983). These forms of learning also occur in primitive invertebrate nervous systems. In contrast, representational and abstract memory develop normally only if structures in the more recently evolved forebrain are intact. Many researchers now believe that information is stored in the same brain regions where it is processed. If they are correct, then lesions impairing memory must either have destroyed both the storage of particular kinds of information and their processing (which means their encoding and retrieval) or have impaired the non-specific modulatory processes that help to strengthen storage, but are not directly involved with information processing.

Oakley's taxonomy is a provisional one and will probably have to be radically revised in the light of future evidence. Finding brain regions that store specific kinds of information is the first step. It can be pursued through lesions and through studies correlating learning with measures of brain activity. The inputs, outputs, internal structure, and physiology of the critical regions then need to be analysed in order to gain more insight into the way in which the stored information is registered, retrieved, and, most importantly, represented. It is quite likely that some separate regions have almost identical internal structures, so the kinds of memory they store may be registered, retrieved, and represented in very similar ways. Only when the structures are radically distinct are they likely to mediate two basically different kinds of memory. In concrete terms, all cortically stored memories are probably similarly organized because the architecture of all cortical regions is basically the same. Thus verbal and visual memories of recent events, which are very probably stored in the cortex, will most likely not be organized very differently. In contrast, cortical and brain-stem structures are differently organized, so memories stored in these two regions are probably fundamentally distinct. Thus verbal memory and conditioning (which is probably stored more in brain-stem regions) may be organized in radically distinct ways.

All taxonomies that postulate a hierarchically arranged set of memory systems presuppose that the brain is organized, at least partially, in a modular fashion. A module performs a specific series of operations on information received from a limited group of sources or one source. It is popularly supposed that much of perception and motor co-ordination is mediated through the activity of large numbers of modules, connected in series and in parallel. Within this framework, the task of neuroscience can be construed as identifying exactly what each module does and how the modules interact with one another to mediate complex functions, such as perception. In a recent formulation, Fodor (1983) has argued that not all the brain is modular. His argument is that modules operate in isolation from the rest of the brain. Apart from their specific inputs, their operation is not affected by information available to many other brain regions. Similarly, they communicate the final product of their processing to only one or a small number of other brain regions. Such isolation enables modules to process rapidly. In Fodor's view, modules have neuronal architectures that reveal their manner of information processing. Humans and animals, however, also have the ability to form beliefs about the outside world. Fodor argues that any information is potentially relevant in assessing the validity of beliefs and that a modular arrangement does not allow information to be made available in this way. He therefore proposes that the brain must contain a non-modular region in which all parts are highly interconnected, so that any subregion can obtain information from any other subregion. In his view, the neuronal architecture of the non-modular region does not reveal the functions of separate parts. Indeed, he believes that functions are not localized, as they are in the brain's modular zones.

The Fodorian non-modular region resembles, in some ways, the central executive with access to all consciously retrievable memories. In chapter 5, it will be suggested that the processes of this central executive may be mediated by the frontal lobes of the brain and that the executive can be envisaged as a planning system. It will be argued that this system may well have separate, modular components. Belief in the non-modularity of such a system is therefore highly controversial. There are other reasons for doubt. First, it is implausible that the central executive should have unlimited access to information relevant 'in principle' to belief validation. Second, it is unclear why a modular brain should not be able to validate beliefs in the way required by Fodor. Third, the degree to which modules work in isolation from the rest of the brain probably varies along a dimension, so that some processing units will receive information from many more sources than others and communicate their outputs to many more regions. It is certain that many brain regions regarded by Fodor as modular have two-way connections with several other regions.

Whether or not it can be extended to include all higher level processes in the brain, however, Fodor's concept of modules as encapsulated processing units suggests the existence of one kind of memory ignored by Oakley's (1983) taxonomy – procedural memory. If information is stored within the regions where it is processed and only the final products of modular processing are communicated to the rest of the brain, which will include the central executive, then modules will acquire information that is also encapsulated. Such information would be inaccessible to direct awareness, so that it could not be reported verbally or experienced as imagery and would be revealed only indirectly by changing the output of the module that contains it. This view of procedural memory is attractive, but unproved. Its corollary is that declarative memories must be directly communicable to the central executive or whatever system mediates consciousness.

Consolidation and modulation:
the microscopic aspects of storage

If lesions of a particular brain structure impair learning and memory for information of a given kind, and the structure shows selectively increased activity when such information is registered or retrieved, then it is plausible to argue that the information is stored in that structure. To confirm this argument, it is necessary to show that neurons in the structure undergo physiological changes that could mediate storage. This represents one important type of research into the microscopic bases of memory – that is, analysis of the changes that underlie stable memory (and short-term memory, if it exists). Two other related lines of research have also been pursued. The first is concerned with the nature of and the time course followed by those physiological and biochemical processes triggered by learning and necessary for the formation of stable memory. These processes, known as consolidation processes, must occur if any long-term trace is to form. The second line of research has grown out of the first and concerns a less specific set of modulatory processes that determines the extent to which consolidation processes occur and hence influence the strength of the resultant memory.

Consolidation and modulatory processes have been investigated by two main approaches: the application of specific disruptive and facilitative treatments at various times after learning to examine the effect on subsequent memory, and the analysis of the changes that appear to be the specific consequences of learning rather than of its incidental concomitants, such as motor activation. Both these approaches are fraught with methodological problems, and their use has not yet given rise to a clear consensus. For example, some workers believe that consolidation is completed usually in less than a second, whereas others believe that it continues for hours, days, weeks, or even years. No one denies, however, that a sequence of changes – consolidation processes – occurs when stable memories are formed.

Despite the lack of agreement in the literature, four points are worth making. First, nearly everyone believes that stable memory depends on structural changes, probably at synapses, that alter the way signals are routed through the brain. This belief is consistent with the somewhat more controversial view that after learning has occurred, new kinds of protein must be synthesized in the neurons undergoing structural changes. Blocking protein synthesis in neurons at the time of learning impairs later memory, and protein synthesis is specifically increased by learning, although the interpretation of these findings is very tricky (for a recent review, see Davis and Squire, 1984). Second, it has proved hard to determine whether effects of treatments on memory are caused by actions on consolidation or on modulatory processes. In general, modulatory processes are held to be results of emotional or other kinds of arousal and to include activities such as the release of adrenalin from the adrenal medulla. The release of this and similar hormones is believed to somehow influence the effectiveness with which storage processes occur. As the intensity of these activities increases at the time of learning and shortly afterwards, there is initially an improvement in memory, but at higher activity levels there is a deterioration.

The third point is a theoretical one that has already been briefly discussed and is central to this book. It concerns the question of whether it is possible to find deficits of storage where registration and retrieval are unaffected. The brain systems that mediate modulatory processes are likely to be distinct from those responsible for storing and processing particular kinds of information. For example, they will include regions controlling the release of hormones, such as adrenalin and noradrenalin. In contrast, consolidation processes for particular kinds of information will occur in those brain regions where the information is also stored. It is easy to imagine that lesions confined to a modulatory system

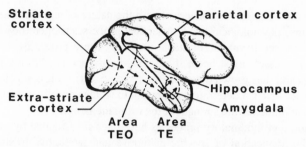

Figure 1.1 Visual information is received first in the striate cortex. It is then projected in parallel into several extra-striate cortical systems, which encode attributes like colour and movement. There are projections from these regions in parallel to the parietal association cortex, which encodes spatial information, and also to areas TEO and then TE, which probably encode shape information and object representations, respectively (see chapter 7). Memory of visually presented objects may be stored, at least partly, in area TE, but effective memory involves activity in projections from area TE to the hippocampus and, possibly, to the amygdala as well. These are limbic system structures that lie within the medial temporal lobe (see chapter 6 and later in this chapter).

might produce selective storage deficits for only those kinds of information whose storage is affected by the modulation. If, however, a lesion selectively affects a system in which occurs the consolidation processes for a particular kind of information, then most researchers would believe that registration and retrieval of that information will be just as affected as its storage. It is argued in accordance with Occam's razor that if a brain region encodes a particular kind of information, that information will be stored in the same neurons that represented it during encoding. The alternative would be for the information to be sent elsewhere for storage. But this would be very wasteful of neural space relative to a system where information is represented and stored in the same neuronal sites. Because the wasteful system would also be more vulnerable to lesions, it is unlikely to have been selected by evolution. It is hard to see how the further brain region would not be concerned with processing aspects of the information as well. One complication of the view that storage and processing sites are identical is the problem of deciding which neurons are involved in representing the information in question. For example, if a person is shown a new car, a whole set of neurons in the posterior neocortex are activated in turn, but it is probably only neurons in the temporal lobe that represent the car (Figure 1.1). Damage to this region may prevent not only storage of the new information, but also the ability to achieve similar representations on future occasions. It is unlikely that relevant storage changes occur more posteriorly in the neocortex than the temporal lobe because the posterior regions mediate earlier visual processes necessary for achieving the representation of the car. Lesions of these posterior regions would disrupt the ability to recognize the car but not because they destroy the stored memory of it. It seems likely that memory for a given kind of information is stored in only the part of the brain system that is necessary for processing that information. Most probably, storage will occur in those parts of the system concerned with the later stages of processing where the information is represented. The general warning is, however, clear. We should be very careful before concluding that a lesion has just impaired storage, leaving registration and retrieval untouched.

The fourth point is that if there are different kinds of memory, stored in different parts of the brain, then the structural changes that mediate their storage, and hence the associated consolidation and modulatory processes, may differ radically. The presence of such differences would be a strong indication that fundamentally distinct kinds of memory were served by the two regions. There is, in fact, some evidence that representational memory and simpler kinds of memory, such as conditioning and habituation, not only are controlled by separate brain regions, but also are dependent on different kinds of change at the neuronal level.

Evidence about the kind of change within neurons that may underlie the ability to store representational memory has been gathered by Lynch and his colleagues (Lynch & Baudry, 1984). High-frequency electrical stimulation, applied for brief periods to a pathway that runs from the cortex to the hippocampus within the temporal lobe, leads to an increase in the sensitivity of the hippocampus to later stimulation. This increased sensitivity is known as long-term potentiation (LTP). LTP may persist for several weeks or even months under some conditions. Lynch's group believe that the raised sensitivity is caused by a change within hippocampal neurons at those sites (the synapses) where the hippocampal neurons receive chemical messengers (transmitter molecules) released by the cortical neurons that stimulate them. This post-synaptic change involves an effective increase in the number of receptor sites on the synapses for the transmitter molecules (the more sites there are, the more transmitter molecules will be 'captured' and the greater will be the sensitivity of hippocampal neurons to incoming messages). The change may also be associated with a modification in the shape of the hippocampal side of the synapses, and depends on the activation of a proteinous enzyme, called calpain, whose activation is, in turn, caused by raised calcium concentrations, triggered by the intense excitation of the receiving neurons, resulting from the initial electrical stimulation. Calpain degrades a structural protein, called fodrin, changing the synapse's shape by releasing hidden receptors. Lynch and his co-workers have some evidence that this calpain-dependent mechanism is found only in the forebrain and may be confined to mammals. Furthermore, they have found that the drug leupeptin, which interferes with the calpain-dependent mechanism and blocks LTP, also impairs memory for a spatial task and an olfactory discrimination without affecting escape and avoidance learning. It might be speculatively argued that whereas the first two tasks are examples of representational memory, mediated by the forebrain, the last task is a form of conditioning, mediated by evolutionarily older brain structures.

This viewpoint is polemical. For example, some people believe that LTP depends on pre-synaptic as well as post-synaptic changes. More importantly, the evidence implying that an LTP-like change provides the basis of storage for representational memory needs much further support. Nevertheless, the evidence is suggestive that complex memory (probably including, at least, episodic and semantic memory) is stored via a process, that is at least partly dependent on post-synaptic changes and the calpain-dependent mechanism. In the hippocampus, the excitatory amino acid neurotransmitter glutamate stimulates the neurons involved in LTP. There are at least three kinds of glutamate receptor, identified by the different drugs that block or excite them, one of which is the post-synaptic NMDA receptor. This receptor seems essential for the development of LTP because a drug that blocks it also blocks LTP and, interestingly, impairs performance on a spatial memory, but not a non-spatial memory, task (Morris, Anderson, Lynch, & Baudry, 1986). Interestingly, the drug does not disrupt LTP and spatial memories that have already been acquired, so activation of the NMDA receptor seems to be essential for only the creation of the plastic changes that underlie LTP and spatial memory rather than for their maintenance (Morris, personal communication). The NMDA receptor is activated only when the post-synaptic neuron is depolarized and does not seem to be involved in normal neural transmission, so blocking its operation by a drug prevents LTP and spatial learning without affecting normal synaptic transmission. The LTP memory change may therefore occur only with high levels of neural activity, whereas normal processing may occur at lower levels. This may make it particularly susceptible to modulation. There is indeed evidence that LTP is modulated according to an inverted U-shaped function by the influence of hormones, such as adrenalin (Gold, 1984). If this kind of modulation occurs, then complex memory may be disturbed by lesions that selectively block modulation, leaving processing unaffected. Other lesions might prevent the high levels of neural activity necessary to trigger the calpain-dependent mechanism. For example, a biochemical lesion that selectively disrupted NMDA receptors might well leave the registration and retrieval of the information, processed by the hippocampus, intact, but prevent its storage – a truly selective storage deficit. Processing of complex information might be relatively unaffected.

The cellular bases of simpler kinds of learning, such as habituation and classical conditioning, have been explored using invertebrate model systems. Best known is the work of Kandel and his colleagues with *Aplysia,* a marine mollusc with a nervous system composed of only a few thousand neurons (for a review, see Hawkins & Kandel, 1984). Invertebrate systems are sufficiently invariant for neurons with specified functions to be identified in different individuals. In *Aplysia,* habituation is found to be caused by a decreased release of neurotransmitter from sensory neurons in the critical pathway. The change is a pre-synaptic one; that is, it occurs within the neurons that release transmitter molecules at their synaptic junctions with the receiving neurons. Sensitization is a form of learning in which decreased responding to one stimulus (habituation) is reversed by the unrelated presentation of another and strong stimulus. It is associated with an increase in the duration of action potentials in the same sensory neurons that release less transmitter when there is habituation. There is a flow of calcium ions into the neurons, so that more transmitter is released. Longer term sensitization that occurs after several presentations of a strong stimulus and may last for days appears to depend on changes at the same pre-synaptic locations because it is linked to increases in the size and number of active zones of sensory neuron synapses – that is, changes in structure. Both short- and long-term sensitization, however, involve pre-synaptic facilitation, which means that relevant sensory neurons release more transmitter molecules for a given strength of the stimulus.

More recently, Kandel and others have found that classical conditioning may depend on a minor modification of the mechanism that mediates sensitization. When the sensory stimulation caused by the conditioned stimulus is paired with a sensitizing stimulus (the unconditioned stimulus), there is a particularly large activity-dependent amplification of pre-synaptic facilitation. This is related to an increase in the influx of calcium ions. Hawkins and Kandel (1984) argue that some of, if not all, the changes underlying classical conditioning are pre-synaptic. More speculatively, they propose that more complex conditioning phenomena, such as latent inhibition, in which the ability of a stimulus to elicit a conditioned response is reduced by presenting it alone prior to the conditioning procedure when it is paired with the unconditioned stimulus, may depend on further modifications of the same pre-synaptic mechanism. The invertebrate nervous system is very different from the vertebrate, so it remains undecided whether mammalian forms of simple memory also depend on a pre-synaptic mechanism. Even so, similarities between invertebrate and vertebrate conditioning are considerable, and the invertebrate studies support the general position that processing and storage of information occur in the same brain region. The possibility that mammalian complex and simple learning depend on different mechanisms at the neuronal level as well as being controlled by separate brain regions should clearly be taken seriously, although much more evidence is needed.

The picture emerging from these studies is that there are distinct memory systems, found in separate brain areas. Some of these systems will differ with respect to the consolidation and modulatory processes and the structural changes that these processes produce. How many kinds of structural change can mediate storage is completely unknown. Some of the systems will also differ with respect to the organization and coding of the stored information, but this remains to be explored. The last possibility is critical because it will determine the extent to which lesions can selectively impair the processes of registration, storage, and retrieval for a given kind of memory. Not all these dissociations may be found in people in whom brain damage is adventitiously located because such damage rarely corresponds exactly with functional boundaries. In animal models, however, it may be possible to create such highly specific impairments.

Section Four: The neuropsychology of memory

The research on normal human memory and on the physiological bases of memory in animals, reviewed in the last two sections, gives some indications about the kinds of lesion-induced memory deficits that may occur in people. But it has revealed little about the organizational and representational processes that may be distinct in the different kinds of memory. Development of a neuropsychology of memory may help answer these questions.

The first stage in this development is the construction of a 'periodic table' of memory pathologies. In principle, this means constructing a list of memory deficits, each of which cannot be broken further into subdeficits by smaller lesions. There is no algorithm for the achievement of this goal. Deficits that seem indivisible may be shown in future lesion studies to comprise several components. Even if this is not found in people, chemical or other more specific lesions in animals may show there to be several distinct deficits. Guidance is mainly through intuitions about the likely unity of the functional deficits and the homogeneity of the brain tissue destroyed. All lesion studies of memory basically follow the method of dissociations – single, double, or preferably multiple. The aim is to show that lesion X impairs memory A, lesion Y impairs memory B, lesion Z impairs memory C, and so on. It then needs to be shown that smaller lesions within areas X, Y, and Z cause mild impairments or no impairments of A, B, and C, rather than deficits describable as subcomponents of A, B, and C.

The programme cannot be fulfilled unless the nature of the functional deficit is properly analysed. This analysis faces two severe difficulties. First, deficits in humans are rarely completely pure, so incidental functional impairments must somehow be separated from those impairments that are causally related to the memory deficit. For example, short-term memory deficits are often associated with poor initial processing of the information for which there is bad memory. It has been argued, however, that such processing impairments are incidental to the memory deficit because in otherwise similar cases, it has been claimed that processing is normal. The problem of cases being confounded with incidental functional impairments can be reduced by selecting 'pure' cases. One way of doing this is to select for detailed analysis only those patients with generally good cognitive functioning and in whom brain damage is known to be localized in a small region. It is also unwise to identify memory syndromes, even initially, solely in terms of certain lost functions because the preserved functions are equally important. The second problem faced in analysing memory syndromes arises because such analysis involves the comparison of poor patient memory with good control-subject memory. A number of artefacts may occur when such comparisons are made; they are considered more fully in chapter 6.

Memory deficits have, then, been initially characterized in terms of the kind of memory that is most obviously disturbed. At this stage, they have also, where possible, been characterized in terms of the brain region whose damage seems to cause the deficit. This is a wise precaution because if more than one lesion can produce the crudely described deficit, further analysis may well reveal there to be separable functional disorders. At the crude level of description, several broad kinds of memory syndrome can be identified. First, there are several disorders in which short-term memory for a number of kinds of information is poor. Second, there are disorders, caused by cortical lesions, in which several kinds of previously very well-established semantic memory are compromised. Such disorders may

Table 1.3. *List of putative elementary memory disorders*

Type of disorder	Responsible lesions	Nature of deficit	Comments
1. Short-term-memory deficits	Posterior association neocortex	Poor recall and recognition on immediate tests	Several disorders, affecting distinct kinds of information
2. Disorders of well-established memory	Posterior association neocortex, particularly left temporal cortex	Failure to access previously well-established semantic information	Several subvarieties, affecting distinct kinds of information and, possibly, retrieval or storage
3. Frontal lobe memory problems	Prefrontal association neocortex	Poor recall of information that requires planned and effortful processing; poor memory for temporal order	Possibly several disorders caused by distinct lesions; it is unclear whether all result from inadequate effortful processing
4. Organic amnesia	Limbic system; medial diencephalon; basal forebrain	Poor new learning, and forgetting of memories acquired pre-traumatically, with good intelligence and short-term memory	Possibly subvarieties; for example, limbic system but not diencephalic lesions may cause faster forgetting
5. Poor memory for skills, conditioning, and perhaps priming	Basal ganglia; cerebellum; perhaps association neocortex	Very poor acquisition of skills, conditioning, and priming	Perhaps should form three groups of elementary disorder for skills, conditioning, and priming, each of which probably has subvarieties; much more research is needed

The table briefly outlines the main putative elementary memory disorders. It should be noted that, in reality, all probably comprise clusters of elementary deficits and that group 5 should perhaps, when more is known, be divided into three separate groups.

also be associated with reduced priming. Third, lesions of parts of the frontal lobes may impair memory for aspects of temporal judgements and also affect the elaborative processing of meaningful information, so that poor memory for complex material is found under some conditions. Fourth, there is the organic amnesia syndrome, in which limbic system and diencephalic lesions cause a complex deficit in semantic and episodic memory. Subvarieties of this syndrome also exist. Thus left hemisphere lesions of the limbic system or diencephalon cause selective verbal memory deficits, whereas right hemisphere lesions of these structures cause selective sensory memory deficits. Lesions that disconnect parts of the neocortex from the limbic system may cause similar amnesias, specific to verbal or sensory information, and, possibly, even more specific deficits, such as amnesias for faces and colours. Fifth and much less adequately researched, basal ganglia, cerebellar, and other subcortical lesions may cause selective deficits in skill learning and memory and in conditioning (see Table 1.3 for an outline of the elementary memory disorders).

To confirm and extend the initial characterization of these five types of memory syndrome, further analysis has been and still is essential. Such analysis has several components. First, it must be shown that other kinds of memory are or can be normal in the presence of the observed deficit. For example, it has been seen as very important in organic amnesia research to show that short-term memory and, more recently, skill memory and priming can be normal. The matter is of particular interest with short-term memory deficits. Their association with long-term memory deficits for information of the kind for which a short-term deficit exists is an open question. Such an association would mean that all information reaching stable memory must first pass through the short-term system. A lack of association would mean that information passes into the two systems in parallel. If an association obtains, then selective short-term deficits for a given kind of information could be distinguished from selective long-term deficits, solely in terms of the fact that memory loss would be apparent immediately after information has been received.

Second, in some sense, it needs to be shown whether the memory deficit is caused by a crude information-processing deficit. The significance of a processing deficit depends on the nature of the memory impairment being proposed. Thus a disorder would not be regarded as involving derangement of a short-term memory storage system if it arose because of an initial processing disturbance sufficiently severe to cause very poor memory. If a patient is partly colour blind or unable to discriminate phonemes well, he or she is likely to have poor short-term memory for colours or words. The same point applies, in general, to long-term memory deficits. For example, it is usually taken as a criterion of organic amnesia that memory is worse than would be expected on the basis of measured intelligence. This criterion is founded on the well-supported belief that memory for complex information is better in those with superior intelligence. In contrast to organic amnesia, however, frontal lobe memory syndromes may essentially involve a certain kind of processing deficit. It is, of course, controversial to what extent and in what way frontal lesions impair intelligence.

There is, in fact, no clear dividing line between deficits that are selective failures of memory and those in which the memory failure is a secondary consequence of a processing failure. Pure storage breakdowns, if they exist, are unequivocal examples of the first category. In contrast, a gross cognitive disturbance associated with poor memory is a clear example of the second category. For example, a blind man would not remember visual stimuli, but would not be said to have a visual memory deficit. In between lie registration and retrieval failures that affect primarily memory, leaving non-mnemonic functions relatively intact. The frontal lobe memory syndrome is of this kind. In this book, we will count all disorders as memory deficits unless they involve a crude processing failure that is responsible for the memory loss.

The third component of memory-deficit analysis concerns further delineation of the breakdown pattern in the syndromes with a view to attaining an exact description of the underlying functional deficit. For example, with organic amnesia, this stage of analysis involves an attempt to see whether registration, storage, or retrieval is affected and whether the failure is specific to only some kinds of complex information. This tricky kind of analysis lies at the heart of the book's next few chapters. Some people would add a fourth component of analysis – that of determining what functional role(s) the impaired kind of memory might serve. For example, it is of interest with short-term memory disorder patients to see whether the memory loss affects things like sentence comprehension and mental arithmetic.

Once a provisional 'periodic table' of memory disorders has been constructed, it will be feasible to begin examining how the brain regions damaged in memory syndromes mediate the lost functions. This examination advances the analysis of the precise nature of the functional deficits undertaken in drawing up the provisional 'periodic table'.

Some basic neuroanatomy

Before starting the more detailed analysis of the possibly elementary memory deficits, some background in the relevant basic neuroanatomy will be provided to set the scene. Most of the disorders considered involve complex information, which is processed in the more recently evolved regions of the forebrain. The visible part of the human forebrain comprises the left and right cerebral hemispheres, joined by connecting fibre tracts, such as the 200 million myelinated fibres of the corpus callosum. The outer surface of the hemispheres is between 1.5 and 4.5 mm thick and consists of layered sheets of neurons. This is the cortex, which in humans mainly includes the most recently evolved neocortex. The cellular architecture of the six layers of neocortex varies from region to region, and this variation seems to relate quite closely to the kinds of information processing for which each region is responsible. Neocortex is usually divided into sensory, motor, and association areas. Sensory cortex is the initial receiver of information from the eye, ear, or bodily senses. For example, striate cortex, lying in the posterior cerebral cortex, is the primary receiving area for visual information. Motor cortex sends fairly direct signals to the peripheral nervous system to control movement. It lies in the anterior half of the cortex, just in front of the Rolandic fissure. In addition, there are two large regions of association neocortex: a posterior region, known as parietotempero-occipital (PTO) cortex; and the prefrontal cortex, lying anterior to the motor cortex (Figure 1.2). Association cortex plays a crucial role in the processing and storage of complex episodic and semantic information. PTO association cortex is important in interpreting sensory information in a meaningful way and receives inputs from sensory cortex (see Figure 1.1). Sensory information is transmitted from the primary sensory receiving areas of the

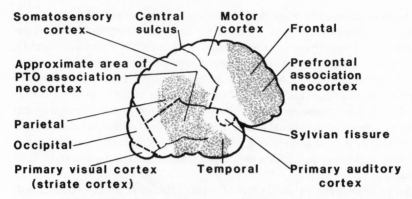

Somatosensory
cortex

Central
sulcus

Motor
cortex

Frontal

Approximate area of
PTO association
neocortex

Prefrontal
association
neocortex

Parietal

Occipital

Sylvian fissure

Primary visual cortex
(striate cortex)

Temporal

Primary auditory
cortex

Figure 1.2 The approximate locations of the PTO and the frontal association areas on the right cerebral hemisphere are indicated by the stippled regions. The locations of the four main lobes of the cerebral hemispheres are also given, as are the locations of the primary sensory receiving areas of neocortex and of the motor cortex.

neocortex to surrounding association neocortex, where distinct sensory attributes are encoded at separate sites. For example, visual information is transmitted in parallel from the striate cortex (the primary sensory receiving area for visual information) to a number of association neocortical areas, where information about stimulus orientation, colour, motion, and binocular disparity (relevant to depth perception) is encoded. Information about these and other separately encoded sensory attributes may be integrated in other regions of PTO association cortex. For example, the inferotemporal cortex seems to be important for encoding information about visually presented objects; parts of the superior temporal cortex are important for encoding information about faces; and parts of the parietal cortex are important for encoding information about objects' positions. The central point is that many sensory attributes are encoded, both in parallel and sequentially, in separate parts of PTO association neocortex, and it will be argued in chapter 4 that storage of these attributes occurs in the same sites as those that encoded them. As will be discussed in chapters 3 and 4, lesions in different PTO regions may selectively impair not only certain kinds of short-term memory, but also memory for many kinds of previously well-established semantic information. PTO cortex interconnects with prefrontal cortex, which is generally believed to mediate planning of cognitive processes carried out in PTO cortex and elsewhere in the brain. Prefrontal cortex lesions disturb planning and also memory in ways that are still ill-understood. Better understanding will probably depend on appreciating that the prefrontal cortex is a heterogeneous system comprising many functional units.

Within the cerebral hemispheres, beneath the neocortex, lie two important, interrelated systems of structures: the limbic system and the basal ganglia. The limbic system structures – such as the hippocampus, amygdala, septum, and cingulate cortex – form a circle on the inner surface of each hemisphere, surrounding the junction with the diencephalon (which comprises the thalamus and hypothalamus) (Figure 1.3). As will be described in chapter 7, both the hippocampus and

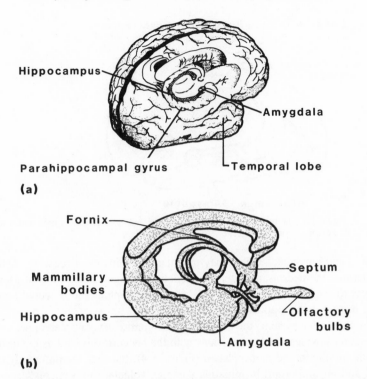

Figure 1.3 (a) The disposition of the limbic system within the medial temporal lobe.
(b) The connections of the hippocampus and amygdala to the septum and diencephalic
structures, such as the mammillary bodies.

the amygdala, which lie within the medial temporal lobe of the brain, project to
different structures in the diencephalon. The hippocampus projects to the anterior
nucleus of the thalamus both directly and indirectly via the mammillary bodies,
which lie in the posterior hypothalamus immediately above the roof of the mouth.
The anterior thalamus projects to the cingulate cortex, an evolutionarily old cortical structure within the frontal region of the hemispheres. Similarly, the amygdala
projects both directly and indirectly, via the bed nucleus of the stria terminalis,
to the dorsomedial nucleus of the thalamus, the major projection nucleus to the
prefrontal cortex. There is evidence that organic amnesia is caused by lesions of
the hippocampus and amygdala within the medial temporal lobe, by lesion of the
projection sites of these structures within the diencephalon, and possibly even by
lesions of the diencephalic structures' projection sites within the prefrontal cortex (a region sometimes referred to as ventromedial prefrontal cortex). It is also
notable that both hippocampus and amygdala receive inputs of processed sensory
information from overlying posterior association cortex and also send projections
back to these cortical regions. Amnesia is also believed to be caused by lesions
of the cholinergic neurons of the basal forebrain. These neurons have their cell
bodies in three nuclei, deep in the forebrain, and project to the neocortex, hippo-

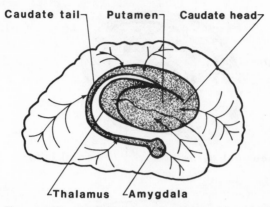

Figure 1.4 The relationship between neocortex and basal ganglia is indicated, showing the extent of cortical projections to the basal ganglia.

campus, and amygdala, where they modulate the activity of receiving neurons by releasing the neurotransmitter acetylcholine. The nucleus basalis of Meynert projects to the neocortex and amygdala, and the septum and diagonal band of Broca project to the hippocampus.

Like the limbic system, the basal ganglia comprise several interconnected nuclei that have widespread connections with the neocortex as well as connections with the midbrain and diencephalon (Figure 1.4), but they are differently organized and are important in initiating complex voluntary movements. Evidence is growing that lesions in parts of the basal ganglia disrupt the acquisition and retention of skills. Very little is known about the effects of lesions in brain-stem structures on learning and memory, although recent lesion studies with rabbits suggest that the cerebellum (Figure 1.5), on the upper side of the brain-stem, helps mediate memory for those kinds of conditioning involving precisely timed motor responses. The cerebellum has also been postulated to play a role in skill acquisition.

The rest of the book will proceed as follows: Chapter 2 critically assesses current testing procedures for giving a preliminary description of memory disorders in the context of the need to distinguish motivated forgetting from memory failures that are caused by brain damage and to characterize less well-understood memory disorders in terms of the elementary memory deficits. The next chapters are concerned with the 'periodic table' of memory disorders. Chapter 3 discusses short-term memory deficits. Chapter 4 reviews the evidence about semantic memory failures caused by cortical lesions. Chapter 5 discusses the nature of the memory deficits caused by frontal lobe pathology. Chapter 6 assesses the kinds of memory that are preserved in organic amnesia, the kinds that are impaired and why, and whether the syndrome should be regarded as unitary. The next chapter examines animal models of amnesia and what is known about biochemical factors that contribute to amnesia. This is intended to serve as an introduction to an examination of the inputs, outputs, and physiology of the brain regions damaged

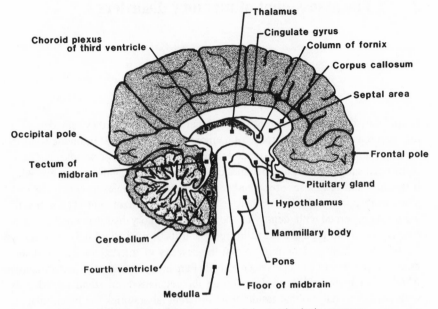

Figure 1.5 The location of the cerebellum relative to other brain structures.

in organic amnesics. For the other elementary disorders, such discussions will be briefer and confined to the chapters in which the disorders are initially considered. Chapter 8 discusses memory problems that have been less extensively researched and characterized. These include possible deficits in memory for skills, habits, and conditioning, as well as other neurological and psychiatric conditions, such as Parkinsonism and schizophrenia, where memory problems have been identified but not well studied and that may either include more than one of the elementary memory disorders or possibly even involve a new kind of elementary memory disorder. Those readers who wish to get an overview of the book's main conclusions can turn first to the final chapter, which outlines the general view of information processing and storage that emerges from the analysis of the elementary memory disorders.

2   The assessment of memory disorders

People may do badly at different kinds of memory tasks, and they may do so for different reasons. It is the purpose of memory assessment to ascertain the ways in which a subject's memory is poor and the causes of this poor performance. Clinicians need such assessments to help them see how patients will cope in everyday life, what their prognoses are, whether there are any therapies to which they are likely to respond, and whether there is any response to treatment. Theoreticians are most concerned with identifying the range of memory disorders and their specific causes. Both groups need valid, reliable tests of particular kinds of memory for which normative data exist so that the severity of the deficits can be determined. But whereas clinicians need tests that tap everyday memory performance, which exist in several equivalent forms, theoreticians need standardized tests with normative data so that results from different laboratories can be compared. Furthermore, as theoreticians seek to identify new kinds of memory disorder, they need to develop their own special-purpose tests to compare the performance of a patient on these tests with that of a group of matched control subjects. The theoretical aim is to identify elementary memory deficits that cannot be subdivided into further simpler disorders and to see what, if any, kinds of brain damage cause them.

The problem that the theoretician faces is that most memory disorders are messy, are poorly understood, and involve several kinds of elementary memory breakdown that arise for many reasons. Because the full range of elementary memory deficits has not yet been identified, the theoretician cannot ignore these messy and poorly characterized kinds of case because one or more of their component memory deficits may not have been previously described. If they exist, these currently unknown elementary memory deficits may be found as only one component of a poorly understood and complex condition that is associated with memory problems. Nevertheless, as indicated in chapter 1, a number of putative elementary organic memory deficits have been located and may be found in relative isolation. Such identifications minimally require it to be shown (1) that only one kind of memory is affected, (2) that the deficit is not caused by other kinds of cognitive deficit, (3) that the deficit is caused by a specific kind of brain damage, and (4) that it is not even partly caused by a functional memory disorder – that is, a memory disorder not caused primarily by brain damage, but by motivational factors of which the patient often denies any knowledge. For example, there is a rare disorder, known as multimodal agnosia, that may be caused by a selective failure to retrieve semantic information about objects when information is presented visually, tactually, and possibly auditorily. Patients with the disorder

36

are unable to name objects or indicate their uses by non-verbal means when the objects or drawings of them are presented via the affected senses. To make a selective memory-deficit interpretation likely, however, it needs to be shown that no other unrelated memory problem is apparent and, more importantly, that other cognitive deficits capable of explaining the agnosic problem are absent. These include sensory loss, intellectual deterioration, altered attention, and aphasic disturbances that might impair comprehension of instructions. All these disorders could explain an apparent agnosia without the need to postulate a failure to access previously well-established semantic memories about objects when those objects are presented via the affected senses. To establish that the disorder is organic in origin, it should be shown that it is associated with a specific brain lesion. Current knowledge cannot conclusively exclude the possibility that the disorder has a functional component (that is, the patient is, for some reason, motivated to perform poorly), but it can at least be determined whether patients have anything to gain by the presence of their impairment.

Adequate assessment of organic memory disorders from a theoretical viewpoint therefore requires a good range of memory tests, a range of tests of other cognitive processes, means of identifying brain lesions or dysfunctions, and some means of determining whether patients are motivated to perform poorly on memory tasks – that is, have functional amnesias. Currently, normative and special-purpose tests of memory and cognitive functions are drawn mainly from theories derived from studies of intact people. In the future, tests may need to be devised to measure unexpected kinds of deficit detectable only through open-minded inspection of patients. Analysis of brain lesions and dysfunctions is carried out in several ways. In some cases, post-mortem analysis of patients' brains can be performed. This can not only identify the extent of brain lesions precisely, but also determine whether certain kinds of biochemical disorder were present. Patients may not come to post-mortem, however, for some years after their last psychological assessment, so it may be hard to know whether or not some of their organic damage was of more recent origin. Fortunately, techniques for assessing patients in life have been revolutionized in the past 15 years. First, Computerized Axial Tomography (CAT) was developed. In CAT scans, X-ray pictures are taken in different positions round the head so that a computer can convert these signals into a series of brain slices. Darkness of shading on each cross-sectional slice indicates the density of brain tissue at that point. Because damaged tissue differs in density from healthy tissue, the technique can locate lesions (Figure 2.1). Although CAT scans are safe and non-invasive, their resolution does not approach that of post-mortem analysis, and the technique is relatively insensitive to slow atrophic changes. More recently, techniques for identifying brain lesions in living subjects have been further improved with the advent of Magnetic Resonance Imaging (MRI). Like the CAT scan, MRI is non-invasive, analysing the radio waves emitted by brain regions when an imposed magnetic field fluctuates, so as to compute very clear slices of healthy and diseased tissue (Figure 2.2).

CAT and MRI help identify damaged brain regions with increasing precision,

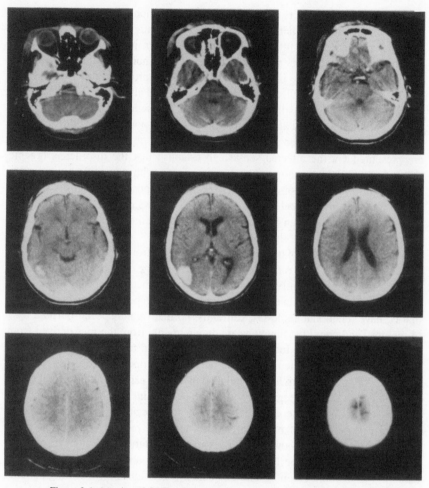

Figure 2.1 A series of CAT scans of a patient with a lesion in the right parieto-occipital area (see central scan). The lesion contains blood, which absorbs more radiation than does the surrounding tissue and so appears white. Left and right are reversed. The upper-left scan shows a section through the eyes and the base of the brain. (Courtesy of J. McA. Jones, Good Samaritan Hospital, Portland, Ohio, from Carlson N. R., *The psychology of behavior*. Allyn & Bacon, Boston. Copyright 1985.)

but they do not reveal biochemical disorders or whether metabolism is unaffected in apparently normal brain regions. The technique of Positron Emission Tomography (PET) can be used to measure abnormalities of neuronal metabolism as well as other features of the brain's biochemistry. Measurement of neuronal metabolic-activity levels can be achieved by the injection of a radioactive form of glucose that is not metabolized and so accumulates in active neurons. The radioactive glucose, which has a half-life of a few hours, breaks down by emitting

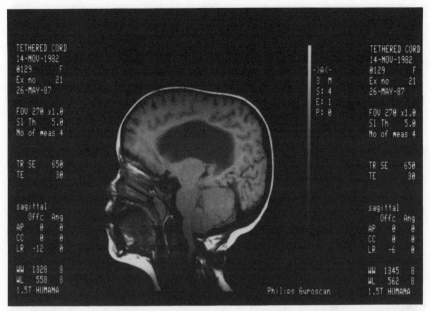

Figure 2.2 Philips and Picker Medical Systems 1.5 Tesla MR sagittal head image of a child. The spinal cord is tethered in the upper cervical region at the site of the meningocele with associated caudal positioning of the medulla. Note the dilatation of the third and lateral ventricles. (Courtesy of Philips and Picker Medical Systems.)

positrons that are picked up by detectors placed around the head. Brain slices are then computed; their colour or shading indicates the level of metabolism in different brain regions (Figure 2.3). The PET scan can also be used to measure cerebral blood flow, which usually correlates with neuronal metabolism. It has thus become possible not only to determine whether particular brain regions are truly normal functionally, but also to identify which brain regions become active when volunteer healthy subjects perform various memory and other cognitive tasks. More recently, PET-scan techniques have been further modified in order to image transmitters and their receptors in living brains. If this development proves successful, it should be possible to identify specific transmitter abnormalities in living patients.

The term 'functional amnesia' is unfortunate because organic memory disorders are associated with the loss of specific psychological functions. 'Psychogenic amnesia', an alternative name that is sometimes used, is less liable to this particular confusion. These amnesias are motivated in that they are describable as the forgetting of the disagreeable. But the precise mechanism of the motivated forgetting is unclear. Unlike the organic memory problems, functional amnesias can sometimes be reversed through the use of hypnosis or sodium amytal therapy. Using these techniques and knowing whether the patient has a reason for forgetting provide the main means of determining if an organic memory problem

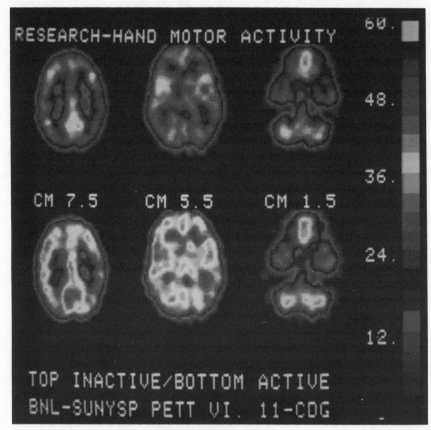

Figure 2.3 A series of PET scans of the human brain. The scans in the top row show a person at rest, whereas the scans in the bottom row show the same person whilst clenching and unclenching his right fist. These latter scans reveal increased uptake of (^{11}C)-labelled 2-deoxyglucose in the cerebellum and left frontal cortex (in the region of the primary motor cortex), which indicates increased metabolic activity in these regions. Arrows point to the active regions, which in the original scan would have been shown in red because PET scans generally use a colour code. (Courtesy of the Brookhaven National Laboratory and the State University of New York, Stony Brook, from Carlson N. R., *The psychology of behavior*. Allyn & Bacon, Boston. Copyright 1985.)

is confounded with a psychogenic overlay. This problem will be further discussed in the next section, which briefly outlines the main kinds of memory deficits.

A brief outline of known memory disorders

It is convenient to divide memory disorders into three main groups: the putatively elementary memory deficits; neurological and psychiatric disorders associated with usually not very well-understood memory deficits; and the functional, or motivated, amnesias. The first two groups make up the organic memory disorders; one key issue with respect to these is the extent to which the neuropsychiatric memory problems can be analysed in terms of the elementary memory disorders. The five subgroups of putative elementary organic memory deficits have already been listed in chapter 1 (see Table 1.2), so will not be discussed further here. It should be remembered, however, that each subgroup probably contains a number of different, although closely related, kinds of memory deficit, each caused by a specific kind of brain lesion. Because they include deficits in short-term memory, failures in retrieval and storage of previously well-established semantic information, failures in memory caused by poor organization of encoding and retrieval, organic amnesia (which may itself comprise several closely related, but more elementary memory deficits), and several disorders that involve poor retention and learning of skills and various forms of conditioning, it is important to see whether the less well-characterized memory disorders of the second group involve kinds of memory deficit that differ from those of the first group or can be understood as compounds of elementary deficits.

The neuropsychiatric conditions that have been associated with poor memory are discussed in chapter 8 and their main features are illustrated in Figure 8.1. They include psychiatric disorders (such as schizophrenia and depression), neurological disorders of movement control (such as Parkinson's disease and Huntington's chorea), and both normal and clearly pathological ageing (as occurs with the various kinds of senile dementia, in which there are wide-ranging reductions in cognitive abilities). In all these disorders, poor memory is merely one component of a complex syndrome, and in many of them, it is not a particularly prominent one. The main reason for mentioning them here is in connection with the analysis of the elementary organic memory deficits. Detailed examination of the neuropsychiatric conditions associated with memory problems should reveal that the observed memory deficit results from a crude cognitive failure, that the observed memory disorder comprises several of the putatively identified elementary memory deficits, or that one of its components is a previously unidentified elementary memory deficit. Unfortunately, no systematic attempts have been made to see whether the memory deficits found in the relevant neuropsychiatric conditions correspond to the elementary memory disorders and to identify the kinds of brain damage with which they are associated. Some attempt to do this is made, however, in chapter 8. As elementary memory deficits are defined in terms of the precise memory functions impaired and the lesions responsible for such impairments, any attempt at analysing the memory problems linked to certain neuropsychiatric conditions must be based on a clear characterization of the memory deficits and lesions commonly associated with each condition. In addition, such an analysis should be based on careful assessments of related cognitive impairments that might explain the observed memory failures, and try to exclude the possibility that the memory failure is the result of motivated forgetting – that is, functional amnesia.

Whereas the first two groups of memory disorders are associated with some degree of brain damage or brain disorder, the functional amnesias, which constitute the third group, may be found in the complete absence of any detectable brain damage. These functional amnesias can conveniently be divided into three kinds, which appear to result most often from emotional shocks (see Schacter, 1986). The first kind is a functional retrograde amnesia in which the victims lose their personal identity and nearly all their autobiographical memories. This loss is often accompanied by a fugue state in which the victims are unaware of having suffered a memory loss, so they may assume a new identity oblivious of their former life. Their ability to learn new information is unimpaired, however. Indeed, functional anterograde amnesias (in which the ability to learn and remember new information is impaired if memory is tapped by recall and recognition) are exceedingly rare. Second, there are limited functional retrograde amnesias (defined as impaired recall and recognition for information acquired pre-traumatically), in which there is usually forgetting of a specific event. This is best illustrated by criminals who fail to remember their crime (most often murder) or the details linked to it. As with the first kind of functional retrograde amnesia, although the forgetting is presumably motivated by a desire not to recall unpleasant or undesirable things, this motivation is supposed to be unconscious. If the motivation is conscious, then the person is play-acting or malingering. It can be very hard to determine whether this is happening, especially if the actor is skilful, although it is very important to do so, particularly in legal cases. The same difficulty of distinguishing between consciously and unconsciously motivated forgetting applies to the third kind of functional amnesia – multiple personality disorders. In multiple personality, several, often very different personalities coexist in one body. It is common for one personality to claim to have no memory of the actions of another, who is 'in control' at another time. Such amnesias are sometimes one-way and sometimes mutual. Individuals who show multiple personality are found to have had very disturbed and neurotic childhoods.

Several points need to be made about the functional amnesias. First, very little systematic research has been carried out on them. The number of experimental studies performed to date probably does not exceed five. Second, although functional amnesias without detectable organic involvement have been reported, the importance of such involvement is still a matter of contention. For example, apart from the association between amnesia for crimes of violence and heavy drinking, it has been claimed that there is a greater than chance association between multiple personality and epilepsy (see Benson, Miller, & Signer, 1986). This is not to say that functional amnesias must really have organic causes, but that some apparently functional cases may have an important organic component. The proportion of cases with an organic component is difficult to determine. With multiple personality, for example, there may be many cases in which epilepsy is subclinical and has gone undetected. The third point relates to the first two and concerns the causes of the functional amnesias. Some light may be thrown on this issue by the phenomenon of hypnotic amnesia. The evidence suggests that lightly hypnotized subjects consciously try to repress what they have been instructed to forget until the instructions are cancelled. More deeply hypnotized subjects do the same thing, but are not conscious of doing so. This suggests that the pattern and mechanism of forgetting seen in malingering and functional amnesia are the same, except that the relevant processes are not accessible to consciousness in functional amnesia. It also suggests that the observed pattern of forgetting will conform to the functional forgetters' view of the way their memory works. For example, recognition of 'forgotten' material may be no better than recall because the usual superiority of recognition over recall is not appreciated by the functional amnesic.

One of the concerns of this chapter is to identify how functional and organic memory problems can be distinguished from each other. This is hardest to do when both functional and organic causes underlie a memory problem. For example, in a case of multiple personality where there is also epilepsy, both types of cause may be involved. The occurrence of a fit is often accompanied by a switch from an aggressive, suspicious personality to a more placid, calmer one, and the two personalities are unaware of each other. When the fit affects the limbic system, the activity of the system's structures may be radically different after the fit. Because the limbic system plays a role in the control of emotion, the changes in its activity may offer a partial explanation for the personality change, and state-dependent forgetting could partly account for the personalities' mutual lack of awareness. If the limbic system is not working properly, this may further contribute to the amnesia that the personalities have for each other. Indeed, temporal lobe epilepsy is known to cause mild memory problems. Even so, it is likely that these organic impairments provide merely a fertile soil on which functional amnesia can grow rather than a complete explanation of all the memory failures. What is needed is some means of determining the extent to which functional amnesia results from organic impairments.

Differentiation between functional and organic memory disorders is further discussed in the next section, which focuses on the kinds of cognitive and memory tests that are necessary for determining the sort of memory deficit that is present, but here the main bases for any distinction will be given. There are three such bases. First, if there is a functional component, then it should be possible to ascertain that the patient has some motivation for not remembering. Perhaps the events in question were very unpleasant, or by showing amnesia, the patient may avoid what, at some level, he judges to be an even more unpleasant consequence. Second, as already mentioned, the pattern of memory breakdown will correspond to the patient's beliefs about the way memory works. This is clearly valuable only when the beliefs are wrong, as will be discussed in the next section. Third, when an amnesia is functional, the lost memories may be recovered when the relevant emotional traumas are resolved, or they may be manifested in nightmares or under hypnosis. Spontaneous recovery is not in itself discriminatory because some organic memory disorders are transitory. These are, however, the three bases on which tests to discriminate between functional and organic memory problems can be founded. The rationale of these and other tests used in memory assessment will now be discussed.

The tests needed for assessing memory

Assessment of other relevant cognitive abilities

If a patient has poor memory and one wishes to gain a theoretical understanding of what has gone wrong, it is necessary to discover what is wrong and why it has gone wrong. The two aims are related. Fulfilment of the first involves measuring the severity of the impairments in memory and other forms of cognition, and fulfilment of the second involves locating any brain damage, seeing whether it relates to the cognitive symptoms, and determining what psychological deficits underlie the memory disorder. In order to achieve these aims, it is desirable to analyse memory deficits either as elementary disorders or as compounds of such disorders. To do this, it may be essential to give a wide range of psychological tests, particularly those tapping different aspects of memory. Some of these tests may be suggested by the form taken by known or suspected elementary memory disorders, but investigators must observe patients carefully in case they have a previously unknown memory deficit. The analysis of elementary memory disorders assumes that the deficits are organic in origin, so it is also necessary to check that they are not functional in nature.

Good memory depends, in part, on the ability to encode material distinctively so as to relate it to other information already in memory. This ability is compromised both by lesions that impair various aspects of intelligence and by any condition that reduces motivation or changes consciousness so that the victim does not exert effort normally and does not engage in elaborative processing. Impairments in intelligence or motivationally induced reductions in elaborative processing are also likely to affect retrieval of long-established memories. Any complete assessment of memory should therefore include not only some appraisal of the patient's emotional and motivational state, but also tests of intelligence, such as the Wechsler Adult Intelligence Scale (WAIS). The WAIS not only gives an overall measure of intelligence, but also consists of a series of verbal and visuospatial subtests that help give an indication of which processes are most affected. Selective impairment on these subtests would predict that memory for certain kinds of material might be differentially affected. For example, poor performance on the visuospatial subtests of the WAIS would be compatible with differentially poor memory for visual material. Such expectations follow from the many observations showing that healthy people with higher intelligence do better on memory tests (see Mayes, 1986). At present, however, the only memory test *battery* about which there is information relating performance levels to intelligence in intact people as well as in brain-damaged people is the Wechsler Memory Scale (WMS). (Scores on the recently developed Rivermead Behavioural

Memory Test, which taps kinds of memory more likely to be used for everyday purposes, such as those for appointments and names, probably correlates less strongly with intelligence, but, currently, this claim is not supported by the critical evidence provided by observations of healthy people.) The WMS battery comprises seven subtests that tap subjects' orientation (the ability to locate oneself in time and space), information about public figures, mental control (the ability to recite rapidly and without error well-learnt sequences of items, such as the letters of the alphabet), short-term memory, story recall, recall of visual forms, and recall of paired associates. It is not a very sensitive test of long-term memory ability and does not even measure recognition. In healthy people, correlations of about 0.8 have been reported between WAIS and WMS scores. It can be calculated from this correlation and the standard deviation of WAIS and WMS scores that a WAIS–WMS discrepancy of 20 or more points would occur by chance less than 5 times in a 100 in a healthy person.

Several points arise from this discussion. The first one is general; where possible, memory tests should have established norms for healthy people of different intelligence and of different ages. The memory scores of patients can then be compared with those of normal subjects of appropriate age and intelligence. If norms do not exist, then it is essential to compare the scores of patients on a special-purpose test with those of an appropriate control group. The second point relates to what an appropriate control group is. This is best illustrated by an example. Both organic amnesics and cortically lesioned patients are likely to have difficulty with the acquisition of new material. But whereas organic amnesics show worse memory than one would expect from their measured intelligence, which may well be unaffected, cortically lesioned patients show aspects of intelligence that are reduced from their pre-morbid levels and memory performance that would be predicted from the new level of intelligence. Severity of organic amnesia is therefore measured by comparing patients with healthy controls, matched on current level of intelligence and for age, whereas severity of the memory deficit in the cortically lesioned patients should be measured by comparison with the performance of a group of age-matched controls whose intelligence matches that found in the patients before they suffered brain damage (in other words, the patients' pre-morbid intelligence). Some indication of pre-morbid intelligence can be obtained from the National Adult Reading Test (NART), which taps reading skills that should have been well established pre-morbidly and whose level should be a function of pre-morbid intelligence. In some patients, unfortunately, the cortical lesions disrupt such previously well-established memories, in which case investigators must rely on estimates based on knowledge of the patients' previous occupation and level of attainment. For example, as there is some evidence that scores on the NART underestimate the pre-morbid intelligence of organic amnesics with an aetiology of chronic alcoholism (Crawford, personal communication), such estimates should be checked by comparison with patients' previous occupations and achievements.

The third point follows from the previous one and concerns the relationship between performance on memory tests and on intelligence tests. There are many popular models of the cognitive processes that constitute intelligence, but one useful broad distinction is between fluid and crystallized intelligence. The former comprises those non-routine and flexible modes of thinking that are relevant to the solution of novel problems, whereas the latter comprises those more routine and stereotyped modes of thinking that depend on previously established knowledge and skills. Crystallized intelligence fares much better than fluid intelligence against the ravages of age and, indeed, is generally less affected by most kinds of brain damage. Nevertheless, some PTO association cortex lesions seem to disrupt it differentially. Because fluid and crystallized intelligence are likely to contribute to encoding and retrieval processes in different ways, it is desirable to measure them separately. Tests of established knowledge, such as the WAIS vocabulary subtest from the verbal scale, tap crystallized intelligence, whereas tests of more flexible thinking, such as the similarities subtest from the same scale (in which subjects have to identify similarities between objects like flies and trees) and both verbal and non-verbal versions of AH4, tap fluid intelligence. Use of tests like these will make it possible to determine which type of intelligence is a better predictor of normal memory and what effect disruptions of each have on patients' memory.

Care must, however, be taken in interpreting correlations between scores on memory and on intelligence tests. For example, the WAIS contains a memory test – the digit-span task – also found in the WMS, which is bound to inflate the correlation between the two tests. Even so, genuine correlations should be expected not only because most memory tasks require elaborative processing skills of the kind that is tapped by intelligence tests, but also because solving the sorts of problem found in such tests depends on the ability to retrieve both established memories and recently acquired information. Indeed, spuriously low correlations between memory and intelligence tests will be reported when the normative sample includes organic amnesics as well as healthy people because the patients' memory is not predictable from their intelligence alone.

The fourth point is concerned with the assessment of the kinds of cognitive deficit that result from lesions of the prefrontal association cortex. Whereas PTO association cortex lesions may sometimes disturb crystallized intelligence, frontal lesions are believed to affect the ability to plan cognitive activities, such as encoding and retrieval. It would seem likely, therefore, that such lesions should disrupt fluid intelligence, although there is little direct evidence for this possibility. There is more evidence that frontal lesions disrupt elaborative encoding and retrieval and hence cause a decline in memory. Assessment of possible frontal deficits is therefore essential to determine the precise causes of a memory problem. Useful information is provided by the various brain-imaging techniques, but they are not sufficient to prove that there is a planning deficit because the frontal lobes are functionally heterogeneous and lesions in some parts may not affect planning or memory. Available tests will be discussed in chapter 5, but it should be noted here that the specificity of these tests is a polemical matter. Performance on them may be poor because of other cortical lesions, may not be affected by frontal lesions in some patients who have clear planning problems, and is influenced by the patient's level of general intelligence. For example, performance on the Wisconsin Card-Sort Test, which taps the ability to form and shift cognitive set in an object-sorting task, may be maintained at a high level in a frontally lesioned patient with planning difficulties through the compensatory use of superior verbal ability and other cognitive skills (Heck & Bryer, 1986). The relationship between the frontal lobes and the different kinds of intelligence remains mysterious, but norms for tests like the Wisconsin should be based on the performance of healthy people with different levels of intelligence.

The last point to arise from the correlation between tests of memory and tests of intelligence is that there should be people with no evidence of brain damage who do markedly worse on memory tests than they do on intelligence tests. On statistical grounds, one would expect 5 healthy people in 100 to show a WAIS–WMS discrepancy of 20 or more. The memory profiles of these people should closely resemble those of organic amnesics over the range of special-purpose tests on which these patients perform distinctively despite the absence of any evidence of brain damage. The necessary research has not yet been done, but if it confirms the above suggestion, it would raise an interesting possibility – that the amnesic syndrome may occur not only because of overt brain dysfunction, caused by lesioning, but also because some people inherit limbic and diencephalic memory structures that are subnormal in size and/or efficiency. This possibility might be tested by MRI and PET investigations. Similar proposals have been made with respect to developmental dyslexia and may well be applicable to the other memory disorders.

Intelligence and memory are interacting abilities. The latter depends on the former because how we think determines how we encode new information and retrieve already stored information. Like memory, intelligence comprises an as yet unspecified number of component processes, and the relationship of each of these processes to memory is currently not well understood. The situation will be improved only if future work on patients and healthy people measures as many components of intelligence as is practicable and relates memory-test scores to these measures. The relationships among intelligence, memory, and mood are similarly poorly understood. In addition to assessment of patients' memory and intelligence, some measures of mood are required if the causes of the memory deficits are to be fully grasped because it is known that mood affects memory.

Assessment of anterograde amnesia

Tests of the ability to acquire and remember new information need to tap all those kinds of memory that brain damage is believed to disturb. In addition, investigators have to be alert to the need to devise new special-purpose tasks. Because these tests will be considered in more detail in later chapters, they will only be outlined here. Ideally, a patient should be given tests of each of the kinds to be outlined to demonstrate as much where performance is normal as where it is impaired.

First, it is important to measure short-term memory, using a simple task like the digit span, as in the WAIS and WMS. If performance is poor, then further tests should be carried out to ascertain whether short-term memory for other kinds of material is also affected, whether processing of the relevant kinds of material is disturbed, and whether rehearsal processes are normal. These tests are required to determine if the deficit is one of short-term storage for the relevant kind of material or if it has some other explanation. Most such tests need to be devised by the investigator.

Second, different kinds of material should be presented for learning, sometimes followed by recall and sometimes by recognition tests. Minimally, there should be tests of verbal and difficult-to-verbalize material (such as faces) because material-specific memory failures are known to occur. Since some of these failures may be very specific, it is necessary to devise a number of special-purpose tests to establish the degree of specificity. For example, to prove that a patient has a problem confined to memory for faces, it would be necessary to test memory for similar material that normal people find equally difficult to learn, such as different makes of car or species of bird. Although it is difficult to give recall tests for difficult-to-verbalize material, recall as well as recognition should be examined when possible (patients might, for example, be required to draw recently presented abstract shapes). It has been claimed that several conditions lead to greater impairments in recall than in recognition, including depression, schizophrenia, and frontal lobe and possibly some thalamic syndromes (see Mayes, 1986). Indeed, recently it has been reported that organic amnesics are also more impaired at recall than at recognition (see Hirst et al., 1986). It is easier to determine that recall is disproportionately poor if recognition is normal, as it may be after most frontal lobe lesions. If, however, a patient's recognition is also impaired, two approaches are still possible. The first involves construction of recall and recognition tests that are equally difficult, are equally reliable, and have similar standard deviations in samples of normal people. Then if the patients perform farther below the normals on recall, they probably have a disproportionate recall deficit (see Calev, Venables, & Monk, 1983). The second approach involves matching patients and controls on recognition by testing the controls after fewer learning trials or after a longer delay, and then examining whether the patients still do worse on recall when the controls are tested under the same conditions. Ideally, both approaches should be combined because tests differing in difficulty, reliability, and variability also differ in their ability to discriminate between normal and impaired memory (see Mayes, Meudell, & Pickering, 1985). This has not yet been done, however, to confirm that recall is more impaired than recognition in schizophrenic, depressive, and frontally lesioned patients. As the preparation of tests that are matched for difficulty, reliability, and variability is extremely time consuming, it is also unlikely to be done. A less demanding alternative would be to use a variant of the second approach and demonstrate a cross-over interaction in which a lesioned group does better than the controls at recognition and worse at recall. A similar procedure could be adopted for other pairs of tests that may not be completely matched.

Recall and recognition are usually tested immediately after the stimuli to be remembered have been presented. This procedure is, nevertheless, supposed to tap long-term memory because the learning list usually greatly exceeds the short-term memory span. The distinction between short- and long-term memory is, however, a blurred one, so it is not always clear whether a test is supposed to be measuring short- or long-term memory ability. For example, the Brown-Peterson task typically requires subjects to recall only three items at a time so that the short-term memory span does not appear to be exceeded. But recall is usually tested after a delay that may vary from 3 sec to 1 min, which is filled with distracting activity, so many would argue that performance depends on long-term memory. The matter is of some theoretical importance because some organic amnesics are impaired on this task but not on the digit-span task.

One aspect of memory that the Brown-Peterson task seems to address is rate of forgetting. Despite popular belief in the variability of rate of forgetting, it is extremely difficult to find any variables (such as degree of original learning) that convincingly affect this aspect of memory. It is, however, believed by some that certain brain lesions result in accelerated forgetting rates, so it is important to devise appropriate measures for how fast recently acquired information is forgotten. The chief problem in devising such measures is that patients with memory problems often perform much worse than their controls even at the shortest test delay and may, indeed, do no better than would be expected by chance. Tests of forgetting rate have typically coped with this difficulty by varying the exposure of items that make up the learning series, so that memory performance is matched at the shortest delay. For example, if the lists are composed of pictures or words, controls might be given 0.5- or 1-sec exposures per item, whereas amnesics might receive exposures from 4 to 20 sec. Typically, tests of forgetting rate have matched amnesic and control recognition at about 75% correct after a 10-min delay and then examined recognition after 1 day and 1 week. (Future work should attempt to match recognition at much briefer delays because pathologically accelerated forgetting may be most prominent in the period immediately after presentation.) Although this procedure is valid for comparing forgetting rates in different groups of amnesics for whom exposure times can be matched, it is open to serious criticism when this cannot be done. In most studies, amnesics are given much longer exposure times than controls, and since delay is timed from the end of the list, the average item-to-test delay is much longer for the patients. Patients' initial recognition levels are therefore underestimated so that the procedure is likely to give an artefactually low estimate of their rates of forgetting, particularly for patients who have very long exposure times. This problem is further discussed in chapter 6, but one way of controlling for the artefact would be to determine the exposure needed to give acceptable recognition for the most amnesic subject and then ensure that all subjects have the same delay between item presentations. For controls, this delay would be filled by a brief item presentation proper and a longer period filled with irrelevant distractor activity. This ensures that the average delays between item presentation and test would be matched across subjects. There is no evidence that spaced learning slows the rate of forgetting.

Faster forgetting has been claimed in schizophrenics as well as in temporal lobe amnesics, but in both cases the claim needs to be properly authenticated. If the claim is true, it supports the idea that some memory problems arise from deficits in processes that are quite independent of intelligence and mood and may indeed be caused by deficiencies in storage processes. There is even some evidence in healthy people that individual differences in memory may be partly caused by differences in forgetting rate. Thus it has been found that delayed tests of visual memory are more weakly correlated with WAIS scores than are immediate tests (see Mayes, 1986), which suggests that a rate-of-forgetting factor as well as encoding and retrieval efficiency play a role in normal memory tested after a delay. Finally, tests of forgetting rate should ideally employ both recall and recognition procedures because it has been claimed that some patients show faster forgetting, but only with recall tests (Calev et al., 1983; Jetter, Poser, Freeman, & Markowitsch, 1986). This kind of claim is important and clearly needs rigorous examination.

Tests of three other aspects of memory are important in the assessment of anterograde amnesia: memory for background contextual information, which normally falls on the periphery of attention; those kinds of memory, particularly priming, that are preserved in organic amnesia; and sensitivity to interference in long-term memory. These are discussed in detail in chapter 6, but some methodological points will be raised here.

If organic amnesia were caused by a specific failure in contextual memory, then such memory should be disproportionately bad in amnesics. Investigators therefore need to compare contextual memory with recall or recognition of target items on which attention was focused during learning. If both are impaired, it is hard to reach any conclusion. Studies have usually tried to match memory-impaired patients with controls on target memory by testing the latter at a greater delay (or after less learning time) and seeing whether controls still show better contextual memory. Care must be taken to keep other factors constant when this procedure is used, and the contextual and target-memory tests should also be matched for difficulty and reliability when possible to ensure that they are equally sensitive in the identification of deficits. These points also apply to tests of priming and interference. It is important to match priming tests with their comparison recall or recognition tests, so that there is equal sensitivity to deficit. The same point applies to tests of interference; that is, baseline list and interference list should be matched on sensitivity to deficit. But it is also necessary to match amnesic and control subjects on learning of the baseline list. For example, in a proactive interference paradigm, amnesics may need five times as many trials to learn the first list to the same level as controls. If they are more susceptible to proactive interference, then after the same number of trials with the second list, their level of learning should be significantly lower than that of the controls. It is possible to argue that when this procedure is not used (and no published study has ever used it), the greater sensitivity of amnesics to interference is a result of their poor memory rather than related to its cause.

Assessment of retrograde amnesia

Unlike anterograde amnesia, retrograde amnesia not only may be caused by brain damage, but also may occur as a functional memory failure. The broad distinctions between functional and organic memory failures have already been listed. Recently, Schacter (1986) developed a procedure that may help further our ability to discriminate between the two causes of retrograde amnesia. The procedure is based on the idea that the form taken by functional amnesia depends on the subject's beliefs about how memory works and that these beliefs may sometimes be wrong. In Schacter's study, two groups were read a passage from a novel or saw a video-taped documentary and were later asked questions about parts of the learning material that they would have been unlikely to remember without specific directions during learning. The first group were genuine forgetters and received no directions, whereas the second were conscious simulators, who received directions about the information that would later be tested and were told to pretend that they could not remember. Transcripts of the retrieval attempts of both groups were shown to some psychologists and psychiatrists, who were unable to discriminate between genuine and simulating forgetters even when they felt confident that they could. When they had made their free-recall attempts, both groups of subjects were asked to estimate their chances of recalling if they were given certain hints. These judgements are known as feeling-of-knowing ratings, and the simulators' feeling-of-knowing ratings were significantly less confident than those of the genuine forgetters. In other words, they erroneously believed that hints would have little effect in aiding the recall of partially forgotten material.

Three points need to be made about Schacter's study. The first is that although there is a significant difference on feeling-of-knowing ratings between genuine and simulating forgetters, the difference is not great enough to allow confident discrimination in an individual case. Furthermore, a knowledgeable simulator should behave just like genuine forgetters, so the procedure's sensitivity is subject to the simulator's degree of sophistication. The second point is that the procedure contrasts the performance of conscious malingerers and genuine forgetters rather than that of functional and organic amnesics. It is, however, reasonable to postulate that the mechanisms of functional amnesia and of conscious malingering are very similar and that functional amnesics would also show low confidence on feeling-of-knowing ratings. This possibility has yet to be tested. The third point is that feeling-of-knowing judgements are part of what is known as metamemory, which is a subject's knowledge about memory in general and the operation of his memory in particular. The fact that normal people have some erroneous metamemorial beliefs therefore provides a means of distinguishing between functional and organic retrograde amnesias, even though the means is imperfect. Assessment of metamemory in patients is also justified on other grounds, as there is evidence (to be discussed in chapters 5 and 6) that frontal lobe lesions disrupt the ability to make accurate metamemorial judgements.

Other formal tests for distinguishing between functional and organic retrograde amnesias clearly need to be found. One possibility is that memory may be made apparent in functional amnesics when tested by indirect means. Indirect memory tests may deceive the mechanisms underlying motivated forgetting. Care will have to be taken in developing such tests, however, because there is some indication that even with organic amnesics, evidence of memory may be apparent in some indirect tests that is lacking in direct tests of recall or recognition. For example, as will be discussed in chapter 6, recent research suggests that organic amnesics show differential changes in skin resistance when viewing words that they do not recognize just having seen. A second possible basis for the development of discriminatory tests would be available if functional retrograde amnesia affected different kinds of information from that affected by organic retrograde amnesia. There have been hardly any experimental studies of functional retrograde amnesia, but Schacter, Wang, Tulving, and Freedman (1982) did examine one such case. It involved a young man who was suffering from a severe retrograde amnesia that recovered 4 days later, except for a more persistent memory loss for the 12-hour period preceding his hospital admission. He showed dramatic forgetting of autobiographical information during the attack, but very little disturbance of more semantic material. Thus nearly all the personal memories that he produced in response to cue words, such as *book,* were dated by him as occurring after his hospitalization, whereas after his recovery most such memories were dated as being far older, something that was also found with control subjects. In contrast, his memory for information about famous people was apparently normal. There is, however, reason to suppose that the test of autobiographical memory was more sensitive than the test of semantic memory, so it is unclear whether this pattern of performance might not also have been found in organic amnesics. Thus we have some way to go before reliable formal tests will be able to distinguish between functional and organic retrograde amnesias, although informal assessments are reasonably good. The ability to make this distinction is particularly important in cases where retrograde amnesia is found in isolation and there is evidence of brain damage. These cases are discussed in chapter 6, but the key issue is whether the brain damage directly causes the memory failure or whether it merely provides a fertile soil for the manifestation of a functional amnesia.

In addition to distinguishing between organic and functional deficits, assessment of retrograde amnesia has several aims. These include whether pre-traumatic memory is impaired with both recall and recognition tests, whether the deficit affects both episodic and semantic memory, whether it affects pre-traumatically acquired skills, and whether older memories are less affected than more recently acquired ones. A number of objective tests have been constructed that probe recall and recognition of public events, people, or television shows that had an impact over a fairly short period of time to ensure that memories for them were acquired pre-traumatically. Such tests tend to be parochial (since few items receive universal, but temporally limited coverage), need regular updating, and differ in their sensitivity to retrograde amnesia. Wilson and her colleagues (see Wilson & Cockburn, 1988) have recently developed a test that asks patients to give prices of various common items, such as milk, petrol, cigarettes, and bread. Their results indicate that organic amnesics typically give estimates that are based on prices that are years out of date. The test has the advantages of being easy to update, sensitive to even short periods of retrograde amnesia, and applicable to young amnesics (for whom many of the public events, television shows, and people in the other questionnaires would have occurred or been around before they were even born). It is, however, a moot point whether the kind of memory tapped by both Wilson's and the other tests is episodic or semantic. Attempts have been made to test episodic memory unequivocally either by giving a structured interview about the patient's autobiography or by getting the patient to produce personal memories in response to a series of concrete word triggers (for example, think of a memory connected with a book). One difficulty with these procedures is that it is almost impossible to determine whether the memories produced by these procedures are genuine or confabulated. Because there is considerable theoretical interest in the question of whether equally rehearsed episodic and semantic memories are differentially affected in organic amnesia, the validation procedure for these episodic tests should be developed. One possibility would be to rely on relatives' validation of patients' putative personal memories.

The most difficult requirement that retrograde amnesia tests have to meet is the one necessary if they are to determine whether pre-traumatic memories are less affected simply because of their age, which has been believed by many ever since Ribot first made the claim toward the end of the nineteenth century. Ideally, such a test should sample in an equivalent way across past time periods so that events from different time periods are learnt equally well and then forgotten at the same rate. A minimal criterion for the meeting of this condition is that normal subjects should remember older items less well and that older subjects should do better on the older items than younger subjects, who did not experience the events when they first occurred. In practice, it seems highly likely that older items have been more rehearsed. If memory for them is less disturbed in organic amnesia, this is more likely to be because rehearsal protects against the deficit caused by the lesion than because of unknown spontaneous changes that occur as memories age. The issue is of great theoretical importance, and there is, therefore, a need to develop test items whose rehearsal is unlikely after initial learning. Tests are much more likely to fulfil this requirement if they tap memory for difficult-to-verbalize material, such as faces that the patient may have briefly encountered at various stages of his or her life.

Conclusion

Memory disorders can be divided into three groups. The first two are caused by brain lesions and comprise the elementary memory deficits and those neuropsychiatric disorders in which memory is disturbed. It is likely that the memory deficits found in the latter kinds of disorder are either *single* elementary memory deficits mixed with other unrelated cognitive and mood disturbances or *several* elementary memory deficits possibly mixed with unrelated cognitive and mood disturbances. Both these groups of memory disorders must be distinguished from the functional amnesias, in which forgetting appears to be in some way motivated, albeit often without the patient's awareness. In order to identify the elementary memory disorders, characterize them clearly, and determine what deficits in psychological processes underlie them, it is essential to use a wide range of neurological and psychological tests. The neurological tests should indicate where neural tissue has been lost and where apparently intact brain regions are not working properly. This knowledge helps ascertain whether a disorder is elementary or is likely to be further subdivisible, and provides a starting point for using what is known about the inputs, outputs, and physiology of affected regions to guide thinking about the psychological deficits that underlie the disorder. The psychological tests have several aims, including assessment of patients' pre-morbid and current cognitive abilities, ascertainment of their prevalent mood state, description of the range and severity of their anterograde and retrograde amnesias, and determination of whether their organically caused memory problems are compounded by functional amnesia. The tests enable the investigator to identify which processes are working normally, which are not, and the extent to which the malfunctioning processes are affected. This knowledge is vital if the deficit is to be specified as one affecting the storage, encoding, and/or retrieval of particular kinds of information. One message of this chapter is, however, that many available tests are inadequate, so claims about elementary memory deficits must be treated with care. The evidence about these deficits will now be reviewed.

3   Disorders of short-term memory

Normal people forget some information in a few seconds but remember other things for years. It is widely believed that the information that is forgotten in seconds has been held in a limited-capacity short-term store and has not been transferred to a more stable, large-capacity long-term store. Of course, forgetting is a continuous process, and normal people forget things after seconds, minutes, hours, days, weeks, months, and years, but researchers do not propose that there are hundreds of stores to cover all these delays. Indeed, most workers believe that one kind of memory store is sufficient to explain all forgetting that occurs with delays of more than a few seconds. So why is belief in a separate kind of short-term store from which information is lost in seconds so widespread? As discussed in chapter 1, there are now psychologists, such as Wickelgren (1974), who argue that all the phenomena of rapid forgetting can be explained in terms of the properties of a single storage system. The evidence, based on studies of normal people, that immediate memory is affected differently from longer term memory by such variables as type of encoding and learning time can just as easily be interpreted in terms of a single storage hypothesis as it can in terms of the existence of separate short- and long-term stores. The short-term-storage hypothesis probably derives its appeal from two factors. First, rapid forgetting is something of which we are all very aware and distinguish from stable, long-term memory, which gives plausibility to the feeling that there is a discontinuity between rapid and slower kinds of forgetting. Second, many physiological psychologists believe that consolidation processes take time to complete and so create stable, long-term storage of information. Before this comes about, the information must be held in a separate kind of storage – in other words, the short-term store.

What weight should be given to these two factors? The answer is that probably the first is an example of where our biased awareness may lead us to possibly erroneous conclusions, but the second is of much more interest. There is, however, one problem with it. Whereas hypotheses about short-term memory storage concern the storage properties of neural systems, consolidation processes operate at the level of the single neuron and concern the changes, particularly at synapses, that lead to long-lasting changes in the connections between individual neurons. Although plausible, it needs to be shown that there is a significant correspondence between processes at the levels of single neurons and of neural systems. Relevant evidence is unlikely to come from the study of intact people because the hypothesis is about storage processes, rather than those of encoding and retrieval. It may be provided by neuropsychological study of brain-damaged subjects, who show deficient immediate memory, and of organic amnesics, who show very poor long-term memory, but may perform normally on tests of immediate memory. The case for the existence of separate short-term storage would be greatly strengthened if it could be shown that some patients have poor immediate memory despite displaying completely normal processing and rehearsal of the kind of information for which immediate memory is poor.

It is therefore of interest that several apparently selective short-term memory disorders have been reported in patients following damage that usually affects PTO association neocortex. This is consistent with the working-memory hypothesis of Baddeley and Hitch (1974), which proposes that several independent short-term stores exist, each holding a specific kind of information. Thus some patients have been reported to show an impairment of auditory–verbal short-term memory (see Shallice & Warrington, 1979); some have shown selective reduction in visual short-term memory for verbal and non-verbal material (Samuels, Butters, & Fedio, 1972; Warrington & Rabin, 1971); some have shown selective reductions in visuospatial short-term memory (De Renzi & Nichelli, 1975); and one patient has been reported with what is argued to be a short-term memory deficit selective for colour information (Davidoff & Ostergaard, 1984). In all these cases, a memory impairment is apparent very shortly after information has been presented.

Several important questions must be asked about each proposed short-term memory impairment and any others that may yet be discovered. First, is each kind of deficit really specific to just one kind of information, such as phonologically coded sounds or colours? Second, does the impairment affect only immediate memory for the relevant kind of information, or is long-term memory for that information also badly impaired? Third, does the impairment in immediate memory for the relevant kind of information occur because there is a storage deficit or because of an encoding or a related kind of processing failure? Fourth, does the impairment affect any other aspect of cognition, such as reasoning or comprehension of speech and writing?

These questions are to some extent interrelated, so ideally research should be designed to answer all of them. Thus it is important to know how many kinds of selective short-term memory deficits there are because this should indicate how many kinds of independent short-term stores exist. But in order to demonstrate that there is a separate short-term store for a specific kind of information, it is vital to show two things. First, it must be shown that some patients have poor immediate memory for that kind of information and that their immediate memory is normal for other kinds of information. Second, it must be shown that the cause of this poor immediate memory is a storage deficit, which can be done only by demonstrating that encoding and other related processes are normal. If some aspect of information processing were defective, then almost immediate forgetting of that kind of material would be expected, even if there were only one kind of store, regardless of the length of time for which things are remembered. For example, if a patient shows poor immediate memory only for colours, this would not require the postulation of a short-term store specific for colours if the poor memory turned out to be caused by a subtle deficit in colour perception.

It was postulated by Atkinson and Shiffrin (1971) that information is transferred from short-term storage into long-term storage. If this serial-transfer view is correct, a patient with poor immediate memory for a specific kind of information should also have poor long-term memory for the same kind of information. This prediction does not, however, clearly distinguish the serial-transfer hypothesis from the view that there is only one memory store responsible for rapid and slow forgetting. But it has been argued that when information is processed, it is passed in parallel into short- and long-term stores (see Shallice & Warrington, 1979). This view clearly predicts that it should in principle be possible to find some patients who show poor immediate memory but normal long-term memory and others who show normal short-term memory but poor long-term memory, and this has indeed been claimed (see Shallice & Warrington, 1979). This prediction cannot be derived from the single-store view without making some rather implausible assumptions; so if it were met, further support would be provided for the existence of a separate short-term store for the kind of information affected.

Whether short- and long-term memory are arranged in series or in parallel, the short-term store would maintain continuity of memory before the long-term store became fully operative. The serial-transfer hypothesis implies that short-term storage is in some way essential if long-term storage is to take place. For example, if, as some people believe, short-term storage depends on reverbatory activity in the neural system that encodes the relevant information, then this activity could trigger later consolidation processes that cause structural changes at synapses. The probability that these later consolidation processes will occur might depend on the intensity and duration of the reverbatory activity, which, in turn, might depend on psychological processes like rehearsal. If, however, short- and long-term memory are arranged in parallel, then some other function or functions must be found for short-term storage unless it is to be regarded as a kind of psychological appendix – that is, redundant. Even if the serial-transfer view were correct, other functions might be found for the short-term store, as, indeed, the working-memory hypothesis claims. Patients with selective short-term memory deficits offer a useful means of examining whether short-term storage plays a role in the perception and interpretation of complex material and in reasoning.

The only short-term-memory disorder that has been intensively investigated is the deficit in auditory–verbal short-term memory. Patients with this disorder have been studied so that provisional answers to the four questions listed above can be given, although final answers are not available. The next section therefore considers auditory–verbal short-term memory deficits in some detail. The third section briefly reviews the anatomy of this disorder and of the other short-term memory disorders about which less is known. The remainder of this section outlines what is known about these other disorders.

Davidoff and Ostergaard's (1984) single-case study of a man with apparently selective impairment of his short-term memory for colours addresses all the important questions mentioned above, except whether or not long-term memory was also affected in their patient. They showed that the patient could remember visually presented shapes over delays of up to 8 sec, even though he was prevented from using verbal recoding of the shapes. When given a similar test with colours, he was impaired at immediate test and then forgot faster than his controls. He even forgot faster than controls who were matched to his immediate test performance by being shown the colours for one-fifth as long. His visual short-term memory for colours was therefore clearly deficient. Although the patient's colour perception was found to be anomalous, the authors argued that poor perception could not underlie his poor memory because they carefully checked that he was able to discriminate the colours used in the memory tasks by giving him sorting tasks that he performed perfectly. This does not, of course, exclude the possibility that a subtle processing failure, which did not significantly affect the patient's colour-discrimination ability, underlay his poor performance on the memory task, but does at least exclude the idea that a crude processing failure explains such performance. Finally, the patient had a colour anomia; that is, he was unable to name colours accurately when examples were shown him on cards. He was, however, able to name objects well and could point to named colours. The authors argued that his colour anomia was caused by the failure of short-term memory selective for colour. In their view, sensory inputs can reach the 'colour lexicon' only via the short-term store specific to colour, and naming can be achieved only if the correct entry is made to this store. If they are right, then one cognitive role of this store is to enable colour naming to be made accurately.

The evidence presented by Davidoff and Ostergaard (1984) certainly makes a prima facie case that their patient had a storage deficit specific to colour, which caused his colour anomia. Although the evidence favouring the storage-failure view is not compelling because subtle colour-processing deficits cannot be excluded, it is strengthened by the finding that the patient forgot colour information faster than his controls. Even here, however, it is possible that the controls were rehearsing the colour information in a way impossible for the patient. Nevertheless, although the patient's colour-naming ability was impaired, his rapid forgetting of colour information could not have been caused by poor verbal rehearsal because the relevant tests used difficult-to-name hues and performance was not disrupted in the normal subjects when verbal rehearsal was prevented. Therefore, if the patient's rehearsal was impoverished, this could only be because of his deficient use of a visually based code. More seriously, one cannot be sure that the deficit was one of short-term memory alone, as long-term memory for colour was not tested in this patient. Almost certainly, it would be very poor unless the colours had been correctly recoded in verbal form. But this was a process at which the patient was very poor, even had the hues been easy to name for normal people, which they were not. It might be argued, therefore, that the patient indeed had a deficit in storing colour information, but that the failure was of a single store mediating both short- and long-term memory. To prove that the patient's primary deficit was in a short-term store for colour, one would have to find other patients who do well on the memory tests at which Davidoff and Ostergaard's patient did badly, but show very poor longer term memory for colours. The relevant patients are organic amnesics, who have not yet been given short-term-memory tests for colour. It should not be assumed that their performance will be normal because Warrington and Taylor (1973) found that amnesics' immediate memory for pictures of faces was deficient, whereas their immediate memory for randomly positioned dots was normal. Interestingly, they argued from this that there is a short-term memory for dots and presumably many other non-verbal visual stimuli, but there may be only one memory system for faces. It remains to be seen whether the same argument might apply to colour as applies to faces. If it does, then amnesics will show poor immediate memory for colours, and Davidoff and Ostergaard's patient will not provide an argument for the existence of a separate short-term memory store for colours.

Belief in the existence of a short-term store for visually presented material, like dots, is based mainly on a study of four patients who had immediate visual memory spans of fewer than two items, regardless of whether they were numbers, letters, or shapes (Kinsbourne & Warrington, 1962). These patients had normal immediate auditory memory spans, and later work by Warrington and Rabin (1971) has shown that brain lesions can independently disrupt immediate visual and auditory memory. These visual short-term memory disorders have, however, been little studied. It is uncertain how specific they are, whether or not they might be caused by subtle failures of visual analysis or other encoding or retrieval failures, whether they are accompanied by longer term memory disorders for the same material, and whether they are associated with other cognitive impairments. Lack of systematic study leads to a similar degree of uncertainty about the other reported short-term memory disorder – that of spatial memory. A typical task at which patients with this disorder fail is the Corsi block test. In this, the examiner points to a few identical and randomly positioned blocks, and the subject then has to repeat what has been done. Patients' span for this task is reduced. Nevertheless, it is found that they can perform normally at some 'long-term' spatial memory tasks, such as learning a spatial maze. Conversely, there are patients who are very bad at the spatial maze task and yet are normal at the Corsi block task (see Newcombe, 1985). This double dissociation is interesting, but it does not compare short- and long-term memory for similar forms of spatial information, and therefore does not enable one to conclude that patients with short-term memory deficits for spatial information have normal long-term memory for the same kind of material. Short- and long-term memory for similar kinds of spatial information might be tapped by comparing performance on the normal form of the Corsi block test with a supraspan version in which subjects have to learn to repeat a series of block positions beyond their immediate span. Normal supraspan learning has been found in one patient with a reduced span (Young, personal communication).

From a theoretical point of view, the major interest in studying the short-term memory disorders is the evidence they may provide favouring the existence of a number of specific short-term stores. To provide this evidence, it is essential to show that the poor immediate memory is not caused by deficient initial processing of information or a failure to rehearse it later. If longer term memory for the same kind of information is also bad, it is important to show that organic amnesics (who are terrible at long-term memory tests) perform normally on immediate-memory tests at which the short-term memory patients fail. Studies of patients with poor immediate memory for colour, a range of verbal and non-verbal visual stimuli, or spatial location have started to broach these issues, but do not yet offer compelling evidence favouring the existence of matching short-term stores.

Impaired auditory–verbal short-term memory

Background

The most widely used short-term memory test is the immediate-memory span task. In this task, a list of words, digits, or letters is read at a fixed rate to the subject, who tries to repeat them back in the same order immediately the list has been presented. In normal people, the number of items that can be correctly repeated correlates with intelligence and depends on the kind of items that are being repeated. For example, normal people can repeat between five and nine digits with a mean score of seven, whereas the mean score for common words is around five. Many aphasics show reduced immediate-memory spans, but it is unclear whether their poor performance has anything to do with bad memory. For example, Broca's aphasics, who have severe problems with speech output and articulation in particular, may show reduced spans because their articulation is slow and frequently inaccurate. Similarly, Wernicke's aphasics, who show drastic impairments of speech comprehension, may show reduced immediate-memory spans because they do not fully understand what they are meant to be doing. There are, however, patients whose speech and comprehension lie close to normal limits, but who nevertheless show immediate-memory spans of one or two items. These patients are known as conduction aphasics. Although their speech is generally fluent and effortless, in most cases it is occasionally contaminated by phonemic paraphasic errors. These are simple distortions of words in which sounds are omitted, added, or repeated. They also show a mild comprehension problem when tested on a sensitive test of speech comprehension known as the Token Test. Their major deficit, however, is a striking problem with the repetition of auditorily presented verbal material.

It has been found that despite having auditory immediate-memory spans of only one or two items, some conduction aphasics' short-term memory for meaningful sounds, like jangling keys, falls within normal limits, provided their normal controls are prevented from recoding the sound verbally (see Shallice & Warrington, 1979). Also, unlike normal people, the patients show an immediate-memory span for visually presented verbal items that is greater than their immediate-memory span for auditorily presented verbal items. The visual span is probably not totally normal in the patients because control subjects can recode the visually presented items into an auditory code. This strategy would not, of course, help the patients.

The deficit therefore seems to be specific to auditorily presented verbal material (see Shallice & Warrington, 1979).

As well as showing auditory–verbal immediate-memory spans of only one or two items, conduction aphasics do badly on other tests of immediate memory. First, they do badly when given recognition tests of auditory–verbal span, even though their spans are larger when tested in this way than when recall is required (Strub & Gardner, 1974), because normal subjects show a similar advantage. The recognition test involves subjects' making 'same–different' judgements about successively presented short lists. Similarly, when subjects' auditory spans are assessed by asking them to point at written equivalents of auditory list items, some conduction aphasics are still impaired (Basso, Spinnlerm, Vallar, & Zanobis, 1982). These findings clearly support the view that the patients have a genuine immediate-memory problem rather than merely a difficulty with speech output in repetition tasks. They do not show that the failure is one of short-term storage.

Second, some conduction aphasics show reduced recency effects in free-recall tasks. In this procedure, subjects are read a list of unrelated words, longer than their memory spans, and are then immediately asked to recall the words in any order they choose. The superior recall that normal subjects show for the first list items is known as the primacy effect, whereas their superior recall for the last few items is known as the recency effect. Although patients show normal primacy effects, their recency effects are reduced (see Shallice & Warrington, 1979). The size of the recency effect is reduced in normal subjects if they do not recall the last list items immediately. But a failure to retrieve the last list items immediately cannot explain the poor recency effects shown by all patients, since one patient, P. V., still showed a reduced recency effect even when instructed to recall the last list items first (Vallar & Baddeley, 1985). Although both span tasks and the recency effect involve immediate memory, there is some evidence that they may be mediated by slightly different processes. Thus if during auditory span tasks, normal people are required to perform irrelevant articulatory tasks, such as repeating the word *the*, their spans may be reduced from about eight to around five or six. In contrast, such articulatory suppression has no effect on the size of their recency effects (Vallar & Baddeley, 1984). It is therefore plausible to argue that immediate-memory span depends on a limited-capacity store for phonologically coded information and on the refreshment of the contents of this store through an articulatory rehearsal process. In the terms of the working-memory hypothesis, mentioned in chapter 1, auditory span depends on both a passive phonological store and an active articulatory rehearsal loop. There is certainly evidence that span may not depend greatly on a semantic store or semantic encoding because Warrington (1975) found that patients who no longer understand the meanings of many common words, owing to cortical atrophy, still show word spans that are no smaller for such words than for words they still understand (Figure 3.1). The recency effect, however, depends on only the phonological store. If this is correct, then at least some conduction aphasics must be suffering from some problem with their phonological stores. It could be that the input to this store is degraded,

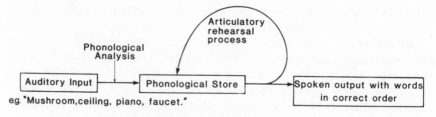

Figure 3.1 A simplified model of how subjects perform auditory-span tasks. The model works without the help of semantic analysis and semantic memory. Use of semantic analyses and memory *can* markedly enhance performance on span tasks, but in the typical digit-span task, they are probably not used.

that the store itself is damaged in some way, or that the output from the store is impaired. The same patients may also have a problem with articulatory rehearsal, and evidence relevant to this will be discussed later.

Some workers, including Vallar and Baddeley, have argued that the above evidence strongly favours the view that some conduction aphasics have a deficit that is selective to short-term storage of phonological descriptions of items. If this view were correct, then a third task at which these patients are impaired might throw light on the nature of the storage deficit. This task is the Brown-Peterson test (chapters 1 and 2), which requires subjects to recall a subspan set of auditorily presented items after a variable interval, filled by a distracting activity that is intended to minimize rehearsal opportunities. Conduction aphasics show more rapid forgetting on this task even when they are required to remember only one word (see Shallice & Warrington, 1979). Because a single word falls within the limits of even their diminutive memory spans, it has been argued that they are suffering from pathologically fast forgetting from their short-term phonological stores. On this argument, the size of this limited-capacity store might not need to be pathologically reduced to explain their poor performance on immediate-memory tasks, but this possibility would require further proof. The faster forgetting might result, in fact, from a failure to show any rehearsal of the single item. In contrast, normal subjects might achieve some surreptitious rehearsal.

The evidence from the Brown-Peterson task does not, therefore, provide compelling support for the view that some conduction aphasics have a deficit in short-term phonological storage, let alone that the deficit is one of pathologically fast forgetting. Such compelling support will be achieved only when it is shown that the patients are not suffering from a deficit in the encoding of phonological information or from a deficit in their ability to rehearse such information. If they have a rehearsal problem, then rapid forgetting in the Brown-Peterson task would be predicted because normal subjects probably rehearse recently presented items in spite of having to perform a distracting task. A problem with rehearsal would prevent conduction aphasics from benefiting in this way, and their disadvantage would increase as the delay became longer.

Despite their very poor performance on tests of longer term memory, organic amnesics show normal immediate-memory spans and normal recency effects, and some have been reported to perform normally on the Brown-Peterson task (see Mayes & Meudell, 1983). In contrast, some conduction aphasics, in spite of their poor auditory immediate memory, can perform within normal limits on long-term memory tasks, such as learning lists of word pairs (for example, *table–cricket*) over several trials, learning lists of unrelated words, or recalling the gist of recently presented stories (see Shallice & Warrington, 1979). In general, patients are able to recall the gist of auditorily presented sentences, even though they are unable to recall them verbatim (unlike normal people). For example, a patient told the sentence 'The old man sank gratefully into the yellow chair' might repeat 'The old man was tired; he wanted to sit in the chair'.

It has been argued that this evidence supports the view that conduction aphasics have a selective deficit of short-term memory. This argument is based mainly on the evidence that organic amnesics show normal immediate auditory memory and would therefore appear to have normal short-term storage for this kind of information. But the argument does not compel belief in the existence of a phonological short-term store. As will be discussed in chapter 6, amnesics may have normal short-term memory because their poor memory for contextual information does not affect immediate memory, which is 'context free'. If this account were correct, then the disorder experienced by conduction aphasics could be a deficit in a single memory-storage system that is specific to phonological information. Whereas amnesics might fail to retrieve phonological information from the single store except at very short delays, when retrieval of context is not needed, conduction aphasics might be poor at retrieving phonological information from the single store at all delays because they are suffering from another type (or other types) of impairment, perhaps of the single store itself. This conclusion appears to conflict with another argument that has been based on the above evidence, which is to the effect that the normal performance of conduction aphasics on long-term memory tasks proves that auditory information is processed in parallel into short- and long-term memory stores. This second argument is, however, even less compelling than the first. There is no evidence that patients can recall words exactly after a delay when they are unable to do so immediately after presentation. If their deficit is in the immediate recall of phonological forms, then the appropriate test is to see whether they can recall such forms after a delay. This would be most effectively assessed by using a learning task with spoken nonsense words that can be encoded only phonologically. It seems very unlikely that the patients would perform normally on such a task. Indeed, it has been shown that one patient, at least, is grossly impaired at learning spoken 'nonsense' words across multiple presentations, as is typical of long-term memory tasks (Baddeley, personal communication). What patients do seem able to do quite well is to access the meaning of spoken items in spite of their poor phonological memory, and this ability may be sufficient to underlie their apparently normal performance on some long-term memory tasks.

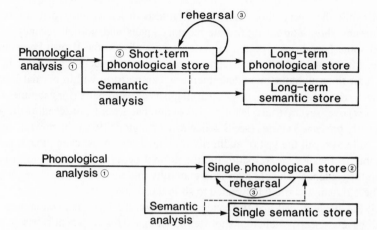

Figure 3.2 The upper model postulates separate serially connected short-term and long-term phonological stores and a distinct long-term store for semantic information, whereas the lower model postulates a single phonological store and a separate, but similar semantic store. Information can be maintained in the short-term phonological store or the single phonological store either by a direct, privileged rehearsal route or by an indirect route that reconstructs the phonological input from its corresponding semantic interpretation. Both models allow immediate memory deficits to result from (1) a failure of phonological analysis, (2) a failure of phonological storage, or (3) a problem with the privileged rehearsal route.

The evidence considered so far suggests that conduction aphasics show deficits in immediate memory for auditory material that probably arise because there has been a selective failure of phonological memory. Preserved phonological memory does not seem that essential for the extraction of meaning from spoken materials, so long-term memory for gist and even unrelated words may be normal. It is not yet clear that the deficit requires the postulation of a separate short-term store for phonologically encoded items. Resolution of this issue will depend partly on discovering why organic amnesics perform normally on the tasks at which conduction aphasics are impaired. It is also unclear whether the patients' deficit should be described as one of storage, initial encoding, or rehearsal. The possibilities are illustrated in Figure 3.2. This considers two models of memory for phonological and semantic information, each of which seems compatible with available evidence. Model A has separate short- and long-term stores for phonological information and a separate processing route from phonological analysis to a long-term semantic store. Model B also includes this route into a single semantic store, but allows for only a single phonological store. The duration of retention of information in this single store is a function of how well stored it is, which may depend on processes like rehearsal. Both models number three processes or stores, impairment of which could underlie the poor immediate memory of conduction aphasics. They also include a rehearsal route from semantic analysis to the phonological store, which is considered further when possible rehearsal deficits are discussed. Since a storage deficit can be established only by exclusion, evidence concerning possible initial processing and rehearsal problems will be considered in more detail.

Do conduction aphasics have a processing deficit?

Paraphasic errors are found not only in the spontaneous speech, but also in the repetitions of most conduction aphasics. This second kind of paraphasic error could be caused by a subtle impairment of phonological analysis, which is also responsible for the immediate-memory disorder shown by conduction aphasics. The occurrence of paraphasic errors and of an immediate-memory disorder might, however, be independent deficits that often appear together in patients because they are caused by lesions to closely adjacent neocortical regions. If this hypothesis is correct, then it should be possible to find conduction aphasics who show poor performance on tests of immediate auditory–verbal memory, but who do not make any paraphasic errors either in spontaneous speech or in repetition. Such patients have been reported (see Vallar & Baddeley, 1984). Their existence not only excludes the possibility that one kind of processing deficit underlies all patients' poor immediate memory, but also strongly suggests that these patients cannot be suffering from poor memory that is specific to the way items are articulated. Of course, it could still be argued that patients who do make paraphasic errors are not deficient in their initial processing of phonology, but that they have poor memory for the articulatory form of words they wish to say or repeat, as well as for phonologically encoded information.

Although some patients show poor immediate memory despite not making paraphasic errors, it might be that their deficit is caused by a kind of initial processing failure that does not lead to paraphasic errors. Some support for this notion has been provided by Allport (1984), who gave one patient a test that required her to make 'same–different' judgements about normally spoken syllables. Even though the demands of the task should not have exceeded the patient's diminished span, she performed badly on it. This finding accords with Allport's view that the system that stores phonological forms in long-term memory and the system that is responsible for immediate auditory memory are one and the same, provided one assumes that phonological encoding involves comparing inputs with what is in long-term phonological storage, so that lesions must affect short-term and long-term phonological memory and processing all together. Vallar's case P. V. has, however, been reported to show no deficits on the 'same–different' task (Vallar & Baddeley, 1985). It might in Allport's defence be argued that this task is very easy and that harder tests of phonological discrimination would be failed by all conduction aphasics. For example, 'same–different' judgements might be required with synthetic speech in which factors like voice-onset time are manipulated. Nevertheless, even if subtle phonological processing deficits were shown to be present in all conduction aphasics, it would need to be proved that the deficits were causally related to the memory disorder rather than unconnected to it. It seems implausible that very subtle processing deficits could lead to an immediate-memory disorder as severe as is found in some patients.

Do conduction aphasics have a disorder of rehearsal?

The essence of Allport's (1984) position might be maintained if it could be shown that any case of poor immediate auditory–verbal memory in conduction aphasics with apparently intact phonological processing is associated with an impairment in the covert or overt articulatory rehearsal of items in memory. Such a rehearsal process might depend on a system independent of that responsible for the long-term storage of phonological information and for phonological analysis. Indeed, it has been proposed by Kinsbourne (1972) that the repetition deficit in conduction aphasics is caused by a disconnection between speech input and speech output, the effect of which would be a reduced capacity to engage in articulatory re-hearsal. According to this view, the initial phonological representations of speech inputs may be adequate, but this information is not normally transferred to ar-ticulatory processes that are also intact. Despite this disconnection, there is no reason why spontaneous speech should not be intact, and paraphasic errors need not necessarily occur in repetition because the articulatory processes should be unimpaired.

This hypothesis has received some support from research on the patient P. V. The research depends on a short-term memory phenomenon known as the word-length effect. It is found that immediate auditory memory is longer for lists of short words than for lists of long ones. This effect is usually explained as a result of the fact that long words usually take longer to articulate than short ones, so that fewer can be rehearsed in a fixed period of time. If memory for recently spoken items cannot be refreshed by rehearsal, then it is likely to be lost; this will happen more with long words because they are rehearsed more slowly than short ones. When normal subjects are made to perform an irrelevant articulatory task, such as repeating the word *the* whilst listening to items that they must later repeat, then the word-length effect is abolished. This finding supports the view that the word-length effect depends on the different rate at which long and short words can be rehearsed. It is therefore of interest that in contrast to normal people, the patient P. V. does not show the effect even when not given an articulatory-suppression task to perform (Vallar & Baddeley, 1984). Vallar and Baddeley attribute the absence of the word-length effect in P. V. to a strategic choice not to use rehearsal because her phonological memory deficit would mean that there was little to be gained from a subvocal rehearsal strategy. An alternative explanation is, however, perhaps more plausible. In line with Kinsbourne's (1972) suggestion, this is that in P. V. there may be partial disconnection between adequately analysed phonological information and intact articulatory processes. On this view, rehearsal may be possible but extremely slow, so patients may not even try to engage in it. If the word-length effect depends on rehearsal, then they should not show it.

Articulatory suppression in normal people not only abolishes the word-length effect, but also reduces the immediate-memory span for digits from seven or eight down to five or six (Vallar & Baddeley, 1984). This reduction is, however, small compared with the span of one or two digits that can be found in some conduction aphasics. This could mean either that these patients have another impairment apart from their deficit in rehearsal or, as Vallar and Baddeley propose, that their lack of rehearsal is a strategic choice and that the basic deficit is one of storage. One does not have to draw this conclusion because the articulatory-suppression technique may not disrupt rehearsal as effectively as the lesion in some conduction aphasics. More effective means of suppressing rehearsal may reduce normal people's spans to the level shown by conduction aphasics.

Although the marked reduction of subvocal rehearsal, caused by a partial disconnection between adequate phonological representations and intact articulatory processes, may explain the reduced auditory memory spans and rapid forgetting of single items in the Brown-Peterson task exhibited by some patients, it is hard to see how it can account for their reduced recency effects. It has been argued that the recency effect does not depend on subvocal rehearsal, but merely on the effectiveness of passive phonological memory. If, however, conduction aphasics have a partial disconnection between their phonological representations and their articulatory processes, then they may take longer than normal people to articulate the last items on a list that they are recalling. During this additional time, they may forget the items that constitute the recency effect. This suggestion might be tested by delaying normal people's list recall for a comparable period of time, during which they have to be prevented from subvocally rehearsing.

Although this test has not yet been performed, there is some evidence that there are two routes through which repetitive rehearsal can be achieved, and the faster of these is compromised in conduction aphasics. The evidence comes from two sources. First, McCleod and Posner (1984) have investigated the way that normal people repeat what they hear, using a dual-task study in which two tasks are performed simultaneously. They found that in normal subjects, the verbatim repetition of a spoken word does not disrupt and is not disrupted by the simultaneous execution of a matching task with visually presented letters. In contrast, there is mutual interference between the visual letter-matching task and a task in which subjects produce an associate for a spoken word (for example, *high* in response to *low*). McCleod and Posner argued that this result implies that the kind of mapping of articulatory rules onto phonological representations involved in verbatim repetition depends on a privileged route that uses little or no attentional effort. In contrast, producing associates to spoken words, which involves mapping articulatory rules onto a transformation of the phonological representation that must require access to semantics, is a non-privileged effort-demanding process. This second route is probably slow and effortful because semantic representations have to be accessed from the phonological ones before a response can be generated.

If McCleod and Posner's view is correct, then normal people could repeat auditorily presented verbal material either by using the direct privileged route, which maps articulatory procedures straight onto phonological representations, or by using the slower, less direct route, which derives words' meanings from their phonology and then produces an articulation based on this semantic representation. This second route for rehearsal is shown as the dashed line in Models A and B of Figure 3.2. According to Kinsbourne's (1972) disconnection hypothesis, the privileged route for rehearsal should be disrupted in conduction aphasics, but the indirect route may well be intact. Friedrich, Glenn, and Marin (1984) have provided some support for this suggestion. They found that their conduction aphasic patient E. A. showed mutual interference between the repetition task and McCleod and Posner's visual matching task, unlike normal people. They therefore argued that E. A.'s repetition relied on the indirect route because the privileged route was disrupted. If they are correct, one would expect patients like E. A. to be very slow at repeating back single spoken words.

McCarthy and Warrington (1985a) have reported clinical evidence that suggests the indirect route is intact in conduction aphasics. They compared a group of conduction aphasics with a group of transcortical aphasics. Unlike conduction aphasics, transcortical aphasics show poor comprehension but preserved repetition. This pattern of symptoms suggests that transcortical aphasics can map phonological representations onto articulatory procedures, but cannot use them to access word meanings, whereas conduction aphasics suffer from the reverse impairment. Support for this idea was found when repetition of verbal material that differed in degree of meaningfulness was compared across the patient groups. Although repetition in the conduction aphasics was worse, they benefited more than the transcortical aphasics from repeating more meaningful material. Although not conclusive proof, this finding is consistent with the idea that conduction aphasics can use their ability to access meaning from phonology to help them rehearse and hence improve their ability to repeat spoken material.

Research on immediate auditory–verbal memory in conduction aphasics has proved fruitful, although it still faces many unanswered questions. Some patients undoubtably have a genuine memory impairment that cannot be discounted as an artefact of poor speech comprehension or output. The disorder seems to be a fairly selective one, affecting phonologically encoded information. Immediate phonological memory is disrupted, but it seems likely that delayed phonological memory will be as well. Organic amnesics show normal immediate memory for phonological material, which could be because such memory does not require the retrieval of background contextual information rather than because it depends on a separate short-term store for phonologically encoded material. It is not, then, conclusively proved that the disorder affects the output of a separate phonological *short-term* store. Also, there need not be a single explanation for the repetition deficit. Conduction aphasics appear to be a heterogeneous group. There is evidence that one group has one or more kinds of phonological-processing deficiency, which may or may not cause paraphasic errors, but which probably does cause poor phonological memory. A second group shows impaired rehearsal because of a partial disconnection between phonological representations and articulatory processes, which could account for most, if not all, kinds of impaired immediate memory. Finally, there may be a third group, who may analyse phonological information adequately and in whom both routes to repetitive rehearsal are well preserved. The memory deficit in this group would have to be a consequence of a storage failure specific to phonological information.

Effects of the repetition deficit
on other aspects of cognition

There has as yet been only one direct test of the idea that good immediate memory for phonological representations is essential if longer term memory for these representations is to be effective. This does, however, seem likely, as the single direct test suggests. But long-term memory for meaningful material seems to be surprisingly well preserved in patients. It would appear that auditory–verbal inputs can be meaningfully interpreted without having to use a route that obligatorily passes through a phonological store. Instead, meaning may be directly accessed from phonological representations that are not being held in any store. There is, however, a widely held belief that intact auditory–verbal immediate memory is essential for the normal comprehension of some kinds of spoken sentences (see Vallar & Baddeley, 1984). Specifically, it is argued that phonologically analysed words may have to be held in storage whilst the grammatical structure of a series of words in a sentence is being computed. Impaired immediate auditory span should compromise understanding if these computations are lengthy.

Conduction aphasics do have mild comprehension problems on sensitive tests, such as the Token Test, which contains in its later sections a number of long and complex spoken sentences, the understanding of which seems likely to place demands on memory. Sentence length does not seem to be the only variable that affects understanding in these patients, however, because when it is held roughly constant and grammatical and semantic content is varied, some sentences lead to comprehension problems and others do not. Semantically reversible passive sentences, such as 'The lion was chased by the tiger', have been reported to cause patients most difficulty. But it has also been found that short sentences known as truncated passives, such as 'The black cat was beaten', cause considerable difficulty (for a discussion, see McCarthy & Warrington, 1987). At first sight, these findings are at odds with the claim that the conduction aphasics' subtle comprehension deficit is caused by the repetition deficit. If, however, it is assumed that these kinds of sentence take longer to parse than sentences with which the patients have no difficulty, then their problem can still be regarded as a result of their rapid loss of phonological representations. This interpretation postulates that short-term phonological memory is necessary for the parsing, or 'on-line' analysis, of syntactically critical word-order information. A somewhat different view has been advanced recently by McCarthy and Warrington (1987). These researchers examined the sentence comprehension of two conduction aphasics who had reliable auditory spans for digits and words of only one. Despite this, the patients' ability to repeat sentences was relatively preserved. In fact, their ability to recall whole sentences was superior to their recall of three words contained within a sentence, which suggests that sentence recall depends on a level of analysis beyond the level of the individual word. The patients also showed adequate comprehension of both active and passive sentences, in some of which understanding required the analysis of order-dependent syntactic information. The patients were impaired, however, at understanding sentences that violated normal conversational conventions related to the order of event occurrence or the role of a subject or an object in an array. For example, they showed poor comprehension of sentences like 'Before she went to the shops she watered the flowers', which reverses the usual order in which we refer to events. The patients were also poor at making comparative judgements in which they had to answer spoken questions such as 'Which is red, a poppy or a lettuce?'. McCarthy and Warrington argued that with those sentences for which the patients showed poor comprehension, an appropriate cognitive representation cannot be constructed 'on-line' from the linguistic analysis, and in such cases it is vital to backtrack over the information that has just been spoken. This backtracking ability might be dependent on the integrity of short-term phonological memory.

It remains unproved, however, that poor immediate phonological memory does cause the mild sentence-comprehension problems that have been reported in some conduction aphasics. The two deficits might be independent of each other, but caused by lesions to closely adjacent structures. If there is a causal link, then minimally one should expect to see a correlation between patients' immediate-memory span and the severity of their comprehension impairment. Evidence that poor phonological short-term memory is not obligatorily associated with poor comprehension of spoken sentences has been found recently by Butterworth, Campbell, and Howard (1986). They reported that a young graduate student with a digit span of about four was unimpaired on syntactic analysis and comprehension of spoken sentences. The finding is impressive because if short-term phonological memory is essential for the comprehension of certain kinds of sentence, then it should be impossible to find any patient with impaired immediate memory and completely normal sentence comprehension. It could be argued, however, that the student had only a mild deficit and may have developed compensatory strategies. If Butterworth's subject had had a span of one, like the patients of McCarthy and Warrington, instead of four, then she might have shown clear comprehension problems with certain kinds of sentence. Thus the matter cannot be regarded as resolved. Given the rarity of appropriate patients, the causal hypothesis might also be tested by simulating poor immediate memory in normal subjects and seeing whether this deficit differentially affects comprehension of the kinds of sentence that the patients have difficulty understanding. This could be done by giving subjects an articulatory-suppression task to perform whilst listening to sentences or presenting sentences embedded in noise. The hypothesis remains interesting, but unproved. It is also true that at present, we lack any convincing model of how sentence parsing and the labile storage of phonological information interact to produce comprehension.

Neuroanatomy of short-term memory deficits: the role of PTO association neocortex

All the disorders of short-term memory that have been reported have been associated with lesions of PTO association neocortex. This is compatible with the assumption, discussed in chapter 1, that where information is encoded, there it will be stored, although it remains to be seen whether the overlap is so great that selective storage deficits do not occur. Information about colour, space, phonology, and other visual material is almost certainly encoded in this region of the neocortex. Unfortunately, because cases with memory problems and no other deficit are very rare, it is difficult to be sure precisely where the responsible lesions lie within PTO association neocortex. Cases with auditory short-term memory deficits seem to have a common area of damage in the left inferior part of the parietal lobe. This conclusion, drawn from single-case studies, is congruent with the results of a retrospective analysis of over 650 patients, which found that integrity of the left parietal lobe was essential for normal auditory–verbal immediate memory (Warrington, Galton, & Maciejewski, 1985). A lesion location within the left hemisphere would be expected because damage to PTO neocortex in this hemisphere is known to affect not only most verbal abilities, but also phonological processing in particular. There is, however, as yet no theoretical reason to expect a lesion in the inferior parietal lobe rather than in any other region of PTO association neocortex.

The anatomical correlates of impaired visual immediate memory are less well known. Kinsbourne and Warrington's (1962) four cases with reduced visual spans had damage to the posterior left hemisphere, and autopsy data from a later case indicated that the damage might be confined to the tempero-occipital region of the left hemisphere (see Warrington & McCarthy, 1986). Group studies are in good accord with this lesion location, as reduction in visual span for both verbal and non-verbal stimuli is greatest after lesions of left posterior neocortex. There is, however, an apparent conflict with the data of Samuels et al. (1972), which show that right parietal lobe lesions are associated with poor memory for visually presented verbal and non-verbal stimuli in the Brown-Peterson task. The deficit in these patients may have had a different origin. One possibility is that they were suffering from a subtle visual-processing disorder. Nevertheless, it is perhaps surprising that the visual immediate-memory deficit is usually associated with unilateral lesions of the left hemisphere because it affects both verbal and non-verbal material. It could be that the non-verbal stimuli are recoded verbally, but an important role of the left hemisphere in non-verbal processing should not be excluded.

Further support for the view that visual immediate-memory impairments are caused by temporal lobe lesions comes from observations on the famous amnesic patient H. M. This patient had both medial temporal lobes removed to treat his intractable temporal lobe epilepsy. The areas excised included the hippocampus and amygdala within the temporal lobes, but there was also some removal of the anterior part of the temporal neocortex (the temporal pole). H. M. was tested on a delayed matching-to-sample task with visual stimuli. This task required him simply to find a match to a visual stimulus he had been shown up to 30 sec previously. Although he performed well on simultaneous matching, he was impaired at zero delay, had great difficulty at 4-sec delay, and dropped steeply to chance at 30-sec delay (for a discussion, see Horel, Voytko, & Salsbury, 1984). This very poor performance was probably not associated with his limbic system damage, which relates to the long-term memory problems shown by this patient, as two pieces of data suggest. First, evidence from animal studies that will be discussed shortly suggests that it was the lesion in H. M.'s temporal pole that caused his short-term visual memory impairment. Second, this patient's performance on an auditory–verbal delayed matching-to-sample task showed no deterioration with delays up to 40 sec. This would be expected if normal auditory–verbal memory depends on the intactness of the left inferior parietal lobe because this region was untouched in H. M.

Very little is known about the anatomical bases of impairments of immediate memory for spatial location and colour. Davidoff and Ostergaard's (1984) patient, who had poor immediate colour memory, was given a CAT scan that showed him to have a vascular lesion of the left tempero-occipital lobe. The authors felt unable to conclude where the critical lesion lay within this region. Disorders of short-term spatial memory have been associated with lesions of the right posterior neocortex (De Renzi & Nichelli, 1975). There is considerable evidence that in humans, the right hemisphere plays a more important role in visuospatial processing than does the left hemisphere, so this lesion location should be expected. Where the lesion lies within the right hemisphere's PTO association cortex remains an interesting question.

All these lesion sites are in cortical brain regions that receive their sensory inputs over multiple intervening synaptic relays from the primary sensory cortical receiving areas. If the locations are approximately correct, this suggests that only the products of the fairly late stages of processing are stored. There is little evidence from lesion studies to support older theories that placed short-term stores at the earlier stages of processing. It seems likely that more immediate-memory disorders will be found that are specific to highly discrete kinds of information. An enormous amount of parallel processing is performed by different regions of association cortex, many dealing with recognizably distinct kinds information. If storage is an intrinsic property of such systems, one might expect to find highly selective kinds of immediate-memory deficit, provided patients suffered from small enough lesions. The neurological evidence does not yet prove that such immediate-memory disorders are caused by disruption of information-specific short-term storage systems. It has been very difficult to exclude other causes, such as subtle information-processing deficits and reduced ability to use rehearsal. Furthermore, it has been extremely hard to find convincing evidence that the deficits reflect a disturbed output from a separate short-term store, as opposed to a single store for information of the relevant kind. Other human and animal research, possibly relevant to the existence of such short-term stores, will now be briefly reviewed.

Evidence from electrical stimulation and recording studies for short-term memory stores

In epileptic patients who are about to undergo surgery for the treatment of their disorder, it is important to ensure that functionally vital brain regions are not inadvertently removed. One way of achieving this is to stimulate electrically the brains of conscious patients. Electrical stimulation of the cortex and most forebrain areas seems to cause a temporary disruption of their normal functions. Furthermore, the effects seem to be highly specific to the site stimulated. Stimulation of another site only a few millimetres away may have a radically different effect. Verbal functions are particularly easily disrupted by stimulation of many parts of PTO and frontal association cortex of the left hemisphere. Ojemann (1983) and his colleagues have examined the effects of stimulation on subjects engaged in a short-term memory task. Sites were found where stimulation disturbed verbal short-term memory, but had no effect on naming stimuli, reading, identifying phonemes, or mimicking orofacial movements. The stimulation disrupted memory only if it was given either during stimulus presentation or during the brief delay before the memory test. Stimulation during retrieval had no effect. Interestingly, the active sites were located in the left parietal and temporal cortex, but not in the frontal cortex. This corresponds quite well with the evidence from lesion studies and provides further evidence about the specificity of the deficits. It does not show, however, that longer term memory is not also affected.

Ojemann's group has also studied the effects of stimulation of the left thalamus on their short-term memory task. Stimulation at the time of input was found to improve memory relative to non-stimulation control trials, whereas stimulation at the time of retrieval speeded retrieval but increased errors. Stimulation during both encoding and retrieval on the same trial had the algebraic sum of the input and output effects. It was argued that they were exciting a specific activating system, which directed attention to incoming stimuli by modulating the activity of the short-term storage systems of the left PTO association cortex. Some lesions of the left lateral thalamus also disrupt short-term memory, and it was also argued that these lesions disrupt a specific activating system, located in the left lateral thalamus, that modulates the activity of verbal short-term memory systems in the left PTO cortex. Stimulation of the right lateral thalamus was found to affect the short-term recall of spatial information in a similar way. The right lateral thalamus might therefore contain a specific activating system that modulates the spatial short-term storage system in the posterior region of the right hemisphere. These interesting ideas clearly need further confirmation. If correct, they suggest one means by which a lesion could produce a selective storage deficit. It could disturb a process that modulates activity in a storage system so as to improve storage without affecting basic encoding of the stored information.

Despite their significance, studies of the effects of lesions and electrical stimulation on immediate memory in humans have failed to find convincing proof of the need to postulate separate short-term memory systems. Perhaps the most convincing evidence of this need comes from physiological work on non-human primates. Some of this work is not dissimilar in principle to that which has been performed on human subjects. For example, Horel et al. (1984) bilaterally cooled the anterior tip of both temporal lobes in three monkeys in order to produce a reversible lesion. This impaired the monkeys' ability to remember photographs of objects over short delays, which was used to support the researchers' view that this area of the temporal association cortex is important for short-term memory. The activity of single neurons in other parts of the temporal lobe has been recorded when monkeys were performing a delayed matching-to-sample task (see Horel et al., 1984). These neurons showed an increased level of activity during the delay, in which the animals had to remember the stimuli they had just been shown, relative to the activity in the immediately preceding period. Activity of neurons at the anterior tip of the temporal cortex has not yet been investigated, but a similar pattern of activity might well be anticipated.

If there are separate short-term memory stores, they are likely to occupy relatively small neural regions and depend either on a rapidly occurring, but short-lasting physiological or biochemical changes, or on the continued reverberatory activity of the coding neurons in the storage system. The temporal cortex neurons, described above, possibly depend on a reverberatory mechanism to achieve brief storage. Rolls (1986) has reported that neurons in other brain regions also hold a changed pattern of firing during the delay period of short-term memory tasks. For example, neurons in the dorsolateral prefrontal cortex of monkeys hold a pattern of firing in the brief delay during which the animals must remember a position to which they must respond. Some neurons in this region seem to code for the position in which a stimulus has been shown, whereas others seem to code for the response that has to be made. Neurons have also been found in the hippocampus that hold a pattern of firing during the delay period. This firing pattern seems also to code for the response that needs to be made at retrieval. By recording the firing patterns of single neurons, Rolls and his co-workers have also found evidence for the other possible mechanism of short-term storage. They recorded the activity of neurons in the inferior temporal cortex (an area that plays a central role in the later stages of visual information processing) during the delay between the first and second presentations of a visual stimulus. Some of the neurons in this region produced a smaller response when the stimulus was shown for the second time, an indication that they 'remembered' its first presentation. The majority of these neurons only showed this changed response, however, provided there were no other intervening stimuli between the first and second presentations of the target stimuli. Only a few neurons maintained this changed response when there were one or two intervening stimuli. These neurons therefore appear to form part of a short-term storage system for certain kinds of visual stimuli.

Although the animal research using recordings from single neurons strongly supports the existence of short-term storage systems within the association neo-cortex, this does not prove that there are lesions that will selectively disrupt short-term storage but leave all other processes and kinds of memory unaffected. It might be found that all lesions that disrupt a short-term store also prevent the fully normal initial processing of the relevant kind of information and its long-term storage as well. But selective storage deficits would occur if lesions affected brain systems that modulated the activity of the short-term storage system in a way that specifically related to short-term storage processes. In such cases, long-term memory should also be indirectly affected, however, if information is passed serially from short- to long-term storage, although there may well be other lesions that cause long-term memory deficits, but leave short-term memory intact. Organic amnesics seem to suffer from such lesions. Even though long-term storage of the affected kind of information may be in the same neurons that subserve its short-term storage, effective long-term memory for this information may also require the storage of additional contextual information. It is tentatively suggested in chapter 6 that amnesics have a selective problem remembering contextual information, which could explain their normal short-term memory because it may be context free. Where immediate memory in organic amnesics is not normal, as appears to be the case with facial stimuli, it could be that the retrieval of contextual cues plays an important role.

At the beginning of this chapter, it was suggested that one reason for believing in the existence of separate short-term stores is that the structural changes that underlie enduring memory do not take place immediately. Current estimates indicate that these structural changes will not occur in less than 1 min and may take much longer. Immediate memory must therefore be subserved by different storage mechanisms. There may be many such short-term stores for different kinds of information in PTO association cortex. If processing and storage occur in the same sites, however, lesions should disrupt processing and both short- and long-term memory for specific kinds of information. It is unlikely that the neuro-psychological deficits described in this chapter affect memory storage selectively unless they damage a system that modulates storage processes. Even if the critical lesions disrupt modulation, they should affect both immediate and delayed memory. Identification of short-term stores is probably best achieved through direct physiological techniques because it remains implausible that any brain lesion can selectively disrupt short-term storage processes.

4   Disorders of previously
well-established memory

There is a rare disorder that is apparently caused by certain lesions of the parietal neocortex of the left hemisphere, in which patients are unable to point on verbal command, to parts of their own bodies as well as to body parts of their examiner or of a picture of the human body. This disorder, known as autotopagnosia, is often accompanied by other cognitive deficits, such as a general difficulty in naming things, known as an anomia, or a difficulty understanding any words that refer to concrete as opposed to abstract concepts. If autotopagnosia is accompanied by these kinds of problem, then it is possible to argue that it is caused by a general difficulty with word names or an inability to understand the meaning of concrete words. There are cases, however, in which patients can name body parts on their own bodies when these parts are pointed to by the examiner, although they cannot point to their own body parts on command or point to their own body part that corresponds to a numbered part on a picture of a body. These autotopagnosias cannot be caused by verbal deficits, but some patients with this pattern of disorder also have difficulty pointing, on verbal command, to parts of inanimate objects. As such patients are also unable to relate a well-known story in logical sequence, it has been argued that autotopagnosia is caused by a general inability to analyse a whole into its component parts.

A case of autotopagnosia, reported by Ogden (1985), is very similar to the ones that gave rise to the above view, except that her patient was able to point, on verbal command, to parts of inanimate objects, such as a truck, flower vase, and washbasin, and to parts of non-human animate objects, such as a toy elephant. The patient had no anomia, could understand complex verbal instructions, and was able not only to name body parts that were pointed to, but also to describe the functions of named body parts. The flavour of his disorder is given by a test in which he was shown a model face, from which parts like the ears, nose, and mouth were removed. He could name all the parts when he picked them up, but was unable to put them back in the right places. For example, he put the mouth on the top of the head, where a hat should have gone! Ogden concluded that the patient's disorder was caused by the loss of a discrete body image, which normal people call on to indicate how the various parts of the body are related to one another. Although the patient had some spatial problems, they could not reasonably be invoked to explain his autotopagnosia because he had no difficulty pointing to the parts of other kinds of complex material. He also suffered from left–right confusion and was unable to name his fingers or point to those fingers that corresponded to the ones on a model that an examiner had identified, a disorder known as finger agnosia. These and other disorders suffered by the patient are not found in other very similar cases of autotopagnosia, however, so are unlikely to be related to that problem. This, as Ogden suggests, seems to have been caused by a specific deficit in his ability to recall an image of his own or other people's bodies. In normal people, knowledge about body image is based on a very heavily overlearnt non-verbal memory, which can be retrieved with minimal conscious effort. The evidence indicates that certain left hemisphere parietal lobe lesions cause a very specific disruption of this presumably very well-established memory for body image, so that an autotopagnosia occurs. In this chapter, more evidence suggesting that there are many disorders of previously well-established memory will be advanced.

Normal human life depends on our ability to retrieve rapidly information about word meanings and usages, about the properties of the kinds of animate and in-animate things we can perceive through our senses, and about the performance of both motor skills, such as unlocking doors, and mental skills, such as doing quick mental calculations. This ability is built on stable memories that have been strengthened over many years by thorough and frequent practice. It is well known that brain damage can cause a variety of verbal disorders that are referred to as aphasias or dysphasias, depending on the severity of the deficit. By definition, a disorder would not be regarded as a dysphasia if it could be explained entirely in terms of a sensory loss, amounting to deafness or blindness, or of a motor impairment that partially paralyses the muscles involved in speech and writing. Dysphasias are supposed to be specific to those parts of the brain concerned with verbal processes. Similarly, brain lesions can disturb the ability to interpret meaningfully information that is presented to us via the senses, although basic sensory processes seem to be intact and patients can understand the instructions that are given to them. These disorders are referred to as agnosias and are gener-ally thought to be caused by lesions that disrupt the fairly late stages of processing of sensory inputs, a belief that is in good accord with the finding that the lesions that underlie most agnosias lie in PTO association neocortex. Autotopagnosia is an example of a specific kind of agnosia. Brain lesions can also disrupt various kinds of skill. They may disrupt motor skills in patients who show good com-prehension of instructions and preserved ability to execute the basic movements constituting the skill. These disorders are known as apraxias or dyspraxias, de-pending on their severity. More cognitive skills, such as the ability to do mental arithmetic, may also be disrupted – a condition known as acalculia. Finally, there is a rather ill-defined group of dementing disorders in which the victims seem unable to do things that depend on the ability to retrieve a wide variety of previ-ously well-established memories. Dementing patients may often show dysphasic, agnosic, and apraxic disorders as part of their condition, which is consistent with evidence that their brain damage is extensive.

Analysis of the cognitive deficits that underlie these dysphasic, agnosic, dys-praxic, and other skill disorders, and of the lesions that cause them, strongly suggests that they do not result from disruption of the early stages of sensory processing or the final stages of motor output. Rather, processing stages far from sensory input or motor output appear to be affected. In the past, these deficits were usually understood as failures of certain kinds of information processing; but in recent years, there has been a growing tendency to reconstrue them as, at least sometimes, resulting from disturbances of previously very well-established memories (see Warrington & McCarthy, 1986). It is argued that the brain damage either has destroyed the tissue where some of the critical memories were stored or has disrupted the mechanisms through which these memories are retrieved from storage. In order to establish this kind of conclusion, it must be shown that the deficit could not have arisen from a sensory-processing failure near to input or some other kind of processing failure that does not require the retrieval of well-established memories. For example, if a patient was unable to indicate what drawings of common objects actually were and was very bad at copying the drawings, then the agnosia might be explained in terms of a high-level sensory-processing deficit. In other words, the patient was unable to achieve a sufficiently good representation of the drawing to have any chance of accessing his semantic memory about the properties of the object drawn. It would be misleading to call such a problem a memory deficit. Similarly, if a patient could no longer understand the meanings of spoken words and badly confused different word sounds with one another, then it would be misleading to say that he was suffering from a disturbance of memory for the meanings of words. It would be much more likely that he was representing the sounds of the words wrongly, perhaps because of a problem with phonological analysis, and so could not begin to access the part of his memory that stores word meanings. If his problem was one of phonological analysis and the sounds of phonemes have to be learnt and stored in long-term memory, then one could argue that memory for the 'phonological lexicon' had been disturbed. Evidence for such a selective disruption of phonological memory would need to show that the earlier stages of auditory analysis were intact and that there was an effectively normal input to a damaged phonological memory system.

The dividing line between disorders of previously very well-established memories and processing deficits is often hard to draw. For example, apraxias are often caused by lesions of the parietal lobe and sometimes by lesions of the prefrontal cortex. These lesions are frequently associated with disorders of spatial processing and of the sequential organization of acts, respectively. It is plausible to suggest that apraxias involving co-ordination of actions in space, such as the difficulty in putting on clothes, known as dressing apraxia, might be caused by a spatial-processing deficit leading to defective sensory guidance of fine motor behaviour. Equally, disturbances in the ability to perform complex actions, such as lighting a candle with a match, usually called ideational apraxia, could be caused by a loss of the ability to organize sequences of actions. These explanations contrast with those that ascribe the apraxias to an inability to retrieve the plan of a well-practised action so that it can activate the motor system. Even if they are correct, however, they do not necessarily exclude a different kind of memory-deficit explanation. For example, dressing apraxia might be caused by the specific inability to retrieve information about the relationship between the spatial organization of the body and that of immediately surrounding space, an explanation closely allied to that which has been given for autotopagnosia.

Another popular explanation of some apraxic, as well as aphasic and agnosic, disorders is that they are caused by a disconnection syndrome, in which one intact processing system or memory store is disconnected from another intact processing system or memory store. An apraxia of this type could be caused by a lesion that prevents the memory for how an action is performed, such as saluting or lighting a candle, from accessing the motor machinery that finally produces the action, or it could be caused by a failure to access the memory of the action plan in the first place. If an agnosia was caused in this way, then an adequate sensory representation of an object might be achieved, but the lesion would prevent this representation from accessing semantic memories about the significance of that object. A similar explanation has been offered for conduction aphasia, according to which an adequate phonological representation of the spoken input is achieved, but the lesion prevents this representation from gaining access to the speech output system, so that repetition of spoken items is very poor. This is, in fact, Kinsbourne's (1972) account of conduction aphasia, discussed in chapter 3. Although they have not usually been interpreted as memory deficits, some disconnection disorders can be regarded as problems in the retrieval of very well-learnt information. For example, in an agnosia caused by a disconnection, normally adequate sensory cues are no longer capable of leading to the retrieval of semantic information, and this is quintessentially a retrieval failure. Although that information may be accessible to other cues, so there may not be a general failure of retrieval, in the present state of knowledge it is reasonable to regard this disorder as a specific kind of retrieval deficit. This point will, however, be further discussed in the section on storage and retrieval failures, as Shallice (1986) has argued that disconnection problems can sometimes be distinguished from retrieval failures.

Several questions need to be asked when it is claimed that a disorder is caused by disruption of a previously well-established kind of memory. The first, whether the disorder might more appropriately be described as one of processing sensory inputs or motor outputs, has already been considered. The second is whether the disorder involves a disturbance of retrieval, storage, or both. Shallice (1986) has proposed some criteria to differentiate between storage and retrieval failures, which will be discussed later. A third question, perhaps less fraught with interpretive problems than the previous one, concerns the degree of specificity shown by the memory disorders in terms of the kind of information affected. This is an important question because answers to it should guide thinking about the way in which very well-learnt information is organized in storage. The fourth question has been little addressed by research so far and arises out of claims that many of the deficits in previously well-established memories are specific to semantic memory and do not affect the episodic memory system. For example, in some agnosias, patients appear to have lost much of their knowledge about common objects and their significance. This knowledge might be found in dictionaries or encyclopaedias, so it is appropriate to say that it depends on semantic memory.

What is uncertain is whether the lesions responsible for such deficits also disrupt patients' ability to retrieve personal episodes about the objects, information concerning which cannot be retrieved from semantic memory. If retrograde amnesia for such episodes was not found, there would be powerful support for the view that semantic and episodic memory are distinct memory systems, based on different brain regions. Although no one has tested for the possibility of this dissociation, it does seem highly unlikely that it would be found. It would, for example, require that someone could not know what a dog is, but produce all kinds of memories of his or her dealings with dogs. The non-occurrence of the dissociation would not, however, in itself refute the idea that semantic and episodic memory might be partially distinct systems, as will be briefly discussed later in the chapter.

There are two further questions that research on disorders of previously well-established memory should answer. As it is claimed that these disorders involve retrograde amnesia, the first question concerns the possible association of this retrograde amnesia with corresponding new learning difficulties. This question is actually directed at two rather different issues. On the one hand, poor ability to access semantic memories would be expected to impair new learning when this learning normally involves retrieving the affected semantic memories. The acquisition of some new episodic memories might well be poor as the result of the operation of a mechanism like this, and the ability to learn some new semantic information might also be disrupted. On the other hand, it is uncertain whether patients can reacquire the memories that they appear to have lost. If the lesion has disrupted retrieval, will it be possible to learn a new route into the lost information, and if the lesion has degraded the store, can new memories for the lost information be laid down in adjacent brain regions? The second question is simply concerned with the locus of the brain lesions that cause these disturbances in previously well-established memory. Although it is known that lesions of PTO association neocortex usually play a central role in these memory disorders, damage is often widespread so that it is difficult to locate the critical lesions precisely. Precise localization may be vital because the critical lesions may not be in the same sites in different people's brains. If this was found, then when a small lesion selectively degrades the storage of a specific kind of memory, the lost information may well be relearnable and stored in a brain region adjacent to the lesioned one.

Research interest in this area is comparatively recent, so most of these questions have been very incompletely addressed. Most has been learnt about the specificity of the disorders. Evidence about this is discussed in the next section, which also considers, where appropriate, the evidence that the disorders are of memory, rather than of the earlier stages of sensory processing or the organization of motor output. Then we examine the means available for discriminating between retrieval deficits and storage degradation. The ability to make such discriminations is essential if some of the theoretical distinctions discussed earlier are to be testable. After this, we briefly review evidence relevant to the possible distinction between semantic and episodic memory and the problem of new learning in patients. The final section considers the anatomical evidence and other research relevant to the physiology of overlearnt information and discusses some theoretical interpretations of what is currently known.

Specificity in the disorders of well-established memory

Warrington and McCarthy (1986) and others have argued that there is good evidence to support the claim that the storage of semantic memory depends on several at least partly distinct stores, presumably with partially distinct anatomical loci. They have argued for separate storage of different categories of semantic knowledge, such as knowledge of animate and inanimate things, and even for separate stores for the various kinds of visual and verbal semantic knowledge. These claims are based on the belief that many patients show highly specific impairments of different kinds of overlearnt semantic information, and they depend on three kinds of evidence. The first kind of evidence must show that patients with apparently selective memory problems can process the relevant information well enough to provide cues that would normally be effective for accessing the affected kind of memory. The second kind of evidence must show not only that there is a selective deficit for the specific kind of memory, but also that this deficit is not caused by the affected type of semantic memory being merely more complex, less often rehearsed, or harder to retrieve than other kinds of semantic memory. Rather, it has to show that the affected kind of semantic memory is organized differently from the unaffected kinds and so is more likely to be stored in partly distinct areas of cortex. The third kind of evidence, important in some cases, must show that storage rather than retrieval has been disturbed. The discussion of Ogden's (1985) patient with autotopagnosia should have made clear that tests of many cognitive functions are necessary if there is to be convincing evidence that either a selective retrieval deficit or storage degradation exists for a specific kind of information.

Patients with visual object agnosia are very poor at naming or describing the functions of objects, presented either in real life or in pictures. Their deficit cannot be simply ascribed to poor understanding, problems with naming, or basic failures of the early stages of visual processing. Although such patients can usually copy pictures of objects reasonably well, it is not always clear that more subtle deficits in the later stages of visual processing may not be responsible for their problems. For example, Davidoff and Wilson (1985) described a visual object agnosic who made visual as well as semantic errors on a task that required the identification of a named object from a number of object pictures. A visual error occurred when the patient picked out a wrong item that had a similar shape to the correct one, whereas a semantic error involved picking a visually dissimilar, but functionally related item, such as a glove instead of a shoe. Davidoff and Wilson therefore concluded that the deficit was caused by a failure to achieve a proper pre-semantic classification of visual stimuli. They were unable to show, however, why the patient made so many semantic errors; hence his agnosia may have been partly caused by a problem with semantic memory.

Other visual object agnosics do not show any obvious signs of impaired visual processing, so it is more reasonable to ascribe their deficit to a selective difficulty in accessing semantic memory. One of Warrington's (1975) patients, A. B., was able, for example, to perform normally on the unusual-views test, in which subjects are shown pairs of conventional and unconventional views of common objects and asked to indicate whether the views are of the same object or two different objects. When shown the conventional view of a table-tennis bat, A. B. remarked that he had already been shown a picture of that object and had said before that he did not know what it was. Another patient, F. R. A., was equally poor at pointing to pictures of named objects when they were part of a complex scene as when they were isolated (see Warrington & McCarthy, 1986). In both these cases, it is difficult to believe that the visual object agnosia was not caused by a problem with semantic memory.

Evidence that a memory deficit, rather than a perceptual-processing failure, sometimes underlies more specific agnosias as well has been found for prosopagnosia. Prosopagnosics are unable to recognize visually presented familiar faces to which they must have been heavily exposed for years. Such a patient not only may be unable to recognize his family unless he hears their voices, but also may fail to recognize his reflection in the mirror. It has been known for some time that some patients with this agnosia for familiar faces can match photographs of faces taken from different angles, taken in unusual lighting, or when disguised, which indicates that their visual processing must be reasonably intact. More recently, it has been shown that although some prosopagnosics fail to recognize photographs of familiar faces, their electrodermal responses show a clear discrimination between correct and incorrect spoken names corresponding to those faces (Bauer, 1984) or between familiar and unknown faces (Tranel & Damasio, 1985). The patients' autonomic nervous system shows knowledge of the faces that they deny recognizing. In other words, although not lying, the patients behave a bit like criminals might do on a lie detector test. Not all prosopagnosics show selective memory deficits, as did the patients of Bauer and of Tranel and Damasio, suffering instead from perceptual problems. Others, however, clearly do. For example, Hanley, Young, and Pearson (personal communication) have described a prosopagnosic who also has very little knowledge about well-known people, but who was able to show implicit memory about famous politicians and football players he was unable to recognize. These findings suggest either that recognition is independent of another system, which yields only implicit or indirect evidence concerning knowledge of remembered faces, and that only the recognition system has been damaged, or that the recognition system includes the implicit memory system and, possibly, stores additional contextual features that enable faces to be explicitly identified, with the brain damage affecting this contextual store or access to it. The latter hypothesis would predict that there should never be a patient who shows a selective loss of implicit memory for face-like material because such a deficit should also affect face recognition. Both hypotheses presuppose that prosopagnosia is sometimes caused by a memory problem.

Once there is good evidence that a patient has a memory deficit for well-learnt information, the degree of specificity of the deficit has to be determined. For example, it is still controversial whether prosopagnosia is specific to familiar faces or whether it also affects other categories of visual information, the members of which have many features in common, such as cars, birds, or other animals. The evidence on this point is very divided, although Assal and his colleagues (1985) have described a patient who became unable to recognize the cows on his farm by sight, despite apparently being able to recognize the members of his family. There are other reasons for thinking that facial information may be stored in a distinct region of PTO cortex; neurons that seem to respond selectively to faces have been found in the temporal association cortex, and facial-recognition ability develops very early (no doubt a reflection of its great biological importance in an intelligent social species, such as ours). Before discussing the evidence for other category- and sensory-modality-specific memory impairments, it is worth making one additional point. Even if it is shown that an apparent memory deficit is caused by a subtle sensory-processing failure, if the impairment is highly specific this might yet provide some support for the view that the affected kind of information is stored separately from other information. For example, it is hard to see how a patient could have difficulty identifying pictures of animals but not pictures of inanimate objects unless these two categories have partially non-overlapping stores. This would apply even if the deficit was caused by a sensory-processing failure.

For many years, it has occasionally been noted that aphasics may show impairments or preservations of naming and word recognition that are surprisingly category specific. For example, Nielson (1958) noted that knowledge of flower names may be selectively preserved in the face of severe generalized verbal deficits. It is possible to argue that such isolated cases might arise because of peculiarities of patients' past experiences leading to their having had abnormally little or great practice with the knowledge category concerned. In aphasia, it is well established that less frequently used words are more likely to be associated with deficits in word retrieval and comprehension, so demonstrations of category-specific impairments should be based on tests in which words from different categories are matched in frequency. The same point can be made if there are some cases showing selective deficits for a particular category and others showing selective preservation. Goodglass, Wingfield, Hydge, and Theurkauf (1986) have shown just this in a large-scale study of a group of aphasics. In one study, patients were required to name pictures of objects drawn from 16 categories, including birds, tools, insects, colours, and body parts. Deviantly high and low naming scores were found most frequently for letters, and then colours and body parts. Preservation did not seem to be a function of there being easy test items because equally easy items for the patients as a whole, selected from all categories, were less well named than the preserved category items. In a second study, naming and the ability to recognize the names of pictures of items, drawn from 6 categories, were tested in 117 aphasics. Once again, performance was deviantly high or low for colours, letters, and body parts. In addition, as naming and recognition were tested for the same items, it was possible to measure the difference in the success rate with these two measures. Although naming was generally worse than recognition, 13 patients were markedly deviant in failing to recognize items that they could name. This tendency was strongest in the patients for the categories of letters, body parts, and then colours.

The findings of Goodglass and his colleagues suggest that aphasics are particularly likely to show disproportionate impairments and preservations in verbal memory for the categories of letters, body parts, and colours. The body-naming impairments probably have a different cause from the case of autotopagnosia, discussed in the last section, because the patients also did not recognize body-part names normally, which is consistent with there being a verbal deficit rather than one of body images. Goodglass et al. argued that these categories of verbal knowledge are particularly likely to be stored at distinct cortical sites because they have a limited number of members and therefore are cohesive and probably received much practice early in life. It should be remembered, however, that the dissociations they reported were only partial, so there is no proof that these verbal category stores are completely separate from other verbal stores. There are two interpretations of the partial dissociation between recall (naming) and recognition of the words. First, these two forms of retrieval depend on partly separate routes into lexical memory storage and can, to some extent, be separately compromised. Second, recall and recognition may depend on accessing distinct stores of lexical information. For example, there would be one store for colour words accessed by recall, and another for colour words accessed by recognition. No available evidence distinguishes between these two possibilities, but the second would be plausible only if the patients' recall and recognition deficits arose from storage degradation. There is no evidence to support this, and, indeed, Goodglass et al. argue that a retrieval deficit is more likely.

There is some evidence that there may be double dissociations for deficits of verbal knowledge for abstract and concrete words. Just as normal people have more problems with tests of abstract knowledge, so brain-damaged patients usually show greater impairments for abstract than concrete words. For example, deep dyslexics, who have a selective deficit in reading and making sense of written words, are known to have greatest problems with abstract nouns and verbs and with function words, such as *if*. There are, however, patients who show the *reverse* pattern of impairment. For example, patients A. B. and S. B. Y. (Warrington, 1975) were unable to define concrete words that had clearly been within their premorbid vocabulary. Thus A. B. did not know the meaning of *garage,* and S. B. Y. defined *harp* as a thing to measure things with. In contrast, S. B. Y.'s ability to define more common abstract words seemed effectively normal (although a deficit with less common abstract words would probably have been apparent if it had been formally tested). Thus he defined *debate* as an argument and *indignation* as when you are not happy about something or get angry about something. This partial double dissociation suggests that concrete and abstract lexical items may to a large extent be separately stored. Further, one must suppose that the concrete-word store is itself subdivided, as letter, colour, and body-part word knowledge seems more likely to be affected differently by cortical lesions than is knowledge of other word categories.

Other categories of concrete-word knowledge may also be maintained in relatively distinct cortical stores. Goodglass et al. (1986) found one patient who showed a deviantly high score on the naming of animals. Similar observations have been made on two aphasic patients by Warrington and McCarthy (1986). One of these patients had no effective speech, so could be tested only by using a word–picture matching technique. She was disproportionately bad at pointing out named pictures of inanimate objects relative to her ability to indicate named pictures of foods and living things. Warrington and Shallice (1984) have reported the reverse pattern of deficit in four patients who had suffered an attack of herpes simplex encephalitis, from which they had made a partial recovery. The virus had caused widespread damage of the temporal lobes, one effect of which was an organic amnesia. But as well as the amnesia, the patients showed deficits of well-established verbal and visual semantic knowledge, not usually found in organic amnesics. Two of these patients were asked to define common names for animate and inanimate objects. Definitions of inanimate objects were far more accurate. For example, one patient defined *camel* as a bird of some type, but defined *thermometer* as a device for registering temperature. The other two patients showed a similar pattern of performance with a word–picture matching task. It was not shown, however, that any of the patients' knowledge of inanimate objects was completely intact.

Warrington and McCarthy argued that the partial double dissociation that is found for lexical knowledge of animate and inanimate objects may indicate a division in the storage systems for these kinds of concrete-word knowledge. They suggested that objects may be identified mainly in terms of their functional characteristics, whereas animate things are identified mainly in terms of their sensory characteristics. For example, a jug and a vase can look effectively the same, but have very different functions, whereas the functional roles of lions and tigers are practically identical, and yet the animals can easily be distinguished by their physical features. The distinction would imply that functional features of things are stored largely separately from physical features of things. Although there may be some truth in this claim, there are other category-specific memory deficits that are too specific for it to be more than a simplification. Even if one accepts that the categories of letters, body parts, and colours are exceptions to the division of concrete-word knowledge into functional- and physical-feature memory systems, one would not expect to find patients who show disproportionately poor comprehension of the names of small manipulable objects as opposed to large outdoor objects, such as trains, as Warrington and McCarthy (1987) have themselves recently reported in the patient Y. O. T. Y. O. T. also showed a relatively preserved ability to match the spoken and written names of occupations, but was very poor at making such matches for the names of geographical features. Like her grasp of the names of small and large man-made objects, this pattern of performance is difficult to explain in terms of a division of the concrete-knowledge system into functional- and physical-feature memory systems. Nor would one expect to find patients who have a selective deficit in the ability to name fruits and vegetables. Yet a patient of just this kind has been reported by Hart, Berndt, and Caramazza (1985). This patient, M. D., had an anomia that disturbed his ability to name pictures and objects from the categories of fruit and vegetables, although he could name other food objects, and things from non-food categories tested without difficulty. Like many anomics, his deficit was confined to recalling names because he was able to classify fruit and vegetable names into their correct categories when they were given to him. D. M.'s deficit clearly cannot be explained in terms of the dichotomy between functional and physical features because fruits, vegetables, and other foods should all be mainly identifiable through their physical features. If physical-feature information has a distinct storage system, then this system must have further internal divisions. Indeed, Warrington and McCarthy (1987) now speculate that semantic memory for different kinds of object may depend on storage of information from many sensory channels and that the weighting of these channels will differ for the various categories of semantic memory. Thus one might expect that information relevant to these different categories would be stored in distinct, if overlapping, association neocortex regions.

Other highly selective category-specific impairments have been reported. There appears to be at least a partial double dissociation with anomias for proper names and object names. One patient was found to name objects without difficulty, but could name only 3 out of 20 photographs of well-known personalities. Her ability to recall another class of proper names, that of towns, was, however, spared. Another patient showed a general anomia except for the naming of countries, which was selectively preserved (see McKenna & Warrington, 1980). It would seem that not only may proper naming ability be selectively preserved or impaired, but so may be specific categories of this ability. A second kind of surprising and perhaps counter-intuitive deficit was found in some aphasics, whose major problem was with grammatical speech. One such patient showed a disproportionate difficulty in recalling verbs and action words, and a similar, but less severe comprehension difficulty with the same kind of words. This patient's recall and comprehension of proper and common nouns were relatively preserved (see Warrington & McCarthy, 1986). It was indeed argued that the agrammatism arose from the patient's category-specific difficulty with verbs. A third kind of highly specific impairment that involves a type of abstract semantic knowledge has been described by Warrington (1982). She examined an acalculic patient, whose poor ability to do mental arithmetic seemed to result from a selective disturbance in his ability to remember previously well-known arithmetic facts, such as $3 + 8 = 11$. The patient still grasped concepts like 'quantity' and operations like multiplication and division, and no other aspect of his semantic memory was impaired. He could give approximate answers to arithmetic problems, but his ability to make accurate calculations was hampered by his loss of much rehearsed number knowledge, such as the multiplication table.

The cases discussed above indicate that patients exist with highly selective category-specific impairments that affect their ability to remember various kinds of semantic information. It has not been shown in all these cases that the deficit results from either degradation of a category-specific memory store or a difficulty in accessing such a store despite the adequate encoding of cues that are normally effective for this purpose. For example, anomia seems to arise for at least two different reasons. First, it may occur because the objects to be named are not encoded in a completely normal way; because of this failure in sensory processing, which probably occurs at a late stage of sensory processing, well after stimuli have been received at the sensory receptors, patients are unable to name the objects accurately. This kind of anomia is not properly describable as a memory deficit. Second, anomia can occur in cases where the object encoding has been adequate; in such cases, a genuine memory deficit is present. As already indicated, however, even when a category-specific deficit is of the first kind, it provides some evidence favouring the existence of a category-specific memory store. The same cannot be said with respect to the main evidence used to support the hypothesis that there are 'modality'-specific semantic memory stores. This evidence is now discussed.

Shallice (1986) has argued that there are reasons for postulating the existence of several 'modality'-specific semantic memory stores or systems. These include a visual non-verbal semantic system, an auditory non-verbal semantic system, and a tactile non-verbal semantic system, all of which are distinguished from a verbal semantic system. He supports this claim with three independent lines of evidence. The first two lines are amenable to a number of other interpretations, which are, in my view, just as plausible at present as the multiple modality-specific semantic store view, so they will be only briefly discussed. The third line of evidence is the main one and depends on the ability to distinguish between storage and retrieval deficits in semantic memory.

The first line of evidence is based on the characteristics of the modality-specific aphasias. Patients with these disorders are unable to name objects that are presented via the affected sensory modality, although they can name them when presented via the other sensory modalities and can demonstrate how the objects should be used even when they are presented via the affected modality. For example, a tactile aphasic cannot name objects that he can only feel, although he can indicate how they should be used appropriately, even when he can only feel them, and name the objects when he sees them. Such aphasias have been demonstrated for touch, sight, and hearing. Shallice believes that the best interpretation of these syndromes is that a semantic system, specific to the affected modality, has been partially disconnected from the verbal semantic system. Presumably, the knowledge contained in these non-verbal systems is illustrated by the patient's ability

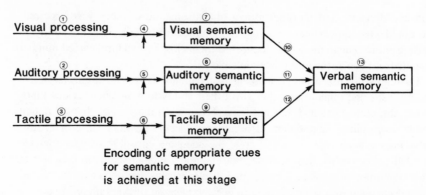

Encoding of appropriate cues
for semantic memory
is achieved at this stage

Figure 4.1 Lesions can affect any of the processes from (1) to (13). Lesions at stages (1) to (3) disturb pre-semantic processing; at stages (4) to (6), they cause retrieval failures after adequate cues for accessing semantic memory have been encoded; at stages (7) to (9), they cause storage degradation in the non-verbal modality-specific semantic stores; at stages (10) to (12), they cause retrieval failures at the verbal semantic store. In addition, some evidence suggests that lesions may cause category-specific retrieval or storage deficits of the four semantic storage systems.

to indicate the use of objects that he cannot name. The relationship of these non-verbal systems to the verbal one, according to this account, is illustrated in Figure 4.1. Other interpretations of the modality-specific aphasias have been advanced. It has, for example, been suggested that naming is subserved by a direct route from sensory input, which is separate from the route that leads into a cross-modal semantic store. Currently, there is insufficient evidence to distinguish between these two and other interpretations.

The second line of evidence is based on priming experiments that have been performed on a patient with semantic access dyslexia (see Shallice, 1986). Patients with this disorder are poor at reading and are unable to access phonology from visually presented words, so that their residual reading ability probably depends on a route that goes directly from the visual form of the words to the semantic system. The patient, who was studied by Warrington and Shallice, was very poor at reading and understanding both letters and words, but showed a striking ability to categorize words that he was unable to read. For example, he was unable to read the word *cereal*, but was able to say that it is something you eat. This patient's ability to read words was significantly improved when he was given semantically related auditory–verbal prompts. This semantic-priming effect was significantly greater for such auditory–verbal prompts than it was for pictorial prompts that were semantically related to the target word. Thus the patient's reading of the word *pyramid* was more likely to be helped by the spoken cue *Egypt* than by a picture of a pyramid. Shallice argued that these priming effects are most plausibly explained by supposing that the patient could not transmit information from a visual semantic system to the verbal semantic one, so that the pictorial cues could not prime the verbal semantic system accessed during reading. In contrast, spoken prompts reached the verbal semantic system normally. Consistent with this interpretation was the patient's inability to name visually presented objects, despite showing a reasonable ability to name such objects from their spoken descriptions. Other interpretations are, no doubt, possible, and although Shallice's hypothesis is provocative and interesting, more evidence is needed from this and similar patients before support for it can be regarded as convincing.

The third and main line of evidence is the finding that patients' deficits in knowledge when tested visually and verbally seem to be independent of each other. This is apparent in two main ways. First, some patients have deficits that are selective to a particular modality. Thus some visual object agnosics have problems with only the meaningful interpretation of visually presented objects. When tested verbally, their semantic knowledge is effectively normal. Conversely, there are aphasic patients, such as anomics, who have no problems in understanding the significance of visually presented objects. There is even a double dissociation that is sometimes, although rarely, found within the visual modality between the ability to read and understand what is read and the ability to appreciate the significance of visually presented objects. Thus a few patients can read for sense but do not understand the significance of objects they are shown, whereas others can grasp the significance of visually presented objects but cannot read for sense. Second, even when patients show poor semantic knowledge whether testing is by visual or by verbal presentation, there is little consistency between their failures and successes for the two modes of testing.

The lack of consistency shown by patients in their verbal and visual semantic memories is apparent in the three patients of Warrington's (1975) study. Although all three patients did badly on visual and verbal tests of semantic knowledge, two of them were worse at the visual tests, whereas the third was worse at the verbal tests. Warrington and Shallice (1984) also examined consistency on visual and verbal tests of semantic knowledge in two of their post-encephalitic patients. Both patients showed category-specific semantic deficits, whether they were tested visually or verbally. Their knowledge of animate objects was equally impaired with these two modes of testing. Similarly, their superior knowledge of inanimate objects was equally good, whether tested visually or verbally. When knowledge of individual items was examined, however, there was little correspondence between the two ways of testing. An item could be failed on the visual test and passed on the verbal test, and vice versa. In other words, a patient's success or failure in defining the name of a common object gave no indication as to whether he would succeed or fail in naming or describing the object when it was depicted in a line drawing. In contrast, if an object was identified on one occasion, then it would probably be identified on a later occasion; similarly, if a name was defined on one occasion, then it would probably be defined on a later occasion. In other words, there was some performance consistency within the visual and verbal modalities, but no consistency between them.

There are two main ways of interpreting these results. The first is that there is a semantic memory system that is accessed by inputs from all modalities and by verbal inputs, but that these access routes are anatomically distinct from one another. Lesions may selectively impair one of these routes, leaving the others intact, as perhaps happens in certain pure cases of agnosia or aphasia, or they may impair more than one pathway, in which case agnosia and aphasia may be found together in one patient. If perceptual processing is left intact, so that patients can encode what would normally be effective cues for semantic memory, then the lesions could be said to have caused a retrieval deficit. This explanation has no ready way of dealing with two features of the evidence. The first is the consistent pattern of patients' performance within modalities across different occasions and their inconsistent performance across modalities. The second is the differential deficit for animate-object knowledge on both the visual and the verbal tests. As the patients' perceptual processing seemed to be intact, it would have to be supposed that the final stages of the visual and verbal routes into the semantic system are anatomically subdivided so that different parts of the pathways project to different parts of the store. Both the visual and the verbal final pathway would have had to be damaged in the same region – namely, the one that projects into the part of the semantic memory system concerned with knowledge about animate objects.

The second interpretation is the multiple modality-specific store view, according to which semantic knowledge is independently represented in visual, auditory, and tactile stores and separately in a verbal store. In Warrington and Shallice's (1984) patients, the lesions would have independently degraded storage in both the visual and the verbal semantic memory stores, so that some knowledge would have been lost and some retained. This is, of course, Shallice's interpretation of the data. The main argument he offers in its favour is that one would expect consistent success or failure in identifying particular items on different occasions only if storage degradation was responsible for the memory deficit. As consistent performance was found only within the visual and verbal modalities, this suggests that visual and verbal information is independently represented. As with the retrieval-deficit interpretation, however, the differential deficit in knowledge of animate things across both modalities can be explained only in an ad hoc manner. Thus it would have to be argued that the visual and verbal stores for animate-object knowledge lie nearer to each other than either does to the stores for inanimate-object knowledge. Such a view is purely speculative at the moment.

It is clear that the need to postulate independent sensory and verbal semantic memory stores hinges largely on the strength of the evidence that Warrington and Shallice's patients and others like them have suffered degradation of their stores rather than a difficulty in accessing information that is stored normally. This evidence is briefly considered in the next section. To summarize this section, several points can be made. First, some agnosic, aphasic, and dementing disorders may be caused partly or wholly by deficits in the retrieval and/or storage of previously well-known semantic memories. The same may be true of the apraxias, which so far have been little studied within a memory context. Second, patients exist who show remarkably specific deficits or sparing of particular categories of semantic memory. These dissociations have been used to support the idea that the semantic memory store is divided hierarchically into a number of semi-independent components, each with a particular location in the neocortex. Thus semantic memory might be divided into knowledge of concrete and abstract words and their objects. Concrete-object knowledge might be divided into knowledge of functions and physical features, which, in turn, might be subdivided. The significance of this structure is discussed in the last section. Alternatively, knowledge of concrete objects may depend on a number of distinct sensory and perhaps other dimensions, and the relative importance of these dimensions may differ markedly with the various kinds of semantic memory, such as that for large and small objects, fruits and vegetables, and colours. The sensory and other information central to the representation of these kinds of memory may be encoded and stored in partially distinct regions of neocortex. Third, patients may show selective impairments with visual and verbal knowledge tests, and even when both are poor, there is no concordance in performance between the two. This has been interpreted by some to support the idea of modality-specific stores. Although it has been suggested that independent semantic stores exist for verbal, visual, auditory, and tactile information, no one has properly discussed whether these stores are meant to hold the same information coded so as to be readable to its input or whether the information they hold differs. As the need to postulate these stores depends on the ability to distinguish between storage and retrieval deficits with semantic information, that topic is now discussed.

Storage and retrieval failures of semantic memory

Five criteria have been proposed by Shallice (1986) to distinguish between storage and retrieval deficits of semantic memory. The first is that storage degradation should be associated with a consistent ability or inability to retrieve particular items of semantic information on different occasions, whereas with a retrieval deficit, the ability to access a particular item of semantic information should fluctuate over time. The argument underlying this distinction is that storage degradation either destroys the memory for a particular item of information or leaves it intact, whereas with a retrieval deficit, access is subject to many local factors that may be present on some occasions but not others. This argument is not, however, compelling. For example, if an item's memory representation is only partially degraded, then its retrieval may fluctuate on different occasions, depending on the operation of local factors. Thus inconsistent retrieval over time may not necessarily indicate that there is a retrieval deficit.

The second criterion is that when a store has been degraded, it should be impossible to improve item retrieval by priming because if the item no longer exists in storage, there is nothing to be primed. In contrast, access to an item may be improved through the use of priming if there is a retrieval deficit. An example of priming was discussed earlier when data concerning Warrington and Shallice's (Shallice, 1986) semantic access dyslexia patient were considered. This patient's ability to read and, presumably, understand words was enhanced when his performance was primed by spoken words or pictures that were semantically related to the word he was having difficulty reading. On Shallice's view, this indicated that the patient had a retrieval deficit, whereas if the primes had not helped, a storage failure would have been indicated. Once again, the argument underlying this distinction is not compelling. If priming is understood as a means of activating the affected memory system, then it may still work if an item's representation in that system is damaged, but not totally destroyed. Unless priming is shown to be completely normal, then, its occurrence need not be incompatible with storage degradation.

The third criterion relates to Warrington's (1975) argument that in cases of storage degradation, item information is lost in a relatively fixed order, with attribute information being lost before superordinate information. For example, a patient with storage degradation who did not know that a canary is a yellow bird that sings would still probably know that it is a living thing. In contrast, if there was a retrieval deficit, Shallice would expect no fixed order of information loss about items. In such cases, the identification of attributes of tested items, given that superordinate information has been accessed, should be no more difficult than the identification of the superordinate initially. This distinction would be compelling if we were sure that semantic memory systems are organized hierarchically, such that when a specific piece of semantic information is retrieved, more general semantic information, under which it is subsumed, would have to be retrieved first. Although theoretically attractive, this view has not yet been proved.

Nearly all the studies of patients, discussed above, controlled for the frequency with which memory items are typically encountered in our culture. This is because less frequently rehearsed items are harder to retrieve not only in many brain-damaged patients, but also in intact people. The fourth criterion is a refinement of this belief. Whilst allowing that patients with semantic memory deficits will be poor at remembering both commonly and rarely rehearsed items, it states that whereas patients with impaired storage will be worse at remembering rarely, relative to commonly, rehearsed items, patients with retrieval deficits will not show this frequency sensitivity. In other words, patients with storage deficits, like intact people, will be sensitive to frequency of item rehearsal, whereas patients with retrieval deficits will not. Shallice's argument behind this claim is unclear, but must depend on the assumption that retrieval problems are insensitive to frequency of item rehearsal. Although it is plausible to suggest that storage deficits should be frequency sensitive because rehearsal probably strengthens storage and increases the number of neocortical regions involved with it, it is harder to see why retrieval deficits should be frequency insensitive. For example, if rehearsal increases the amount of information related to a target item already in storage, then it might increase the number of cues available at retrieval, and so compensate for a deficit that affects the ability to use such cues effectively – that is, a retrieval deficit. The only way a retrieval deficit could be frequency insensitive would be if a lesion selectively affected those retrieval processes that *are* sensitive to frequency. There is no direct evidence for this view, although, as will be discussed, some patients show frequency-sensitive semantic memory deficits and others do not. The criterion is not therefore well supported, although it is hard to see why a patient with a storage deficit should show a frequency-insensitive semantic memory problem.

The fifth criterion also does not discriminate unambiguously between storage degradation and retrieval deficit explanations. It is that slower rates of item presentation will improve access if there is a retrieval deficit, but have no beneficial effect if there has been storage degradation. Once again, this distinction depends on the assumption that degradation either totally destroys an item's representation in storage or leaves it intact. But if there is only partial destruction, then allowing more time may enable the retrieval system to access the 'noisy' memory trace.

It is apparent, then, that each of Shallice's five criteria fails to discriminate unequivocally between storage and retrieval deficits. The discrimination would be more convincing if patients fell into either a 'storage deficit' or 'retrieval deficit' pattern on all five criteria. Shallice (1986) has, in fact, analysed the results on a mixed group of 'semantic memory problem' patients on whom data are available for some of the five criteria, and has argued that the patients clearly fall into two groups. Thus consistent retrieval tended to go with sensitivity to item frequency and reduced likelihood of losing superordinate knowledge about items, whereas inconsistent retrieval on different occasions was associated with insensitivity to item frequency and an equal tendency to lose superordinate and attribute information about items. Three patients fell into the storage deficit pattern, and three into the retrieval deficit pattern; but these patients were not given tests relevant to all five criteria, and the differences were not always very large on some of the tests. Nevertheless, it might be argued that the slightly blurred distinction between the two groups arises because some patients may suffer from both storage and retrieval deficits. Clearly, more test data on more patients are needed before firm conclusions can be drawn, but there is already a suggestion that there may be two patterns of semantic memory impairment, which might conceivably correspond to storage and retrieval deficits.

The major problem is that no agreed hypothesis exists about how retrieval and storage of semantic memory are achieved. It has already been indicated that Warrington and Shallice distinguish between disconnectionist and retrieval explanations of poor semantic memory. The idea of disconnection is a general one, in that any process or store might, in principle, be disconnected by a lesion from any other. But in this context, the disconnection is specifically between the processes that encode the cues that are normally adequate for accessing a particular item from semantic memory and the semantic memory about the item itself. If this link is partly disrupted and made noisy by a lesion, then retrieval will be unreliable. It is hard to imagine other kinds of retrieval deficit unless retrieval processes operate within the store itself and can be disrupted without causing storage degradation. Such processes might direct the set of questions whose answers need to be accessed from the store if the meaning of an item is to be identified. Shallice (1986) suggests that processes of this kind may be compromised in some retrieval deficits and contrasts these with disconnectionist retrieval deficits. He speculates that the directing processes within the store contain no memory of their recent inputs and so have to be continuously supplied with the relevant information whilst they are directing a sequential and related series of questions to the semantic memory store. Whether or not this distinction is real, it is certain that it cannot be tested given our current state of knowledge.

The relationship between semantic and episodic memory

The memory disorders discussed above involve the kinds of information that might well be found in a dictionary or an encyclopaedia – that is, semantic knowledge. As indicated in chapter 1, Tulving (1984) has argued that semantic memory is a distinct system from episodic memory, which is concerned with autobiographical experience. There are, in fact, three possible views about the relationship between semantic and episodic memory. The first is that the two forms of memory are identical and are maintained in one storage system. On this view, the differences between different kinds of semantic (or episodic) memory are at least as great as those between particular kinds of episodic and semantic memory. The second view is that effective episodic memory depends on the storage of semantic information and of a kind of non-semantic information, without which autobiographical experiences could not be retrieved. For example, as will be argued in chapter 6, retrieval of personal episodes may require the retrieval of both semantic material and information about the spatiotemporal context in which that semantic material was experienced. The third view is that semantic and episodic memories are completely separate. For example, well-learnt general knowledge about mountains would be kept in a particular part of the semantic store, but personal memories about a holiday in the Alps would be kept in a totally separate episodic store.

If the third view is correct, one should predict that semantic memory impairments should not disturb pre-morbidly acquired episodic memories with a similar content. For example, losing all one's knowledge about mountains should not impede one's ability to remember that long-ago holiday in the Alps. This seems a most implausible suggestion, but it has not been formally tested. Both the other views predict that if semantic memory is poor, so will be memory for pre-morbidly experienced episodes. Although this seems likely, it has not been tested, and even if the prediction appears to be met, it might be argued that a large lesion has independently compromised both semantic and episodic memory systems. For example, Alzheimer's dementia is associated with extensive loss of pre-morbid episodic and previously very well-established semantic memories (Weingartner, Grafman, Boutelle, & Martin, 1983). Alzheimer's disease is the most common form of dementia, one variant of which may affect people as young as 40, although the most common variant affects people over 65. All dementias cause progressive deterioration of cognitive functions as a result of increasing amounts of brain damage. In the cases of both early- and late-onset Alzheimer's disease, there is progressive atrophy of the PTO and, to a lesser extent, frontal association cortex, which could cause loss of semantic memory, and of the hippo-campus and amygdala in the limbic system, which could cause loss of pre-morbid episodic memory.

If patients show loss of pre-morbid episodic memories, only the view claiming that episodic and semantic memory are identical would predict that they must also show impairments of previously well-established semantic memories. The second view would not predict this because the episodic memory impairment might be caused by disruption of retrieval or storage of non-semantic information, such as that involving spatiotemporal context. Something like this appears to happen in organic amnesics because despite showing a sometimes dramatic loss of pre-morbid autobiographical memories, they often show excellent preservation of well-rehearsed semantic memories. If these amnesics do have problems with well-rehearsed semantic memories, they must be extremely subtle, because most studies fail to find any effects at all. Amnesics do, however, show some loss of less well-rehearsed semantic memories. For example, they have poor memory for little rehearsed information that concerns publicly known facts about politicians and sports figures; such information cannot be regarded as episodic, although it would originally have been experienced in a probably forgotten personal episode, as are all other semantic memories. This dissociation does suggest, however, that less well-rehearsed episodic and semantic information cannot be maintained in exactly the same storage system as well-rehearsed semantic information. It also implies that the third view is wrong because semantic and episodic information cannot be stored in totally separate memory systems.

It can be tentatively concluded, then, that whereas all well-rehearsed semantic information is held in the compartmentalized vaults of the semantic memory system, less well-rehearsed episodic *and* semantic information is held in this system and in a non-semantic system that may contain something like contextual information. What implications does this view have for ideas about the acquisition of new episodic and semantic information? If the relevant parts of the semantic memory system are damaged, then one might expect that it will be difficult to learn new information of both kinds. This follows because the new information will not be encoded in appropriately rich and distinctive ways. It may also be the case that some of the newly encoded information cannot be properly stored because its 'appropriate' storage site or access to it has been damaged. This pre-diction is fairly hard to test because many patients have lesions that extend not only into PTO cortex, so as to affect semantic storage, but also into limbic system structures, so as to cause organic amnesia and hence poor ability to acquire new episodic and semantic information. Nevertheless, Warrington (1975) argued that her three semantic memory patients were not like organic amnesics. They did, however, show very poor ability to acquire most new information. One exception was a test of recognition for recently shown complex representational pictures, on which, unlike amnesics, the patients scored in the normal range. This finding is difficult to assess because one does not know the extent to which normal people would draw on their semantic memory in encoding such pictures. Furthermore, one does not know whether the relevant aspect of the patients' semantic memory was impaired. Nevertheless, one of the patients was clearly impaired at recognizing recently seen words whose meanings she had largely forgotten, so it seems likely that her poor encoding ability did impair word learning. Further studies of this kind, in which new learning tasks are matched to the aspects of semantic memory that are affected, need to be done.

It is, of course, very difficult to show that patients with deficits in previously well-established semantic memories have learning difficulties because of both impoverished encoding and storage-related failures. Whereas it is relatively easy to demonstrate poor encoding of new information, which surely at least partly underlies the deficient learning of Warrington's patients, it is harder to find convincing evidence that poor learning in such patients is caused by a storage problem. Nevertheless, most evidence suggests that even if encoding is poor, there should be only a moderate impairment of learning. As storage failures are most likely to affect learning when patients attempt to reacquire lost semantic information, one should predict particularly severe deficits when patients attempt such relearning. Relevant observations about relearning have been made in only three studies. In the first study, McCarthy and Warrington (1985b) examined the ability of their agrammatic patient to learn the names of pictured actions, such as drinking, that he had not previously known. Being told the correct name improved his naming ability over a few days, but no learning benefits were retained over a period of 2 months. As this patient showed consistency over time in his ability to retrieve the names of particular pictured actions, it could be argued that his storage of the meanings of action words had been disrupted. This may have impeded his ability to relearn this information. In the second study, it was noted by Hart et al. (1985) that their patient with an anomia specific to the categories of fruits and vegetables failed to relearn the lost names over many test sessions. A similar result was found in the third case study, of another anomic (Kay & Ellis, 1987). This patient had a non-specific anomia, showed normal semantic knowledge of things he was unable to name, and could frequently produce part of a name that he could not produce in its entirety. Despite having a normal ability to learn lists of words, this patient proved unable to relearn the names of words he had been unable to produce during initial tests. These two cases of anomia are probably caused by a disconnection between an adequate semantic representation of the to-be-named object and a lexical memory store, but they could be caused by disruption of a lexical memory specific to recall (as has been speculated by Goodglass et al., 1986). Either way, relearning seems to be well-nigh impossible, something that would be unlikely if poor encoding were the only cause.

It would be interesting to see whether relearning is possible in other agnosic and aphasic disorders, especially if it could be determined whether these disorders are caused by storage or retrieval deficits. Ease of relearning lost material might indeed become an additional criterion for distinguishing between storage and retrieval deficits. Much more research will be needed, however, before any confident conclusions can be drawn.

Neuroanatomy of semantic memory and conclusions

Most of the impairments in previously well-established semantic memories seem to be caused by lesions of PTO association cortex of the left hemisphere. It is impossible to locate the critical lesions precisely within this area. Nevertheless, Warrington and McCarthy (1986) have made some preliminary suggestions. First, they argue that deficits in word retrieval are more severe after lesions to the left temporal lobe than they are after lesions to other sectors of the left hemisphere. They cite evidence that shows that oral synonym judgements are particularly affected by left temporal lobe lesions. This evidence supports the view that word comprehension may be specifically compromised by lesions of this lobe. The association is not, however, invariably found. For example, Hart et al.'s (1985) patient with an anomia specific to fruits and vegetables had a lesion that affected his left frontal cortex and basal ganglia (with which the frontal cortex is directly connected), and similar lesions have been found with other anomics. It is possible that the storage and retrieval of word names involve a circuit that includes the left temporal cortex, frontal cortex, and basal ganglia. It might be speculated that within this circuit, the major storage site lies in the left temporal cortex.

Second, Warrington and McCarthy argue that visual object agnosia is also associated with lesions of the left posterior cortex. They cite evidence that lesions of this region cause significantly greater deficits in visual object knowledge than do other cortical lesions. Evidence from single-case studies may indicate that a lesion on the boundary of the parietal and occipital lobes is particularly critical in causing visual agnosia. It must be confessed, however, that many semantic memory deficits are associated with rather diffuse left PTO cortex lesions, so it is impossible to determine whether the disrupted storage is spread over the whole area or just a small part of it. This becomes particularly important when deficits affect just one part of semantic memory, such as knowledge of animate objects or the meanings of colour words.

Although the evidence suggests that the storage of much semantic information may occur within the left temporal lobe region of PTO association cortex, it leaves three important questions largely undecided. The first question is whether different kinds of semantic knowledge have standard locations within PTO cortex in all people or whether the storage location for such information is an idiosyncratic matter, dependent on people's interests, experience, and education. It could, of course, be argued that, contrary to the impression given by the lesion evidence, there is almost complete overlap in the storage locations of different classes of semantic information. The second question concerns the kind of semantic information storage that occurs within PTO cortex of the right hemisphere.

As this region is generally believed to be less involved than the left hemisphere with mediating verbal behaviour, it seems likely that it would be a good site for the storage of modality-specific non-verbal memories if such exist, although the famous split-brain cases of Sperry and his colleagues (see Sperry, 1974) suggest that, at least in some people, verbal semantic material may also be stored there. The two hemispheres of these patients have been surgically disconnected, so it is possible to test the semantic memory ability of the right hemisphere in isolation. In some patients, there is evidence that verbal semantic information is stored in the right hemisphere, probably in the temporal lobes. These patients may not, however, be typical, as their brains may have been reorganized in response to their long-standing epilepsy. There is, unfortunately, little evidence currently available to resolve this issue. The third question is whether frontal association cortex also stores certain kinds of well-established information. It might, for example, store the motor programs for well-learnt skills, although other possibilities should not be excluded – for example, the related one that the frontal cortex may contain the 'scripts' for specific events, such as being in a restaurant (see Newcombe, 1985).

The involvement of the frontal lobes in memory is discussed in chapter 5, so will not be considered further here, and little can presently be said about the role of the right cortex in semantic memory. Some speculations will, however, be made about how semantic memory may be represented in the left hemisphere. It is unlikely that lesions will enable more precise locations of particular kinds of semantic memory to be made. The use of electrical stimulation of the cortex in epileptic patients may offer a brighter prospect. For example, Ojemann (1983) examined the effects on naming pictures of objects when adjacent sites in the superior temporal cortex of the left hemisphere were stimulated. The patient was bilingual, and stimulation of one of the sites affected his ability to name objects in English, but not in Greek, whereas stimulation of the other site affected his ability to name the same objects in Greek, but not in English. This kind of finding, which is not unique, suggests that object names may be stored in different, but adjacent sites in the left superior temporal cortex. It does not, of course, prove this, as the stimulation may have disrupted retrieval from a storage site distant from the point of stimulation. It does, however, strongly imply that the sites are distinct.

There are two radically different accounts of the way in which semantic memory may be organized in people's brains. The first account proposes that we develop such knowledge according to a largely pre-ordained plan; thus different kinds of knowledge have their separate storage sites, which are approximately the same in all people, or would be if all people acquired that knowledge. The second account proposes that storage location is not pre-ordained in this way, but depends on idiosyncratic factors; thus knowledge of animate things may be stored at site A in one person and at site B in another person. Both views presuppose a particular kind of hypothesis about how semantic memories develop, but neither has had any elaborated theoretical underpinning. Recently, however, Allport (1985) advanced a possible theoretical underpinning for the first kind of account that might be regarded as a specific adaptation of Hebb's (1949) famous cell assemblies view.

According to this theory, semantic knowledge is represented by distributed neural activity patterns that are unique to each piece of knowledge. For example, knowledge of a particular spoken word would be represented by activity in a set of phonological detectors. These phonological detectors are known as the attribute domain for spoken words because each word is defined in terms of the phonological sounds that make it up. Memory for each word depends, then, on establishing links among the brain regions that encode the phonemes that constitute the word, so that with the appropriate input, the pattern that represents the word can be reactivated. With repeated practice, the links become so strong that the whole pattern may be activated by what would once have been an inadequate stimulus. The theory bases higher level knowledge of things like object concepts on interconnected patterns of sensory attribute domains. Thus the concept of a telephone would involve activating attribute domains that represent what a telephone looks like, sounds like, and feels like, and how it is used in a whole set of standard routines. Appropriate links among all the appropriate attribute domains would have to be created, so that the network is activated when a telephone is thought about. It will be remembered from chapter 1 that much evidence suggests that sensory attributes are encoded both in parallel and in series, in many separate regions of PTO association neocortex. All these regions receive inputs from primary sensory receiving areas of the neocortex. Depending on the sensory attributes that are linked in an activated network, a semantic memory may be contained in a small cortical region or a very large one.

Allport's (1985) theory has a number of interesting properties. First, retrieval simply involves reactivating the pattern that represents a particular item of semantic knowledge through the presentation of cues that somehow trigger the activation. This idea is very similar to the one presented in chapter 1.

Second, particular components of the attribute domain can take part in many semantic memories. For example, a part of the phonological attribute domain that encodes a particular phoneme may be involved in the representation of any spoken word that contains that phoneme. The key point is that semantic memories depend on the establishment of stable links among those parts of the association cortex that encode the sensory attributes and action programmes that define the relevant semantic memory. The distribution of these attribute encoding regions determines the extent of the storage area for the memory in question. Thus one would expect the concept of a telephone to be stored over a wider area than the spoken-word representation *telephone*. It would also be expected that if concepts were based on somewhat different attribute domains, they would be stored in partly distinct cortical regions. This might apply to knowledge of animate and of inanimate objects, if the former was defined more in terms of sensory attributes and the latter, more in terms of functional attributes, like action routines. One might even predict highly specific dissociations, such as that noted by Ojemann (1983), if, for example, Greek and English spoken words have somewhat different phonemic structures.

A third property of the theory is that the location of different kinds of semantic memory in the brain should be to a large extent pre-ordained, so that similar kinds of semantic memory should be stored in roughly corresponding regions in different people's brains. There is some uncertainty in this statement because the theory claims that the building blocks of semantic and lexical memories are encoded sensory attributes and action routines. It is not known fully how the ability to encode these attributes develops and to what extent location of the encoding structures varies in different people's brains. The location of such structures may be changed in people suffering from early brain damage, as is the case with some epileptics. Even so, the theory does imply that subtypes of semantic memory may have the same reasonably specific locations in most people's brains, although there is likely to be a good deal of overlap in the storage sites for different subtypes of semantic memory.

A fourth property of the theory is that it is capable of predicting category-specific semantic memory impairments, such as those that have been reported. Indeed, Warrington and McCarthy's (in press) recent explanation of such specific semantic memory deficits can be regarded as an application of Allport's (1985) view in that it postulates that different categories depend to varying degrees on the different sensory channels. For example, knowledge of small manipulable objects (such as scissors) may depend more on stored information derived from actions and on somatosensory information and less on visual shape information than does knowledge of large man-made objects (such as buses). As these kinds of information are processed and stored in different parts of association neocortex, certain lesions may disturb one kind of semantic memory far more than another.

A fifth property of the theory is relevant to the relationship between semantic and episodic memory. Distributed memories are able to extract the common attributes of many similar encoded events as an automatic by-product of the encoding of these many episodes. In other words, semantic memories emerge as the common elements in a set of similar episodic memories, even though the entire set of common elements may never have been experienced before in isolation. This property of the theory fits the available facts because it predicts that it should not be possible to lose semantic memories without affecting corresponding episodic ones. But isolated loss of episodic memory should be possible because it may be caused by an inability to retrieve contextual features that uniquely mark individual episodes. If in the early stages of learning, the common elements can be retrieved only through accessing their contextual markers, then the theory would also predict that less rehearsed semantic memories may be lost without well-rehearsed ones being affected. Repeated experience of similar episodes eventually creates such strong links among the common elements that they can be activated independently by several kinds of input.

The distributed memory theory of semantic memory is attractive because it seems to explain many of the disturbances of well-established semantic memory reported in this chapter. In one or two respects, however, it seems to have properties that conflict with some of the claims that have been made on the basis of lesion studies. First, it is difficult to see how it can accommodate the notion of independent modality-specific non-verbal semantic systems and also a verbal semantic system. The concept of a telephone remains the same whether we access it visually, auditorily, or tactually or hear its name spoken. Either the theory needs some modification or the available evidence should be reinterpreted as indicating that lesions cause modality-specific access deficits to a single semantic memory system. Second, the theory predicts that impairments in semantic memory should usually be accompanied by high-level sensory and motor deficits because damage to the sensory and action routine encoding areas probably underlies the semantic memory disturbances. For example, Allport (1985) believes that disorders of auditory–verbal short-term memory (which depends on remembering phonological forms) must be associated with phonological-processing deficits. The evidence against this view was discussed in chapter 3, and, similarly, most of the researchers concerned with semantic memory deficits do not believe that they are invariably accompanied by processing failures other than those directly attributable to the memory losses. Allport does, however, allow that semantic memory storage deficits may also be caused by lesions that break the links that bind together the components of each memory. As such lesions do not damage the sensory and action routine encoding areas directly, high-level sensory and motor processing may be left intact. The notion that the links binding a semantic network can be selectively broken is, however, somewhat implausible. Allport's theory may need to be modified to include non-sensory and action routine attribute encoding components in semantic memory networks. These components could be destroyed or disconnected from their sensory inputs or motor outputs without causing high-level sensory or motor deficits. The matter is unresolved; but although the distributed memory theory may need some modifications, it offers the best framework for understanding the lesion-induced disorders of well-established semantic memory.

5   The memory problems caused
by frontal lobe lesions

The evidence, reviewed in chapter 4, strongly suggests that PTO association neocortex stores many aspects of well-established semantic memory, and probably
also the semantic components of episodic memory. In this chapter, the role in
complex memory of the frontal association neocortex is considered. Although
many issues remain unresolved and much research needs to be done, the role in
memory of the frontal cortex is perhaps best approached by comparing it with
the role in memory of PTO association cortex and of the structures damaged in
organic amnesics. First, both PTO and frontal association cortex receive inputs of
sensory information that has already undergone some processing, and the frontal
region projects to areas that more directly control motor output. If they have
broadly similar roles in memory, then one would expect the frontal cortex to be
involved in storing certain kinds of well-established information. One possibility
is that it may store action plans and 'scripts' that indicate what should be done
in different kinds of situations, such as meeting friends or going to a restaurant.
Strong evidence for a frontal cortex role in these kinds of storage does not yet
exist. The second comparison is with the structures involved in organic amnesia.
Warrington and Weiskrantz (1982) have argued that organic amnesia is caused by
lesions that disconnect the frontal cortex from PTO association cortex. It is not the
links across the neocortex that are severed, however, but those that connect frontal
and PTO cortex via the limbic system and diencephalic structures. The effect of
this disconnection is that amnesics cannot either store or retrieve all those kinds
of information that require elaborative processing and planning during encoding.
According to Warrington and Weiskrantz and many others, the frontal cortex is
very important in the processing of any kind of information where planning is
needed, and the operations involved cannot be entirely routine. It therefore follows that a large frontal lesion should impair elaborative processing of information
and cause a memory disorder practically identical to organic amnesia.

   This discussion indicates that three main views can be adopted about the effects
of lesions of frontal association cortex. First, like lesions of PTO cortex, they
will clearly cause loss of well-established memories of particular kinds. This
position may be correct, but the deficits are not obvious. They still need to
be properly demonstrated. Second, frontal lesions may impair the elaborative
and planned processing of information, so that a condition very like organic
amnesia results. Without anticipating chapter 6 too much, this would mean severe
deficits in the recognition and recall of recently learned material and pathological
forgetting of information acquired pre-morbidly, probably with sparing of the
very oldest memories. The deficit would not be quite identical to organic amnesia

102

because the frontal lesions should impair elaborative encoding, which according to Warrington and Weiskrantz (1982) is unaffected in amnesics. This encoding problem could affect frontal lesion patients' intelligence on certain measures, so that their intelligence might be lower in particular respects than that of amnesics with equivalently poor memory. The third view is that frontal lesions do indeed cause deficits in planned activities like elaborative processing of information, but this does not result in memory disturbances like those shown by organic amnesics.

Although the second and third views are in conflict, there is no reason that deficits in elaborative processing should not arise, at least in part, from disturbances in the storage of well-rehearsed memories that are concerned with the courses of action to follow in various non-routine situations. This is an intriguing and, as yet, untested idea. Its proper examination would, however, require a means of determining whether memories of this kind had been lost. There is already good evidence that frontal cortex lesions do cause various kinds of deficit in the kinds of non-routine behaviour that involves planning. In the next section, this evidence is discussed, together with evidence showing that frontal lesions may also affect mood. This second type of evidence is briefly discussed because it could be that frontal lobe dysfunction is implicated in disorders, such as depression and schizophrenia, associated with memory deficits. In the third section, the effects of frontal lesions on memory are reviewed, and the last section considers whether any of the three views outlined above can accommodate the data.

One major point that must be borne in mind whilst assessing the evidence is that the prefrontal cortex is a very large area of the brain, different regions of which are engaged in somewhat separate functional processes. This notion of frontal functional heterogeneity is, in fact, much more clearly supported by recent work that measures cerebral metabolism whilst human subjects perform a variety of structured tasks (see Roland, 1984) than it is by studies on the effects of frontal lobe lesions. The research on cerebral metabolism suggests that there are at least 17 distinct functional zones in the frontal cortex, which implies that this area comprises a mosaic of interacting modules. Many of these modules may be concerned with different aspects of behaviour relevant to planning, but it does not follow that all are. This point must be borne in mind when considering the evidence discussed in the following sections.

The prefrontal cortex is illustrated in Figure 5.1. The functional map contains a number of regions often referred to in lesion studies, including the dorsolateral cortex, the orbitofrontal cortex, and the frontal eye fields. Each of these regions receives a projection from a different division of the dorsomedial nucleus of the thalamus, the major thalamic projection nucleus of the prefrontal cortex. Behind the prefrontal cortex lie the supplementary motor, premotor, and motor areas and also Broca's area, damage to which may disturb the fluency of speech and writing. In addition to input from the dorsomedial nucleus of the thalamus, the prefrontal cortex receives input from basal ganglia structures, such as the caudate nucleus; from the amygdala; and from structures in the hypothalamus, such as the mammillary bodies. The prefrontal cortex itself sends heavy projections to

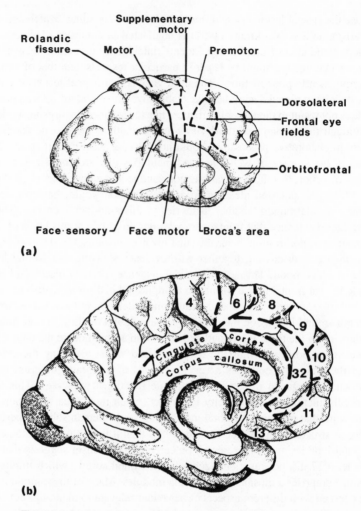

Figure 5.1 (a) A lateral view of the right cerebral hemisphere that shows the main regions of the frontal cortex. (b) A medial view of the left cerebral hemisphere that shows the main cytoarchitectonic zones. Areas 9 and 10 correspond to the dorsolateral prefrontal cortex; area 11, to the orbitofrontal cortex.

PTO association cortex, the dorsomedial nucleus of the thalamus, the hypothalamus, basal ganglia, the amygdala, the hippocampus, and structures in the lower brain-stem. As amygdala and hippocampus are the limbic system structures that project to PTO association cortex, it can be seen how limbic system lesions can subcortically disconnect the prefrontal cortex from PTO cortex. The prefrontal cortex also projects to the cingulate cortex, the position of which is illustrated in the medial view of the brain (see Figure 5.1). Cingulate cortex is sometimes included as a limbic system structure and sometimes as a frontal one. Together with the orbitofrontal cortex, it has been referred to as the ventromedial frontal cortex. As well as receiving projections from the parietal cortex (possibly concerned with spatial information), the cingulate cortex receives a projection from the anterior thalamus, and the orbitofrontal cortex receives a projection from the magnocellular division of the dorsomedial nucleus of the thalamus. Lesions of this thalamic region have been associated with organic amnesia (see, e.g., Aggleton and Mishkin, 1983a). It has therefore been suggested by Mishkin (1982) that lesions of the ventromedial frontal cortex cause amnesia. This view is briefly discussed here, but will be considered more fully in chapter 7.

Effects of frontal lesions on planning, attention, and mood

In 1923, after a systematic study of 200 frontal lesions and 200 non-frontal ones, caused by gunshot wounds in World War 1, Feuchtwanger concluded that frontal lesions had surprisingly little effect on intelligence or even on memory, but did have widespread effects on mood, attitude, and the ability to make plans (see Kolb & Whishaw, 1985). A part of this conclusion was later echoed by the great Russian neuropsychologist Alexander Luria (1973), who believed that the frontal lobes contain the brain system that controls planning. In his view, the frontal lobes are essentially involved whenever mental activity is not routine and requires the initiation and maintenance of a plan as well as the operation of a checking procedure to see whether the plan is working. His evidence for this belief was based largely on the effects of massive frontal lesions caused by tumours, strokes, and head injury (Luria, 1973). He found that patients with such massive lesions tended to be extremely apathetic and seemed incapable of initiating any complex activities, such as searching pictures in order to answer questions or solve problems when the solution could not be achieved by the most obvious route. Instead, appropriate planning behaviour was replaced by irrelevant and illogical activities that Luria called 'inert stereotypes'. These were strong habits linked to situations of the general type in which the patients found themselves, but inappropriate in the particular circumstances. To use a crude analogy, the patients were like a factory without its senior executives. As long as demands were routine, things ran smoothly; but as soon as a novel situation occurred, the demands were not met and the factory workers fell back on inapt, but established routines.

Many of Luria's patients showed very poor memory, and he argued that this was because the encoding and retrieval of complex memory requires a certain amount of processing that is not routine. In other words, the patients' inadequate processing caused their poor memory. Typically, he found that patients could not learn a list of words beyond what they could pick up passively on the first trial. They could learn only passively, and never actively sought to use mnemonic aids. When read a sentence, they could retain it for a minute or two if there was no interference; but if a second sentence was read to them, they became unable to recall the first and instead either repeated the second one *ad nauseam* or produced a sentence that was an amalgam of the two. It is plausible that failures of planning may cause a variety of memory deficits. The evidence provided by Luria for this position is not, however, very strong. This is because his patients with massive frontal lesions suffered extensive damage to other brain regions, particularly the limbic system structures, which are affected in organic amnesia. Evidence based on smaller lesions that are probably confined to the frontal cortex has made clear, however, that damage to this region does impair planning ability. Even so, the effects are subtler than those observed by Luria, and there is a suggestion that differently placed lesions affect different functions. For example, orbitofrontal lesions may reduce the fluency and spontaneity of complex behaviour. This is shown by a reduction in patients' ability to produce words beginning with a certain letter or belonging to a given category within a fixed period of time. In contrast, these patients are less likely to perseverate their responses in a range of test situations characterized by changing demands. The patients who perform worst on this task have lesions in Brodmann's area 9 (see Kolb & Whishaw, 1985). This is a region defined by its cellular features, or cytoarchitecture, that lies in the dorsolateral frontal cortex and in the frontal eye fields, as shown in Figure 5.1. One test on which these patients do particularly badly is the Wisconsin Card-Sort Test, described in chapter 2. This test requires subjects to sort cards according to the colour of the shapes on them, the shapes themselves, or the number of shapes. Patients with lesions to Brodmann's area 9 have great difficulty in shifting from one strategy to the next when it becomes appropriate.

There are several kinds of deficit caused by frontal lesions that can reasonably be described as disorders of planning. First, when performance on a fluency task is poor, the patient is either not initiating or not maintaining appropriate search programmes. Second, when patients show inappropriate perseveration of no longer apposite responses, they clearly have difficulty in switching out of programmes designed for circumstances that no longer apply. Interestingly, some patients show this difficulty even when they can state verbally what the correct solution is. So flexibility can no longer be maintained by verbal guidance. Third, patients with frontal lobe lesions show deficits on problems that cannot be solved using established routines. For example, they do poorly on the Tower of London test (see Shallice, 1982), in which coloured beads, threaded on three rods in several configurations, have to be moved to specified target sites on the same rods in a fixed number of moves. As there is no 'algorithm' for this task, subjects have to construct and modify a plan as they proceed with each problem. Many intelligence-test items can be solved using established routines, so there need be no recourse to novel approaches. This may explain why frontally lesioned patients often do well on standard intelligence tests, even though their ability to think is clearly impaired.

A fourth kind of deficit found in frontal patients has been noted by Luria (1973). He claimed that many patients did not display a normal operation of the activation processes that underlie voluntary attention. In other words, they could not gener- ate the levels of physiological arousal necessary for the initiation and maintenance of cognitive processes that demand attentional effort. As discussed in chapter 1, when two such effortful processes are performed simultaneously, they interfere with each other, so that neither is performed as well as it would have been in isolation. Difficult cognitive tasks require the exertion of considerable amounts effort in order to maintain effective planned behaviour, so patients with this kin of arousal problem should be poor at such tasks. It is not, however, certain that these deficits were caused by frontal lobe lesions. Nevertheless, there are many reports that frontal lobe lesions disturb sustained attention because they increase distractibility. Wilkins, Shallice, and McCarthy (1987) have recently examined the effects of unilateral frontal and temporal lobe lesions on the ability of patients to count a succession of 2 to 11 stimuli. The stimuli were either a series of clicks or a series of pulses, presented to the right or left index finger. When the presentation rate was one stimulus per second, then the counting of the patients with right frontal cortex lesions was least accurate, regardless of the stimulus modality or side of stimulus presentation. No impairment was found when the presentation rate was increased to seven stimuli per second. The experimenters argued that at the slower rate of presentation, when the task was most monotonous, the patients with right frontal lobe lesions were least able to sustain attention voluntarily. Their argument that these patients have a vigilance deficit and not one specific to the cognitive processes underlying counting is consistent with the finding of normal performance at faster presentation rates.

This experiment suggests that patients with bilateral frontal cortex lesions may show poor planning abilities partly because they cannot maintain attention, particularly when tasks become less interesting. Some frontal lesions also seem to impair the ability to show voluntary attentional orienting towards novel or interesting stimuli in the environment. Unilateral frontal cortex lesions often cause a contralateral neglect syndrome in which the patient ignores stimuli in the half of space opposite to the side of the lesion. The patient may bump into objects on the neglected side of space and may show no awareness of sounds or tactile stimuli emanating from this half of space because the deficit is a polysensory one. Neglect is particularly prominent if the lesion includes the frontal eye fields, and it has been argued that this region contains a system that initiates the voluntary direction of attention towards stimuli of any sensory modality that are interesting or novel.

There are some cognitive deficits caused by frontal lobe lesions, however, that are hard to interpret as planning disorders. For example, some patients are very poor at behaviours related to egocentric spatial orientation, which depend on precise assessment of one's body orientation in space. This is shown by their failure to point accurately to those parts of their bodies indicated on a simple diagram, a disorder not dissimilar to autotopagnosia. The patients can, however, use a map to find their way around a room (see Kolb & Whishaw, 1985). Patients with parietal lobe lesions are more likely to show the opposite pattern of impairment. If the frontal lobe deficit in egocentric spatial orientation is a planning failure, the nature of the breakdown has not yet been demonstrated.

Lesions of the frontal cortex cause not only disturbances of cognition, but also mood changes in patients. Famous cases, like that of the dynamite worker Phineas Gage, who had a 3 foot, 7 inch long tamping iron blasted clean through his frontal lobes, made it clear, even in the nineteenth century, that frontal lobe injury may cause dramatic changes in temperament. Gage, who was a foreman, changed from being conscientious in carrying out his plans, to being impatient, profane, abusive, and capricious with no capacity to hold a plan in his head and execute it. More recent research has noted two kinds of persistent mood change: pseudo-depression and pseudopsychopathy. Patients with pseudodepression manifest the outward signs of apathy and indifference – loss of initiative, decreased sexual interest, few overt signs of emotion, and little verbal output – but these symptoms are not accompanied by a sense of depression in the patient. This syndrome is obviously associated with a disturbance of planning. Patients with pseudopsy-chopathy display disinhibited and immature behaviour, characterized by lack of tact, coarse language, promiscuous sexual behaviour, and a marked loss of social graces, although these symptoms are not accompanied by the usual emotional and mental signs of psychopathy. Once again, it seems likely that patients with this disorder have problems sticking to a plan of action (indeed, Phineas Gage appears to have suffered from this syndrome). Lesion location may be an important deter-minant of the kind of mood change found. Thus Grafman, Vance, Weingartner, Salazar, and Amin (submitted for publication) compared the effects on mood of orbitofrontal, dorsolateral frontal, and non-frontal cortex lesions, caused by pene-trating missile wounds, in Vietnam veterans. They found that right orbitofrontal lesions were associated with abnormally increased edginess, anxiety, and depres-sion, whereas left dorsolateral lesions were associated with increases in anger and hostility.

It remains uncertain to what extent these mood changes cause planning difficul-ties and to what extent they might be caused by them or other cognitive deficits. Clearly, these kinds of mood disorder could affect the control of attentional effort, which would affect planning ability. It has not been shown, however, that all cognitive deficits caused by frontal lobe lesions are consequences of planning failures. As long as this remains the case, it might be argued that some of the memory difficulties shown after such lesions could have nothing to do with the in-adequate planning and execution of elaborative encoding and retrieval processes. The kinds of memory deficits that have been observed after frontal lobe lesions will be outlined before returning to this issue.

Memory deficits caused by frontal lobe lesions

The first kind of deficit associated with frontal lobe lesions is a disturbance in the learning of complex material. There is a general belief in this kind of deficit, but there have been few formal demonstrations of it. Luria (1973) reported that patients with massive lesions of the lateral frontal zones could not form stable intentions to memorize new material and hence acquired information in only a passive fashion. As much material can be acquired efficiently only if it is encoded in an elaborative and meaningful way, it is not surprising that the learning of his patients was ineffective. With lists of words, they could pick up four or five items without effort, but thereafter made no progress in learning the remaining items. On similar lines, Signoret and Lhermitte (1976) reported that frontally lesioned patients were very poor at learning weakly associated word pairs, such as *chicken–mountain*. They also showed that the deficit could be largely abolished if the patients were shown how to construct images that formed a link between the two words. For example, it might be suggested that they think of a giant chicken on top of a conical mountain. The experimenters argued that this deficit occurred because, unlike normal subjects, patients with frontal lobe lesions do not use elaborative encoding strategies in a spontaneous way. They can, however, use such strategies if given a detailed plan of how to do so and guided in its use. There is some evidence that bilateral frontal lobe lesions may cause learning difficulties even with more closely related word pairs, whereas unilateral frontal lobe lesions do not have this effect (see Kolb & Whishaw, 1985). Presumably, the pairs were still sufficiently distantly related to make the use of elaborative encoding a more efficient strategy than passive rote learning. This effect illustrates an important point. Bilateral frontal lobe lesions can sometimes have severe effects on function when unilateral lesions have little or no effect.

The work just described suggests that bilateral frontal lobe lesions impair learning when rote approaches to acquisition are less effective than planned elaboration. The evidence that poor patient learning is caused by inadequately planned encoding is, however, very circumstantial. More direct evidence for the claim has recently been provided by Rocchetta (1986), who compared the performance of patients with unilateral temporal lobe lesions and those with unilateral frontal lobe lesions on a categorizing and recall task. The patients were shown a set of pictures, which they had to sort into a number of categories of their own choosing within 5 min. Patients' recall of the pictures was later tested. Those with left or right frontal lobe lesions did poorly at the categorizing task, leaving some pictures completely uncategorized and others only vaguely categorized as 'remainder' items (for example, some pictures might have been classified as 'other animals', rather than as 'birds', 'zoo animals', or 'pets'). They also did poorly at the free *recall* of the pictures. Interestingly, whereas patients with right frontal lobe lesions showed a negative correlation between the number of pictures they left uncategorized and their recall scores, no such correlation was found in patients with left frontal lobe lesions. Rocchetta argued that this difference may indicate that the poor recall of patients with right frontal lobe lesions is caused by inadequate elaborative encoding of the pictures, whereas that of patients with left frontal lobe lesions may depend more on their failure to use elaborative retrieval strategies. This interpretation requires confirmation, but the results do suggest an interesting and unexpected lateralization of function within the frontal lobes. In contrast to the frontally lesioned patients, those with temporal lobe lesions were unimpaired at the categorization task, and only those patients with left temporal lobe lesions were poor at recall. The deficient recall of these patients therefore very likely has a different explanation from the deficient recall of the frontally lesioned patients. This conclusion is particularly interesting because the temporal lobe lesions extended into the limbic system structures, which are damaged in organic amnesics.

A second kind of memory impairment that may be somewhat more controversial than the one just discussed is that frontal lobe lesions disrupt recall more than recognition. Patients with focal lesions of the frontal lobes are generally found to have intact recognition of recently presented material, even though their recall may be quite severely impaired. Although in a large-scale normative study Warrington (1984) has reported recognition impairments in patients with frontal lobe lesions, one cannot exclude the possibility that lesions in some of her patients may have extended into other regions where damage can cause a mild amnesia. Certainly Grafman et al. (submitted for publication) found that their frontally lesioned patients from the Vietnam Head Injury Study did not show recognition problems. Indeed, although dorsolateral frontal lesions caused recall but not recognition problems, orbitofrontal lesions generally had no effect on either recognition or recall. Even if some frontally lesioned patients are poor at both recall and recognition, there is evidence that they are likely to be worse at recall. Hirst (1985) gave patients with both unilateral and bilateral frontal lesions lists of words to learn and after a 5-min delay tested their memory, using a recall test followed by a recognition test. Whereas the unilateral patients were unimpaired on both tests, the bilateral patients did poorly on the recall test. In a second study, Jetter, Poser, Freeman, and Markowitsch (1986) gave frontally lesioned patients lists of words to learn and tested them after either 15 min or 1 day by free recall, cued recall, or recognition. The only test on which the patients were impaired was that of free recall after 1 day.

Several points should be noted about these results. First, it is unclear under what circumstances, if any, frontally lesioned patients show recognition deficits. The issue is unclear because effects may critically depend on the location and extent of lesions and on the sensitivity of the recognition tests used. Recognition may be appreciably impaired only after massive frontal lesions, such as those described by Luria (1973), and such lesions almost certainly encroach on other brain regions, such as the temporal lobes, that are implicated in organic amnesia. The question of test sensitivity was raised in chapter 2. When deficits in recall and recognition are to be compared, if tests are to be equally sensitive, they should be matched on difficulty, reliability, and variability. It must be admitted that it is uncertain to what extent recall and recognition tests used on patients with frontal lobe lesions have fulfilled these requirements. Even so, the second point is that the weight of evidence strongly implies that frontal lobe lesions do affect recall more drastically than recognition, and this is what one would expect if the lesions impair learning by disrupting elaborative processing. There is much evidence that recall depends more than recognition on the ability to interconnect items that are being learnt. This is particularly obvious with the free recall of a list of words. Cueing reduces the dependency of recall on encoded links between items, which may explain why Jetter et al. (1986) found no deficit in cued recall in their patients with frontal lobe lesions. Under certain conditions, recognition may also depend more on elaborative processing strategies, as when complex stimuli like faces are tested after a delay (see Mandler, 1980). It would be interesting to see whether frontal lesions have a worse effect on recognition under these circumstances. Third, the possibility that a memory deficit may develop after a delay following presentation, but not be present on more immediate testing, is supported by Jetter et al.'s results. They interpret this as evidence that frontal lesions cause faster forgetting. This interpretation clearly needs more support, particularly as recall deficits are usually found at fairly immediate test. It would, however, be interesting to see whether recognition deficits become apparent after even longer delays.

A third kind of memory deficit was noted by Hirst (1985) in his patients with bilateral, but not unilateral, frontal lobe lesions. The deficit concerned patients' knowledge of the workings of their memory system and the effectiveness of their memory strategies. This kind of knowledge is known as metamemory and was tapped by various questions about what would determine good or bad memory in different situations. For example, one question asked whether it would be easier to make a call immediately after hearing a telephone number or after getting a glass of water! Patients with bilateral frontal lesions gave atypical answers to these questions. Such a disturbance of metamemory is consistent with Luria's (1973) view that frontal lesions impair the ability to monitor the effectiveness of one's plans. This view is supported by evidence that frontally lesioned patients are poor at estimating the costs of such things as cars, refrigerators, and furniture (see Milner, Petrides, & Smith, 1985). These judgements, like others, such as estimating the length of the average man's spine, at which frontally lesioned patients are also bad, cannot be performed accurately unless the different stages of the plan on which they depend are effectively monitored. As Hirst, like Rocchetta (1986), found that his bilaterally lesioned patients inadequately categorized the words from a word list, it could be argued that the metamemory and categorizing deficits are causally related.

Failure to monitor the effectiveness of plans and actions may also underlie a group of more spectacular retrieval disorders, which constitute a fourth group of memory problems probably caused, at least in part, by lesions of the frontal lobes. The best known of these disorders is confabulation, which is defined as the recall of incorrect, sometimes bizarre, information in response to standard questions. For example, if asked how he came to be in hospital, instead of answering that he did not know, a patient might produce a detailed and fantastic story. Stuss and Benson (1984) reviewed available evidence that strongly suggests that confabulation is associated with frontal pathology, whether it takes a severe, spontaneous, and fantastic form or a milder form, made apparent only by prompting from the examiner. The degree of confabulation did not correlate with the extent of mem-

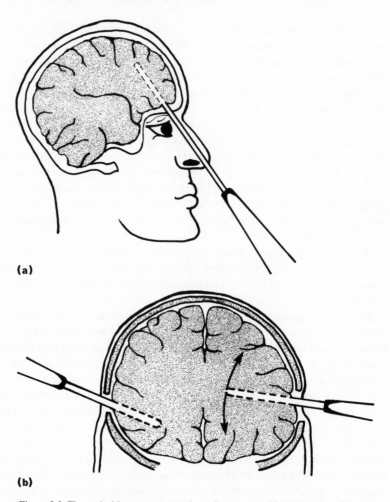

(a)

(b)

Figure 5.2 The typical leucotomy procedures that were used in the heyday of the operation's popularity were very crude. The precise brain damage inflicted on different patients was likely to be highly variable.

ory disturbance, but did relate closely with the inability to self-correct. Frontal pathology has also been linked to reduplicative paramnesia, in which a patient asserts that two or more places, such as hospitals, exist with nearly identical properties, when in fact only one such place really exists. It has also been linked to the very similar Capgras syndrome, in which reduplication concerns close relatives, so that the patient may, for example, look on his wife as an impostor who merely closely resembles his true wife. Although the precise cause of these unusual reduplicative syndromes is uncertain, they probably involve extensive cerebral damage; thus frontal lesions are likely to be a necessary, but not a sufficient, condition for their occurrence. For example, frontal lesions may often cause problems in the integration of different kinds of information (something that probably needs planning and effort), and when these problems are combined with perceptual and memory deficits arising from other brain lesions, then reduplicative paramnesia or Capgras syndrome is seen. In other words, patients misinterpret an unusual experience of what should be a familiar place or person.

A fifth group of effects of focal frontal lesions relates to the sensitivity of patients to high levels of interference during learning. Stuss et al. (1982) tested a group of patients who many years previously had undergone prefrontal leucotomy operations for the treatment of schizophrenia. This operation involves severing the connections between the prefrontal regions and underlying subcortical structures, such as the dorsomedial thalamus (Figure 5.2). Whether or not the operation has any effect on schizophrenia, some of the patients studied by Stuss and his colleagues had undergone a remission of their psychotic symptoms in the years since their operation. It was argued that the major site of damage was in the orbitofrontal cortex. The patients were given a number of memory tests, including the WMS, and the researchers found little evidence of impairment, which is in agreement with the results of Grafman et al. The patients were, however, very bad at the Brown-Peterson task. Specifically, they were poor at recalling triplets of consonants after a delay filled with an interfering task that involved counting backwards by threes from an initial randomly chosen number. Normal subjects probably perform this task by rapidly alternating counting with covert rehearsal during the delay. A disturbance of planning might prevent frontally lesioned patients from rehearsing because they would be unable to interdigitate this activity with the primary activity of counting. It would be interesting to check this idea by giving patients dual tasks, neither of which involves an obvious memory load. For example, if the idea is correct, then frontally lesioned patients should do worse than control subjects at fairly difficult sensory discriminations if they were simultaneously having to perform a difficult counting task.

Another kind of frontal interference effect, which may have a somewhat similar origin to the disturbance in the Brown-Peterson task, was initially reported by Moscovitch (1982). He presented five lists, containing 12 words each, to subjects with unilateral temporal or frontal lobe lesions. Subjects were required to recall as many words from a list as they could immediately after it was presented. Words from the first four lists were drawn from the same semantic category, and recall declined as subjects progressed from the first to the fourth list. This effect is usually ascribed to proactive interference from the semantically related words in the earlier lists. Words in the last list were drawn from a different semantic category, and normal people show improved recall of this list, known as release from proactive interference. Although patients with temporal lobe lesions showed poor recall of the words, they also showed a normal release from proactive interference on the fifth trial. In contrast, patients with unilateral frontal lobe lesions showed far less release from proactive interference, and this particularly applied to those patients who performed worst on the Wisconsin Card-Sort Test, which can be regarded as tapping the ability to form hypotheses and to shift when appropriate from one hypothesis to another. There is some evidence that patients are aware of the change in the fifth list but do not make use of their knowledge. More recently, Freedman and Cermak (1986) replicated Moscovitch's study, using shorter word lists. They also presented five different blocks of five trials each, with a short break between each block. The frontally lesioned patients in their study were divided into two groups: those with memory impairments and those without. Memory impairment was indicated by a patient having a lower standardized score on the WMS than on the WAIS. The differences were, however, very small, and it should be pointed out that the WMS measures only recall. Only the memory impaired frontally lesioned patients showed no release from proactive interference, and this failure persisted across the five blocks of trials. Freedman and Cermak argued that the elaborative processing deficit that caused this failure to show release from proactive interference was probably also related to their patients' poor recall performance. It remains unclear, however, whether the set-shifting deficits underlying poor performance in Stuss et al.'s and Moscovitch's tasks are identical or different.

Neither Stuss et al. (1982), Moscovitch (1982), nor Freedman and Cermak (1986) reported whether their patients made more intrusion errors than their controls. In these studies, an intrusion would be made when a subject retrieved an item from a preceding list rather than from the target list on any given occasion. Similar effects have, however, been claimed by Luria (1973) with word lists and stories. He describes how patients, when read two stories separated in time, were unable to recall the first because they repeatedly recalled the second or blurred the two stories together. Both blurring and repetition of the wrong story constitute intrusion errors. As the patients were able to remember either story when it was presented in isolation, it is possible that the interference effect occurred not because of any basic memory failure, but because the patients had difficulty in deciding whether information came from the first or the second story. This kind of difficulty could be a direct result of another kind of memory difficulty, about to be discussed – a problem in identifying the temporal order in which items are presented, despite being able to recognize them. In other words, Luria's patients might not have been able to tell whether items were drawn from the first or the second story because their temporal discrimination ability was so poor. If so, it is possible that susceptibility to intrusion errors may be caused by different frontal lobe lesions from those that cause the two other kinds of interference effect, described above. Some support for this possibility can be derived from a study by Kapur (1985). He compared two patients' performance on a version of the Wisconsin Card-Sort Test and the Brown-Peterson task, which included a semantic-category shift on its fifth trial. Although the patients' memories were equally bad, one performed well on the Wisconsin task and, on the fifth trial of the Brown-Peterson task, showed normal release from proactive interference despite making many intrusions from earlier trials and perseverating on them, whereas the other performed very badly on the Wisconsin task and, on the fifth trial of the

Brown-Peterson task, failed to show release from proactive interference despite making no intrusion errors from earlier trials.

The sixth group of memory deficits caused by frontal lobe lesions includes poor memory for the temporal order and frequency of events and for the order in which the remembering subject has carried out a series of acts. First, it has been reported by Milner et al. (1985) that frontal patients are poor at judging which of two events was more recent. This has been shown with several tests. Initially, Prisko in Milner's laboratory (see Milner et al., 1985) found poor performance on a delayed comparison task in which a few readily discriminable items were repeated many times. On each trial, the subject had to say whether the second stimulus, shown after a variable delay, was the same as the stimulus shown before the delay. The results suggested that the patients could not keep the trials apart in their minds and could not easily determine which stimulus had been seen more recently. In later work, Corsi (see Milner et al., 1985) presented patients with long lists of concrete words, representational pictures, or abstract paintings. On recency discrimination trials, two previously shown items were presented, and patients indicated which they had seen more recently. For example, one item might have been presented 8 cards back and the other item, 16 cards back. Recognition trials were similar, except that one of the two items presented was novel. Patients with unilateral temporal lobe lesions did poorly on the recognition test, but their recency judgements were unimpaired. In contrast, those with unilateral frontal lobe lesions performed normally on the recognition test, but very badly on the recency judgements. Patients with right frontal lobe lesions scored at chance on recency judgements involving the abstract pictures and badly with the representational pictures. Patients with left frontal lobe lesions did particularly badly on recency judgements involving the verbal material.

Second, Smith and Milner (see Milner et al., 1985) have shown that frontal lesions cause difficulties with frequency judgements. Patients were shown a series of abstract designs or words, with 20 different items in each series. Each design or word appeared once, three times, five times, seven times, or nine times, with the repetitions evenly spaced through the series. At test, each of these items was presented with four others that had not been seen before, and the subjects were required to indicate the number of times each item had been shown in the series they had just seen. Both patients and controls were quite accurate at estimating item frequencies up to three, but patients with frontal lesions seemed to be relatively insensitive to frequencies greater than this. Right frontal lesions particularly affected frequency judgements involving abstract designs, whereas left frontal lesions more seriously affected frequency judgements involving words. Despite these impaired frequency judgements, however, the patients showed normal recognition for the items from the series. Contrastingly, patients with unilateral temporal lobe lesions showed poor recognition but unimpaired frequency judgements.

Third, Petrides and Milner (see Milner et al., 1985) have reported a related deficit with a self-ordered task, in which subjects were given stacks of cards, each having a regular array of stimuli whose position varied from card to card. Subjects had to work through the stacks, touching one item on each card without touching the same item twice on different cards. The same range of stimuli was used as in the recency test, but this time patients with left frontal lobe lesions did very poorly at the task whenever they had to point in sequence to more than six items, regardless of the nature of those items. The patients with right frontal lobe lesions showed only a mild impairment on the non-verbal tests. It is not known why the laterality of the lesion had a different effect in the recency and self-ordered pointing tasks, although it is presumably related to the fact that the 'events' were self-generated in the second task.

Despite finding that unilateral frontal lobe lesions impair memory judgements about event recency and frequency and about self-ordered pointing, Milner's group failed to find any evidence of a deficit in spatial memory (see Milner et al., 1985). Patients were shown several toys, randomly positioned on a grid, and were required to estimate the costs of the real objects represented by the toys. Their ability to replace the toys in their correct positions on the grid was later tested and found to be unimpaired, although their ability to recall the names of the toys, tested immediately before, was impaired. It was argued that when spatial memory deficits have been found in monkeys or humans with frontal lobe lesions, the spatial tests involved trial-to-trial variability. When such variability is introduced, subjects have to be able to retrieve what spatial position was occupied on the most recent trial, an ability that is disrupted by frontal lesions.

Although Milner's patients rarely had lesions that were confined to just one frontal lobe region, she was able to draw some provisional conclusions about the location of the lesions that had the greatest disruptive effect on judgements of recency and frequency and of self-ordered pointing. Whereas lesions of the dorsolateral cortex were sufficient to cause deficits on the tasks, at least for recency discriminations, orbitofrontal lesions had little or no effect. If correct, this conclusion is interesting because lesion studies with animals have found that the temporal organization of behaviour, in general, and the ability to remember the order of occurrence of spatial events, in particular, are disrupted by lesions of the dorsolateral frontal cortex or its homologue. The conclusion is also interesting because of Grafman et al.'s finding that orbitofrontal lesions were not associated with memory deficits in young missile-wound patients, whereas dorsolateral frontal cortex lesions were associated with recall problems. It is possible, but still unproved, that dorsolateral frontal cortex lesions disrupt one function or several closely related functions that particularly affect the recall of recently presented information.

With the possible exception of the Capgras syndrome and the reduplicative paramnesias, all the memory disorders caused by frontal lesions that have been discussed so far apply to memories that were acquired after the onset of brain damage; that is, they are anterograde amnesia deficits. As organic amnesics show retrograde amnesia and a key question is the extent to which this syndrome is similar to the memory deficits caused by frontal lobe lesions, it is important to ask whether these lesions cause retrograde amnesia. The evidence on this important issue is not good because no studies have given objective tests of remote memory to patients with focal frontal lesions, but no additional problems. The closest that existing research has come to this goal is the study of Stuss et al. (1982), which compared the performance of control subjects on a relatively unsophisticated objective test of memory for remote public events with that of a group of schizophrenics, whose disease had largely remitted following a frontal leucotomy that had been performed many years before. There were only five such patients, and although they showed a trend for poorer memory of events that had occurred between the 1920s and the 1960s, this was of borderline significance. Apart from the small group size and history of schizophrenia in the patients, it should be pointed out that no separation of recall and recognition measures was made by the experimenters in their report. This is potentially important because it is more likely that frontally lesioned patients will show retrograde amnesia when their recall is tested. Also, Stuss and his colleagues indicated that the leucotomy operation had damaged mainly the orbitofrontal cortex, lesions of which do not appear to cause anterograde amnesic problems either.

In addition to former schizophrenics with orbitofrontal lesions, patients with Huntington's chorea have been given tests of remote pre-traumatic memory. Huntington's chorea is a genetic disorder in which abnormal involuntary movements and dementia become progressively worse with time. These symptoms are caused by an increasing atrophy of the caudate nucleus in the basal ganglia and of the frontal association cortex. Albert, Butters, and Brandt (1981) assessed the memory of patients with Huntington's chorea for events and faces prominent in the years between 1920 and 1970. They found that the patients were equally impaired at remembering items from all the decades sampled. They did not find this pattern of no sparing of the oldest memories in organic amnesics, who were, however, much more impaired in remembering more recent events and faces. Unfortunately, because Huntington's choreics have lesions in both the caudate nucleus and the frontal cortex, it is impossible to conclude confidently that this pattern of retrograde amnesia is caused solely by the frontal lesion.

If retrograde amnesia does constitute a seventh kind of memory deficit caused by frontal lesions, then it is likely to have several distinguishing features. First, it will probably affect recall more than recognition, as this seems to apply to frontal anterograde amnesia. Second, if the deficit disrupts the ability to use organized and effortful retrieval strategies, then it might be expected to affect all remote memories equally, regardless of their age. This is, of course, what seems to be found with Huntington's choreics. Third, as the retrograde amnesia deficit should be one of retrieval and not storage, then if one accepts Shallice's (1986) criteria for distinguishing between retrieval and storage deficits, patients' success or failure at recalling particular items is likely to vary from occasion to occasion. Fourth, as frontal lesions cause deficits in the ability to discriminate the temporal order of events, frontally lesioned patients might be expected to show particular problems with locating remote remembered events in time. Interestingly, Sagar et al. (1985) have reported that Parkinson patients show exactly this kind of problem. Although these patients showed normal recognition for remote public events, unlike patients with Alzheimer's dementia, their ability to date the events was worse than that of the dements whose recognition *was* matched to theirs. Interestingly, there was also evidence that *recall* of remote events was impaired in the patients. Parkinson's disease is a motor disorder characterized by a resting tremor, muscular rigidity, and slowness in initiating and stopping movements. It has long been claimed that these motor symptoms are accompanied by cognitive deficits. The disease is caused by atrophy (the origin of which is unknown) of dopaminergic neurons, primarily in the substantia nigra of the midbrain. These neurons project to the caudate nucleus in the basal ganglia, which projects, in turn, to the frontal neocortex. There is also evidence that patients with Parkinson's disease suffer atrophy of other dopaminergic neurons, lying near the substantia nigra in the midbrain, and these neurons project directly to the frontal neocortex. In recent years, a number of people have argued that patients with Parkinson's disease will show signs of frontal dysfunction, and in support of their argument it can be said that the patients not only show poor recall and preserved recognition, but also have been reported to perform poorly on the Wisconsin Card-Sort Test and other tests of categorizing ability. Only further research can establish whether these patients truly suffer from a frontal lobe dysfunction. Whatever the answer, patients with focal frontal lobe lesions in several locations clearly need to be systematically tested for retrograde amnesia.

Patients with frontal lobe lesions show other learning problems, which have not been described above. For example, they are often exceedingly poor at learning a path through mazes, an impairment associated with an inability to follow the rules they have been told or to use knowledge of errors to correct their performance (see Stuss & Benson, 1984). Frontally lesioned patients are also very poor at learning associations between arbitrarily related things. Thus they are very bad at learning to associate colours with different movements and at associating colours with spatial positions or abstract designs (see Kolb & Whishaw, 1985). Similar impairments in monkeys are caused by lesions of dorsal and more posterior parts of the frontal lobes. This kind of learning problem is not found in patients with temporal lobe lesions who do badly at standard tests of memory, although patients with early Parkinson's disease do show it if they also tend to make perseverative errors on the Wisconsin Card-Sort Test. This latter finding tends to support the hypothesis that some Parkinson patients may be suffering from a frontal lobe dysfunction caused by the atrophy of dopaminergic neurons that project to that region.

Conclusion

Before discussing the interpretation of the pattern of memory deficits caused by frontal lesions, it needs to be stressed that the identification of many of the deficits is still very tentative. For example, although it is very likely that certain frontal lesions cause a retrograde amnesia, the precise form that this amnesia takes has not yet been systematically explored. Much more research needs to be done before the precise kinds of memory deficit caused by frontal lesions are properly delineated. This delineation will have to take into account the location of the critical lesions. The research reviewed in the previous section seems to suggest that dorsolateral frontal cortex lesions may be more disruptive of memory than orbitofrontal lesions. As lesions in humans are usually widespread, it is possible that the question of localization may be best pursued with animal models. This is uncertain, however, because some of the memory functions affected by frontal lesions, such as metamemory, involve kinds of self-reflective activity currently impossible to test in non-verbal species.

Any interpretation of the memory deficits caused by frontal lobe lesions must raise the following issues. First, are the memory deficits basically the same as those seen in organic amnesics? Second, can all the deficits be explained as results of the impairment of the ability to engage in planned and organized, elaborative-processing activities found in frontally lesioned patients? Third, might these deficits in planning ability be caused, in turn, by degradation in the storage of what might be described as 'action scripts'?

The first question cannot be fully answered before consideration of chapter 6, which discusses the pattern of memory deficits associated with organic amnesia. Nevertheless, some points are fairly clear. Some frontal lesions seem to affect memory little, if at all, and so obviously do not have an amnesic-like effect. Even lesions of the dorsolateral frontal cortex do not seem to cause memory problems that bear a close resemblance to organic amnesia. They are associated with relatively normal recognition, but with poor recall, poor judgements of event recency and frequency, poor ability to monitor self-ordered responses, confabulation, certain kinds of difficulty with interference, poor metamemory, and poor ability to categorize stimuli; amnesics, however, have exceedingly bad recognition, and many show no confabulation, no difficulty with interference of the 'frontal' type, no disproportionately bad memory for event recency and frequency, good metamemory, and good categorizing ability. Amnesics with an aetiology of alcoholism do show difficulties of these kinds, but, as will be discussed in chapter 6, they often have incidental damage to the frontal lobes.

It has been argued by Mishkin (1982), however, that combined lesions of the orbitofrontal cortex and of the cingulate cortex (the ventromedial frontal cortex) will cause a conventional organic amnesia. The evidence for this view is discussed more fully in chapter 7 but one comment will be made here on the human data. It has sometimes been suggested that patients who have undergone rupture and repair of aneurysms of the anterior communicating artery suffer from amnesia because of a lesion to ventromedial frontal cortex. Figures 6.3 and 7.2 illustrate the location of the anterior communicating artery and of the ventromedial frontal cortex, which is believed by some to be one of the brain regions damaged by aneurysms of this artery. In patients with this disorder, a dilated and weakened section of the anterior communicating artery bursts and affects the blood supply of several brain regions, the precise ones depending on the location of the burst and the nature of the repair operation. The disorder is often not accompanied by a permanent amnesia. Most typically, patients show a moderately severe amnesia, together with confabulation and personality change. Although the latter symptoms may be caused by damage to frontal structures, it has been argued by Damasio, Graff-Radford, Eslinger, Damasio, and Kassell (1985) that the amnesia is caused by damage to basal forebrain structures, such as the septum, so that a secondary disruption of the hippocampus (one of the structures damaged in organic amnesia) results. The evidence from human cases that ventromedial frontal lesions cause amnesia is therefore weak. As bilateral frontal lesions sometimes severely impair functions when unilateral lesions have little effect, it might be argued that organic amnesia is caused by only very large lesions that destroy most of prefrontal association cortex. This possibility is probably untestable in humans because massive frontal lesions are almost sure to damage the limbic system and diencephalic structures, lesioned in organic amnesics. There is, however, little reason for believing that large lesions confined to the prefrontal association cortex cause organic amnesia, so it will be provisionally concluded that frontal lesions do not cause the kind of memory deficits seen in organic amnesics. Rather, they cause a milder and qualitatively distinct set of memory disorders.

On the second question, it can be provisionally concluded that at least the majority of memory deficits caused by frontal lesions are associated with planning deficits. These deficits arise when remembering requires the initiation and maintenance of effortful and organized strategies of encoding and/or retrieval, as well as the ability to switch from one strategy to another. Such effortful strategies enable semantic memory to be searched so that previously unrelated items of information can be integrated, an activity that should increase the effectiveness of encoding as well as of retrieval. Different aspects of planning may be mediated by distinct frontal regions, so lesions may have distinct effects on planning and memory, depending on their location. But this remains to be proved. What does seem likely is that the frontal cortex contains modular processing units that enable organized searches to be performed on the semantic memories that are stored in PTO association cortex. The products of such searches may be new semantic memories that will be stored in PTO cortex. More routine retrieval from well-established semantic memory probably does not depend on frontal cortex mechanisms. For example, the sight of a tiger will automatically evoke the animal's name, and its name on other occasions will probably automatically bring to mind an image of the animal.

Although the majority of memory deficits caused by frontal lobe lesions can be seen as results of inadequate effortful processing of information, it is harder to explain the deficits in recency and frequency discrimination in these terms. As briefly described in chapter 1, Hasher and Zacks (1979) have claimed that information about the recency, frequency, and spatial position of events is automatically encoded. In other words, such information and probably other kinds of background contextual information are encoded without the need for intentional direction and with minimal attentional effort. This kind of encoding seems to differ radically from the kinds of intentional, effortful, and organized encoding that is known to be disrupted by frontal lesions. In the view of Hasher and Zacks, it is even impossible to improve the encoding of information that is normally encoded automatically, by bringing it under voluntary control. If Hasher and Zacks are correct, frontal lesions may disrupt memory not only because they impair effortful processing, but also because they impair automatic processing.

It is possible, of course, that automatic and effortful encoding are disrupted by differently located frontal lobe lesions. If Hasher and Zacks are correct, however, automatic and effortful encoding are radically distinct kinds of processing, and it would be slightly surprising that they should be performed by closely adjacent cortical regions. Also, there are certain objections to the view that some frontal lobe regions mediate the kinds of automatic processing postulated by Hasher and Zacks and that other frontal lobe regions mediate effortful processing. First, if the lesions directly disrupt automatic processing, then spatial memory should be poor, but there is evidence that spatial memory can be spared in frontal patients (see Milner et al., 1985). The claim that spatial memory is preserved does, however, need confirmation with different tasks and patients because it has usually been found in patients with unilateral lesions and has only once been reported in patients with bilateral lesions, whereas some other studies have reported deficits. For example, Passingham (1985) has reported that lesions of the sulcus principalis (a region that includes part of the dorsolateral frontal cortex and extends back into the frontal eye fields) cause a spatial memory problem in monkeys. The animals' failure did not seem to result from excessive perseveration or from the use of poor search strategies. It is also known that neurons in the monkey dorsolateral frontal cortex fire in the 2- to 5-sec delay during which an animal must remember the position to which it must respond, and that some of these neurons code for spatial position during the delay. However, although monkeys with dorsolateral frontal lesions are bad at this kind of delayed-response task, there is no evidence that human patients are impaired at similar kinds of spatial short-term memory tasks any more than they are impaired at non-spatial short-term memory tasks, such as the digit span. Furthermore, in humans and monkeys, spatial deficits are not usually apparent unless the tests of spatial memory lack consistency from trial to trial, so that temporal discrimination is probably also required. Future research must ascertain whether frontal lobe lesions in humans ever disturb spatial memory when temporal discrimination is not required.

Second, there has been some criticism of Hasher and Zacks's claim that spatiotemporal information is automatically encoded. The matter is currently unresolved, but many believe that the application of conscious effort by normal people does improve their memory for contextual information of this kind. For example, in my laboratory, it has been found that under certain conditions spatial memory can be improved when subjects' attention is directed towards it. This does not, of course, show that such information is not usually encoded with minimal attentional effort. Even if spatiotemporal information is only habitually encoded automatically rather than essentially so, as proposed by Hasher and Zacks (1979), it might still be necessary to postulate that frontal lobe lesions impair both automatic and effortful encoding processes. There are, however, also claims that memory for spatiotemporal and frequency information is affected by effortful, semantic encoding of target items (see, e.g., Jackson, Michon, Boonstra, DeJonge, & Harsenhorst, 1986). Further work is needed to confirm these claims. If they are correct, they mean that contextual memory must depend in part on the effortful encoding of information about target items. At present, it remains possible that failure to engage in such effortful encoding impairs item memory, and this lowers contextual memory. It has not been shown that contextual memory is brought down disproportionately in such cases, whereas this kind of disproportionate contextual memory deficit definitely occurs in patients with frontal lobe lesions. Until this issue is properly examined, it will remain possible that patients with frontal lobe lesions suffer from memory failures for aspects of context that cannot be explained in terms of deficits in effortful processing.

Like the second, the third objection is fundamental if valid. Frontal lesions could affect recency and frequency judgements not because they affect automatic encoding, but for some other reason that may be more consistent with a planning deficit. There is little direct evidence relevant to this point, but Sagar et al.'s (1985) observations of impaired temporal discriminations in Parkinson patients have been extended to situations where there is a minimal memory load. Not only did these patients' recency judgements not improve when the interval between the recent and the remote event was increased, but the patients were poor at the Wechsler Picture Arrangement Test, which requires pictures to be ordered so as to make a meaningful story. This task clearly minimizes any memory load. As it has been argued that cognitive deficits in Parkinson's disease result from frontal lobe dysfunction, it would be interesting to see whether patients with known focal frontal lesions have a similar problem. If they do, this would be consistent with the view that their poor recency and frequency judgements are not caused by deficient automatic processing, but by the inability to use the products of such processing to make the relevant judgements. Indeed, the difficulty that patients experience with these judgements may not be one of memory, but of ability to use cues that are in memory to direct their decisions effectively.

On balance, the existing evidence supports the view that frontal lesions impair memory because they disturb effortful and elaborative processing of information, rather than because they do this and disturb automatic processing. More research is needed because there are opposing views (see Schacter, 1987a), and the issues concerning automatic processing and contextual memory will probably remain contentious for several years. It seems likely that the frontal cortex acts as a kind of central executive that mediates the various components of planning. This system is particularly important when a situation can be coped with only by behaviours that are not routine. Different frontal lesions seem to disrupt the ability to plan in distinct ways, but more research is needed to clarify this issue.

It remains unknown what causes the deficits in planning in patients with frontal lesions. One possibility relates to the third question raised above. It may be that frontal regions themselves contain stored memories of the procedures needed to carry out acquired plans of action and cognition. The frontal cortex might, for example, store information about what to do in different situations, such as visiting a restaurant or greeting a stranger as opposed to a friend. Information of this kind might be arranged hierarchically, so that it indicates first what to do in a situation in general, and then more specific actions to be performed as contingencies arise. It might also indicate the temporal order in which things should be done (as the frontal cortex may play a central role in making temporal judgements) and when to switch from effortful to automatic processing. Damage to such a storage system might not affect memory except in situations where the stored information is important for directing available processing skills. It might well cause problems with the use of analogies, failure to follow rules, and difficulty with planning sequences of action, all of which result from frontal lobe lesions. The possibility is therefore attractive because it makes frontal association cortex more similar in function to PTO association cortex. It has recently been developed in more explicit form by Grafman (see Newcombe, 1985). If his or related proposals are to be heuristically valuable, they must be able to make precise predictions not made by other hypotheses. This remains to be shown.

6   Organic amnesia

Organic amnesia is a fairly common disorder, but most often the amnesia is intermixed with other cognitive symptoms because the brain damage that is responsible for it extends into regions unconnected with the amnesia, such as the association neocortex. Pure cases of amnesia show four major characteristics, two positive and two negative. First, intelligence, as assessed by standard tests, such as the WAIS, is preserved. Although the fine print of this claim is still disputed by some, patients with exceedingly poor memory have been described with IQs of 140. Subtle and selective cognitive deficits cannot be excluded yet, but there is no real evidence for them. Second, short-term memory, as assessed by digit span and the recency effect, is preserved. Third, there is poor acquisition and retention of new episodic and semantic information (anterograde amnesia). And fourth, there is poor memory for information that was acquired pre-traumatically (retrograde amnesia). As will be discussed in more detail later in this chapter, not all kinds of memory are disturbed in amnesics. It has been claimed that amnesics show preserved learning and memory for certain motor, perceptual, and cognitive skills, for conditioning, and for what was referred to in chapter 1 as priming (i.e., changed or more efficient processing of stimuli that results from having recently perceived them).

The relatively high frequency of the disorder is reflected in the variety of conditions that can cause it. A brief list of its causes includes bilateral surgical removal of the medial temporal lobes in the treatment of epilepsy (bilateral removals are no longer made, but unilateral removals can have the same effect if there is pre-existing pathology in the contralateral temporal lobe), chronic alcoholism, thiamin deficiency, nicotinic acid deficiency, anoxia, carbon monoxide poisoning, complications from viral and bacterial infections of the brain (such as herpes simplex encephalitis and tuberculous meningitis), strokes affecting the circulation of the posterior cerebral or anterior communicating arteries, midline tumours, closed head injury, and probably normal as well as pathological ageing. All these causes usually produce a permanent amnesia, from which there may be little or no recovery over many years.

In addition, transient amnesia can be produced by repeated electroconvulsive shock treatment (ECT), most often used to alleviate depression; and there is a syndrome, called transient global amnesia, that is most common in late-middle-aged and elderly men. This syndrome may be caused by a temporarily inadequate blood supply to the medial temporal lobes, by a kind of epileptic disturbance, or both. Attacks are sometimes triggered by emotional excitement and typically last for some hours. During an attack, the patient may be intellectually intact, but will be disoriented because he cannot work out how he got to be where he is and is unable to retain any new information. After the attack, memory usually returns to its pre-morbid level, so new information is acquired fairly normally. In contrast, although memories of events before the attack occurred return, the period of the attack itself remains a blank.

All these multifarious conditions may cause organic amnesia because they cause a temporary or permanent dysfunction in specific limbic system and diencephalic structures. It is clear from the anatomical evidence that amnesia may be caused by lesions to different, albeit interconnected, structures. Prominent among these structures are the hippocampus and amygdala in the medial temporal lobes, and the mammillary bodies and dorsomedial nucleus of the thalamus in the diencephalon. In addition, there is evidence that lesions of the basal forebrain, which sends cholinergic projections to the hippocampus and amygdala, may cause amnesia, and some have argued that ventromedial frontal cortex lesions do so as well. One difficulty in identifying the lesions that are critical for the emergence of amnesia is that many of the conditions that produce it cause additional damage to other brain-stem and neocortical regions. These lesions may superimpose further memory and cognitive disturbances on the ones caused by the critical lesions. For example, amnesics with an aetiology of chronic alcoholism very often have widespread brain-stem damage and atrophy of neocortex, particularly frontal neocortex, which superimposes other symptoms on the organic amnesia.

The problem of identifying the minimal critical lesions that can cause amnesia is considered in the next section. As several distinct lesions seem to be capable of causing the basic syndrome, this raises the question of whether there may not, in fact, be several subtly different amnesic disorders that are distinguished not only by the brain lesion that causes them, but also by the precise kind of memory deficits that characterize them. In answering this question, care must be taken to separate incidental cognitive and memory deficits from the memory deficits that are intrinsic to amnesia. The issues related to the possibly multiple deficits that have the common name of organic amnesia are assessed in the third section of this chapter. Whatever the final answer to the problem of whether amnesia is a unitary deficit or comprises several superficially similar deficits, the syndrome is associated with a wide range of symptoms that are common to all its forms. The fourth section reviews available evidence about these memory deficits.

The amnesic syndrome is of great theoretical interest for several reasons. First, it can be extremely severe. For example, the famous patient H. M., who had his medial temporal lobes surgically removed in the 1950s, describes his life since as though he were continually waking from a dream, with all the things that have just happened slipping beyond his ability to retrieve them. Other patients lose their sense of personal identity because they can remember little of the past 20 or 30 years of their lives. Thus whatever is disturbed in these patients has to be very important for the development of normal memories. Second, despite their drastically impaired memories, some amnesics function at a high intellectual level, so it is most unlikely that their problem is caused by disruption of the effortful and elaborative encoding and retrieval of semantic information. If it were, then intelligence would inevitably also be badly affected.

Viable accounts of the functional deficit underlying amnesia must be able to accommodate the third reason why the syndrome is of theoretical interest. This reason directly arises from the argument of the last two chapters that well-established semantic memories are stored in the association neocortex, which is undamaged in organic amnesics. Several accounts of the functional deficit in amnesia are consistent with the notion that well-established semantic memories are stored in regions not lesioned in patients with pure amnesia and with the idea that intelligence is preserved in pure amnesics. One such account proposes that amnesia is caused by a specific failure of storage, which implies that the critical limbic–diencephalic structures, affected in the disorder, are not concerned with information encoding and retrieval, but have something to do with the consolidation and/or maintenance of storage. Although there may be such storage-specific systems in the brain, another account of the functional deficit in amnesia obviates the need to postulate that such a system exists in the limbic–diencephalic structures. According to this account, amnesics have an encoding and retrieval deficit for the extrinsic context of events (their background spatiotemporal context and their format context, or manner of presentation), which can dramatically impair the ability to acquire new information and retrieve some older memories. This account is consistent with the preserved intelligence of amnesics and, indeed, their preserved short-term memory (which may be 'context-free'). It is also consistent with the neocortical storage of well-established semantic memories, if it is supposed that aspects of contextual information are stored in the limbic–diencephalic structures lesioned in amnesics and that the ability to remember less rehearsed episodic *and* semantic information depends on the storage and retrieval of such contextual information. In its various guises, the context-memory deficit account of amnesia has been very popular in recent years (see Mayes, Meudell, & Pickering, 1985) so it will be discussed in the final section of this chapter, along with other hypotheses about the functional deficit(s) that underlie(s) amnesia.

The human evidence about the critical lesions in amnesia

Identification of the lesions that are critical for the production of a pure amnesic syndrome has proved very difficult for two main reasons. First, many amnesic patients show not only anterograde and retrograde amnesia, but also deficits in intelligence, planning ability, short-term memory, and atypical memory losses, such as poor recall of information that was very well learnt in childhood. When amnesia is confounded with other cognitive symptoms, it becomes very tricky to isolate the damage that causes only the core deficit of anterograde and retrograde amnesia. Second, there have been very few post-mortem analyses of patients who have received anything more than a cursory clinical assessment of their amnesia. The quality of anatomical data on well-studied cases is, however, gradually being

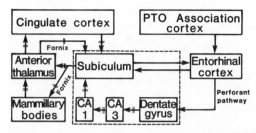

Figure 6.1 The arrows marked with two lines represent the Papez circuit. The hippocampal formation is taken to include all the structures surrounded by the dashed lines: the dentate gyrus; the cornu ammonis, or hippocampus proper, subdivided into fields CA1 to CA4, of which CA1 and CA3 are the most important; and the subiculum, which is the source of nearly all the output from the hippocampus. The figure does not show the projections back from the hippocampus to the overlying association neocortex.

improved as the accuracy of identifying lesions in life, through the use of CAT scans, MRI, and PET scans, has increased. These techniques not only provide means of imaging where brain tissue has been destroyed, but also, in the case of the PET scan, offer a means of determining whether apparently intact brain regions show normal levels of metabolic and, by implication, neural activity in amnesics.

The oldest view of the minimal lesions necessary to cause amnesia is that they involve the hippocampus or other structures that are serially connected to it. These structures and some of their connections are illustrated in Figure 6.1, which shows that processed sensory information from association neocortex reaches the hippocampal structures via the perforant pathway of the entorhinal cortex. After further processing within the hippocampus, the major output of the system is through the subiculum, from which the fornix originates. One fornical target is the mammillary bodies, which project via the anterior thalamus to the cingulate cortex, which, in turn, completes what is traditionally known as the Papez circuit by sending a projection back to the subiculum of the hippocampus. Activity of the hippocampal system is modulated by an input from neurons in the medial septum and closely adjacent nucleus of the diagonal band of Broca, which is cholinergic. These structures lie close to the hippocampus and form part of a basal forebrain cholinergic system of neurons, the other part of which is the nucleus basalis of Meynert, which innervates the neocortex and amygdala (Figure 6.2). In recent years, it has been proposed that organic amnesia can be a result not only of direct damage to the hippocampus or related parts of the Papez circuit, but also of damage to the basal forebrain cholinergic neurons.

Evidence from surgical cases, such as H. M., suggested that the anterior temporal cortex, the uncus (a region of 'old' cortex that lies on the medial temporal cortex and is intimately linked with the hippocampus and other limbic system structures), and the amygdala could be removed without causing amnesia unless the hippocampus was also invaded. It was indeed found that the extent of removal of the left hippocampus is well correlated with the severity of impairment of

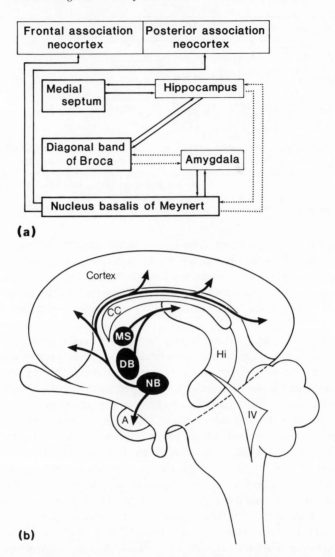

(a)

(b)

Figure 6.2 (a) The heavily outlined boxes indicate the three main structures that constitute the cholinergic basal forebrain. The solid arrows represent what recent research indicates are the major projections between the basal forebrain and the association cortex, and between the basal forebrain and the limbic system. The dotted arrows represent what recent research indicates are projections between the basal forebrain and the limbic system. The research was carried out on non-human primates, but probably applies to humans as well. It can be seen that basal forebrain and limbic system projections are reciprocating ones. Also, the major pattern of linkage is between the medial septum and the diagonal band of Broca in the basal forebrain and the hippocampus in the limbic system, and between the nucleus basalis of Meynert in the basal forebrain and the amygdala in the limbic system. (b) The approximate location of the cholinergic basal forebrain structures and of their main projections in the primate brain. CC refers to corpus callosum; MS, medial septum; DB, diagonal band of Broca; NB, nucleus basalis of Meynert; Hi, hippocampus; A, amygdala; IV, fourth ventricle. (Courtesy of Dr. H. J. Sagar, Royal Hallamshire Hospital, Sheffield.)

verbal memory, and the same relationship holds between the degree of damage to the right hippocampus and the deficit in non-verbal memory (Milner, 1971). There has also been recognition of the fact that post-encephalitic amnesia, particularly that caused by the herpes simplex virus, is associated with damage to the limbic system structures of the medial temporal lobe, most notably the hippocampus. The herpes simplex virus rarely damages the diencephalon, although it often destroys parts of the PTO association neocortex and may affect the posterior orbitofrontal cortex and cingulate cortex. Occlusion of the posterior cerebral artery also typically causes extensive damage to the hippocampus, and although it may often cause additional damage to PTO association neocortex, the diencephalon is less likely to be affected (see Parkin & Leng, 1987). Similarly, it has been argued that amnesics with an aetiology of chronic alcoholism, who are known as Korsakoff patients, do not usually show hippocampal atrophy, but invariably show degeneration of the medial parts of the mammillary bodies (see, e.g., Victor, Adams, & Collins, 1971). It has also been claimed that damage to the fornix, the pathway that links the hippocampus to the mammillary bodies, causes amnesia, although the claim is disputed. It has less often been asserted that focal lesions of the anterior thalamus or cingulate cortex cause amnesia, and the evidence here is fragmentary. Cingulate lesions have been reported to produce a transient amnesia in which memory for temporal order is surprisingly poor, and amnesia has occasionally been reported after anterior thalamus lesions, but, once again, the deficit is usually only transient (see Markowitsch, 1985; Mayes and Meudell, 1983). Finally, it has been argued that when amnesia is found in cases with ruptured aneurysms of the anterior communicating artery, the lesion responsible lies in the septum (and possibly in other cholinergic basal forebrain structures). The location of the affected artery is shown in Figure 6.3. This argument is consistent with the view that amnesia is caused by dysfunction of the hippocampus or structures serially linked to it in the Papez circuit because the medial septum is the source of a modulatory cholinergic input to the hippocampus.

In recent years, the 'hippocampal circuit' hypothesis of amnesia has been severely criticized. Horel (1978) argued that in cases like H. M.'s, many structures other than the hippocampus are damaged, and therefore proposed that the critical damage in that and similar cases is not to the hippocampus at all, but to the temporal stem, which is a white matter pathway linking the temporal cortex to subcortical nuclei, such as the dorsomedial nucleus of the thalamus. Although evidence from a monkey model of amnesia, which will be discussed in chapter 7, indicates that Horel's view is wrong, there have been reports that unilateral and bilateral hippocampectomies, sometimes performed to relieve severe pain, do not always cause amnesia of the kind seen in H. M. (see Markowitsch, 1985).

The role of fornix lesions in amnesia is also in doubt, as Squire and Moore (1979) reviewed 50 cases of fornical lesions and found evidence of amnesia in only 3. In these cases, it was argued that amnesia resulted from additional damage. Victor et al. (1971), in their classic monograph on alcoholic amnesia, attacked the notion that mammillary body lesions are sufficient to cause the syndrome. Five of their cases had atrophy of the mammillary bodies without concomitant

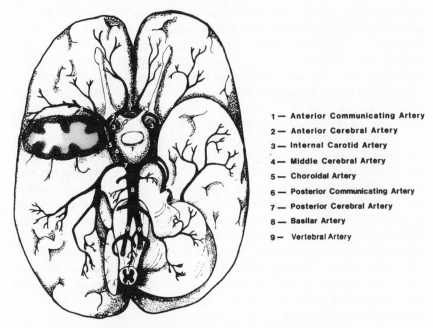

1 — Anterior Communicating Artery
2 — Anterior Cerebral Artery
3 — Internal Carotid Artery
4 — Middle Cerebral Artery
5 — Choroidal Artery
6 — Posterior Communicating Artery
7 — Posterior Cerebral Artery
8 — Basilar Artery
9 — Vertebral Artery

Figure 6.3 This view of the underside of the surface of the brain illustrates its major arterial blood supply. It can be seen that the anterior communicating artery is located beneath the frontal lobe. Nevertheless, aneurysms of this artery may damage not only parts of frontal association cortex, as it has been claimed that they also often damage the medial septum in the basal forebrain. Vascular accidents affecting the distribution of the posterior cerebral artery can also cause amnesia because, as can be seen, this artery supplies structures deep within the temporal lobes, such as the hippocampus.

atrophy of the dorsomedial nucleus of the thalamus, and they reported that these five did not show amnesia in life. Thirty-eight other cases had lesions of both the mammillary bodies and the dorsomedial nucleus of the thalamus, and all of them were reported to have amnesia (although it should be noted that detailed formal tests were not given). Victor et al. therefore tentatively proposed that alcoholic amnesia results from a lesion to the dorsomedial nucleus of the thalamus. As this thalamic nucleus does not receive direct hippocampal inputs and is not part of the Papez circuit, their conclusion was critical of the hippocampal hypothesis of amnesia.

Victor et al.'s alternative to the hippocampal hypothesis – namely, that severe amnesia can be caused by focal lesions of the dorsomedial thalamic nucleus – derived most of its support from cases of alcoholic amnesia. Some cases exist where the brain damage has not been caused by heavy drinking, in which the amnesia has been attributed to dorsomedial thalamic lesions. Perhaps the most famous such case is N. A., who became amnesic (at least for verbal information) in 1960 after receiving a stab wound from a miniature fencing foil. CAT-scan analysis revealed that N. A. had a lesion that included the left dorsomedial thalamus (Squire & Moore, 1979), although the nature of the penetrating wound indicates that other structures (such as the frontal lobes) must also have suffered some damage. Others have argued, however, that the route taken by the foil after it passed through the right nostril made damage to the orbitofrontal cortex and basal ganglia likely, and Markowitsch (1985) has suggested that indirect damage to the mammillary bodies was also likely to have occurred. A careful MRI study of N. A. has now confirmed that this patient does indeed show marked bilateral mammillary body damage as well as lesions to the left thalamus and right anterior temporal lobe (Squire, Amaral, Zola-Morgan, Kritchevsky, & Press, 1987). Von Cramon, Hebel, and Schuri (1985) have recently analysed CAT scans of 11 patients with vascular lesions confined to the thalamus. They found that there was an area of damage, common to all the patients who showed amnesia, that included white matter tracts that linked the mammillary bodies to the anterior thalamus as well as the amygdala to the medial thalamus. The lesion therefore disconnected the mammillary bodies from their thalamic projection nucleus, as might be expected from the hippocampal hypothesis. After surgical removal of the dorsomedial nucleus (sometimes done to relieve pain), memory disturbances have been reported to be transient at most (see Markowitsch, 1985).

The evidence that selective lesions of the thalamic dorsomedial nucleus are sufficient to cause a severe, permanent amnesia is not good. But neither is the evidence that focal lesions of the anterior thalamus or mammillary bodies cause severe, permanent amnesias. One way of explaining these puzzling findings has been proposed by Mishkin (1982), who has argued that a severe, permanent amnesia results only when there is damage to both limbic–diencephalic circuits. One circuit is the hippocampal circuit of Papez, as already discussed. The other runs from association cortex to the amygdala in the medial temporal lobes, from there to the dorsomedial nucleus of the thalamus either directly or via the bed nucleus of the stria terminalis, and from there to the orbitofrontal cortex. Most of the direct support for this hypothesis is drawn from animal models of amnesia, which are discussed in chapter 7 (Figure 7.1 also illustrates in more detail Mishkin's hypothesis). But the human anatomical data relevant to the hypothesis are considered here.

First, the bilateral removals of the medial temporal lobes that were performed in Montreal, and included case H. M., involved resections of the amygdala as well as the hippocampus, and post-encephalitic amnesics almost certainly have damage to both these structures. The view that conjoint damage to both structures is necessary to produce severe, permanent amnesia is consistent with evidence that selective amygdala lesions do not cause amnesia (Sarter & Markowitsch, 1985). One recent case study does, however, suggest that selective hippocampal lesions may be sufficient to cause at least a moderate amnesia. This patient developed amnesia, which was documented by formal tests, after a hypotensive episode that followed cardiac by-pass surgery. Five years later, post-mortem histological analysis showed that he had suffered a bilateral lesion confined to the CA1 field of the hippocampus and that the only other brain damage involved unilateral lesions in the basal ganglia and somatosensory cortex (see Squire, 1986). It was argued that only the hippocampal lesion could reasonably have been linked to the patient's amnesia. This case is important, but it does not by itself prove that amygdala damage would not have exacerbated this patient's amnesia. Mishkin's (1982) hypothesis does allow that damage to either hippocampal or amygdala circuit alone may cause a mild and possibly transient amnesia, but claims that a severe amnesia results from only conjoint damage of the circuits.

Second, in the Victor et al. (1971) study, all the alcoholic patients who had permanent memory deficits also had atrophy of both mammillary bodies and dorsomedial nucleus of the thalamus. In other words, the diencephalic lesion had affected both hippocampal and amygdala circuits. There is, however, some evidence that alcoholic amnesics do not always have lesions of the thalamic dorso-medial nucleus. Mair, Warrington, and Weiskrantz (1979) have described detailed post-mortem analyses of two alcoholic amnesics on whom extensive formal memory tests had been performed over several years. Both patients showed marked atrophy of the mammillary bodies, but in the thalamus, there was only a thin band of gliosis, adjacent to the walls of the third ventricle and medial to the dorso-medial thalamus, in a region called the paratenial nucleus. Although the medial extremity of the dorsomedial nucleus is hard to define, the nucleus did appear to be intact in both patients. In my laboratory, we have recently performed a similar analysis on the brains of two formally tested alcoholic amnesics and found much the same result. The findings do not refute, but may call for some modification of, Mishkin's (1982) hypothesis. The amygdala projects to the paratenial nucleus as well as the dorsomedial nucleus, so it could be argued that the deficit of the four alcoholic amnesics was caused by a conjoint lesion of the mammillary bodies and of a thalamic projection of the amygdala.

As the anterior thalamus projects to the cingulate cortex and the part of the dorsomedial thalamus believed to be damaged in alcoholic amnesics by Victor et al. (1971) projects to the orbitofrontal cortex, Mishkin (1982) has also argued that lesions to this ventromedial frontal area will also cause amnesia. His argument is slightly weakened by the cases just described, although they in no way prove that dorsomedial thalamic damage is unrelated to amnesia. It should also be noted that the circuits contain feedback pathways, so that the hippocampus can influence the association cortex and the mammillary bodies, the hippocampus. It could be, therefore, that lesions of the ventromedial cortex will have little effect on memory. This accords with the evidence, already discussed, that amnesia caused by rupture of the anterior communicating artery probably results from lesions of the septum and other parts of the cholinergic basal forebrain (Damasio, Graff-Radford, Eslinger, Damasio, & Kassell, 1985). If this view is correct, then one would expect that lesions confined to those parts of the basal forebrain that project to only the hippocampus will cause less severe amnesia than lesions that also affect cholinergic projections to the amygdala. This prediction cannot be tested with human patients, but it should be noted that patients with Alzheimer's disease, who are densely amnesic, show a striking loss of cholinergic neurons from all parts of the basal forebrain, so that hippocampal, amygdalar, and neocortical activities are all likely to be affected. These patients show very low levels of the enzymes involved in synthesizing and breaking down acetylcholine (for a discussion, see Bartus, Dean, Pontecorvo, & Flicker, 1985), although reduced levels of other transmitters, such as noradrenalin and somatostatin, are often found as well. In its early stages, Alzheimer's disease may be associated with a relatively selective amnesia, unconfounded with other cognitive deficits, and this may be caused by damage to the basal forebrain cholinergic system that causes dysfunction in the hippocampus and amygdala. Direct hippocampal damage has also been reported, however, so the importance of the basal forebrain lesion is hard to assess in humans.

It can tentatively be concluded that Mishkin's (1982) double-circuit hypothesis is reasonably compatible with the human anatomical data, although these data do suggest that the theory may need some modification. For example, there is no good evidence that selective ventromedial frontal cortex lesions cause amnesia in humans, which raises questions about the precise structures involved in the 'memory circuits'. Knowledge of what these structures are needs to be improved, as Mair et al.'s (1979) work illustrates. Are both paratenial and dorsomedial thalamic nuclei involved in the amygdala 'memory circuit,' or only one? It may even be that other circuits are involved, as Jurko (1978) has reported that whereas neither left amygdala nor left centre median (another thalamic nucleus, lying close to the walls of the third ventricle) lesions alone caused poor verbal paired associate learning, combined lesions did. If this finding is replicable, the relationship of the centre median nucleus to the structures of the Papez circuit needs to be examined. Finally, there is some evidence to suggest that hippocampal lesions may have greater effects than amygdala lesions, and although this does not show that the conjoint lesion does not have a greater disruptive effect on memory, Mishkin's hypothesis may need some modification to accommodate it.

The evidence that amnesia may sometimes be caused by a loss of cholinergic neurons from parts of the basal forebrain raises the interesting possibility that it may occasionally be a biochemical disorder, in the sense that it is partly or wholly initiated by a dysfunction of neurons that release one or, at most, a few kinds of neurotransmitter. It has been suggested that two kinds of biochemical disorder can cause memory problems: a cholinergic disorder and a noradrenergic disorder. In addition to the evidence that Alzheimer's disease and ruptures of the anterior communicating artery are associated with basal forebrain damage, it has been argued by Butters (1985) that alcoholic amnesia is caused by basal forebrain damage. He speculated that diencephalic lesions cause only mild memory difficulties in alcoholic amnesics, but that basal forebrain lesions cause severe problems. This speculation was based on a post-mortem study by Arendt, Bigl, and Tcanstedt (1983), which examined the brains of three alcoholic amnesics as well as of Alzheimer dements, patients with Huntington's chorea and schizophrenia, and chronic alcoholics without amnesia. Only the alcoholic amnesics and the Alzheimer patients showed significant reductions of neurons in the basal forebrain. In fact, the alcoholic amnesics showed an average loss of nearly 50% of the neurons in the nucleus basalis of Meynert, the diagonal band of Broca, and the medial septum, which are the three largely cholinergic nuclei of the basal forebrain. Although these observations support the possibility that damage to cholinergic neurons in the basal forebrain may contribute to amnesia found in chronic alcoholics, Butters's speculation is unlikely to be correct. Mair et al. (1979) reported no basal forebrain damage in their two alcoholic amnesics, and the two brains analysed in my laboratory also showed no significant loss of basal forebrain neurons from the nucleus basalis of Meynert, although there was an indication that metabolical activity in septal neurons had been slightly reduced.

Perhaps the major source of evidence favouring the possibility that a cholinergic deficiency can cause amnesia comes from drug-study findings. Whereas there is evidence that drugs that stimulate central cholinergic function may improve memory in young and old volunteers, drugs that block central cholinergic function impair memory performance (for a review, see Bartus et al., 1985). For example, Drachman (1977) claimed to have modelled an Alzheimer-type dementia in young volunteers, who had received the anticholinergic drug scopolamine. His subjects showed impaired visuospatial intelligence and memory, which was reversed by the drug physostigmine, which boosts cholinergic function when the transmitter is in relatively short supply. As scopolamine affects arousal, it was important that Drachman found that its cognitive effects were not reversed by amphetamine, a drug that increases arousal. The interpretation of drug studies is very complex, and other results have not always agreed with those of Drachman. The drugs are also given systemically, so they act on all cholinergic neurons in the brain, not just those in the basal forebrain. Nevertheless, if cholinergic depletion was confined to the neurons that project to the hippocampus and amygdala, it is plausible to argue that a mild amnesia would result.

The main support for the hypothesis that a dysfunction of noradrenergic neurons contributes to amnesia comes from work on alcoholic amnesics. Victor et al. (1971) reported that lesions of the locus coeruleus in the brain-stem were quite commonly found in their large sample of brains from alcoholic amnesics. This small nucleus, located just above the pons in the brain-stem, sends projections to a very large number of systems in the forebrain, including the neocortex and the hippocampus. It influences these systems through the release of the neurotransmitter noradrenalin. Victor et al.'s observation does not in itself show that locus coeruleus lesions contribute to amnesia because alcoholic amnesics frequently suffer from many lesions, most of which are unrelated to amnesia. The two patients on whom a post-mortem was performed in my laboratory had, however, differed markedly in the severity of their amnesia. The lesions of the less amnesic patient were at least as great as those of the more amnesic patient in the diencephalon and all brain regions, except for the locus coeruleus, where the more amnesic patient had a greater amount of damage. This finding is consistent with a noradrenergic dysfunction contributing to the amnesia in some cases. The idea receives further support from the work of McEntee and Mair (1978), who measured levels of the noradrenalin metabolite 3-methoxy, 4-hydroxyphenylglycol (MHPG) in the lumbar spinal fluid of a group of alcoholic amnesics. They found reduced levels of the metabolite and a correlation of the level with the size of the patients' WAIS–WMS discrepancy, which was used as a measure of the severity of their amnesia. This observation and later work, which found that their patients' anterograde amnesia was partially alleviated by a drug that improves noradrenergic efficiency, is consistent with the view that a noradrenergic dysfunction, caused by locus coeruleus lesions, contributes to amnesia in some, but perhaps not all, alcoholic amnesics.

The cholinergic and noradrenergic dysfunction hypotheses are not incompatible with Mishkin's (1982) dual-circuit view because neurons that release both kinds of transmitter modulate the activity of the medial temporal limbic structures. In addition to the older view that lesions of the hippocampus and some of the structures to which it projects are sufficient to cause a severe, permanent amnesia, another criticism has been made of Mishkin's hypothesis by Markowitsch (1985). His criticism is, in fact, fundamentally one of the general belief that specific cognitive deficits are reliably caused by lesions of particular brain regions. He argued that strict relationships between particular brain structures and amnesia are questionable. As support for this argument, he cites evidence that equivalent brain damage sometimes does and sometimes does not cause amnesia. Among this evidence, he reports the claim that in some cases, bilateral resection of the medial temporal lobes has not resulted in amnesia. The anatomical and neuropsychological bases of this claim need to be assessed further, but in my view, there is currently no other compelling evidence that contradicts the claim that amnesia is consistently caused by certain lesions in all people.

Although brain damage in amnesic patients can usually be identified by CAT scanning or MRI techniques, there are kinds of damage that they do not seem to detect well. For example, patients who have suffered from an anoxic episode probably have destruction of the large pyramidal neurons in the CA1 field of the hippocampus, but this is not apparent with CAT scanning. The damage is, however, revealed by PET scanning when measures of blood flow, blood volume, and cerebral metabolism are taken. In one such patient, it has been shown that there is a reduction in cerebral metabolism (particularly in the medial temporal lobes), but no reduction in blood flow in the medial temporal lobes (see Gazzaniga, 1984). A patient with transient global amnesia showed a similar depression during an attack, which resolved once her amnesic state cleared. PET scanning may therefore be valuable in revealing areas of brain dysfunction not apparent with CAT scanning or MRI.

PET scanning may also be useful in assessing another suggestion of Markowitsch (1985) – that a lesioned structure should not be regarded as solely responsible for the memory deficits observed in a patient because the brain acts in an integrated way. In other words, the function that has been lost or impaired should not be solely ascribed to the lesioned structure, but to the integrated neural system of which it forms a part. This reasonable view, which seems compatible with Mishkin's (1982) notion of dual memory circuits, still leaves one with the problem of identifying the precise function of the damaged region. Each structure in the circuit receives specific kinds of information, processes it, and then sends the results to other structures in the circuit. The problem is to identify what that processing involves. Although animal research offers more opportunity for solving this kind of problem than work with humans, the recent development of PET-scan techniques that measure regional variations in neuronal metabolism may help determine the precise functions of specific brain structures. In fact, measures of both regional cerebral blood flow (which correlates with the level of neuronal activity in a brain structure) and neuronal metabolic activity in amnesics with both diencephalic and medial temporal lobe lesions could be taken to suggest that the memory deficit arises because of inadequate modulation of neocortical activity (see, e.g., Gazzaniga, 1984). Blood flow and metabolism were reduced, relative to controls, in the neocortex and, indeed, globally when the patients were resting, although the metabolic reductions were less severe than those found in the medial temporal lobes. These impairments resolved in the patient with transient global amnesia when her memory recovered, and it is possible that they were caused directly by the disruption of normal function in the medial temporal lobes. Similar study of the patient N. A., whose lesion includes the left dorsomedial thalamus and the mammillary bodies, showed that there was reduced metabolism not only in that neocortical region, but also over the left basal ganglia (which might have been directly damaged) and the entire left neocortex (which could not have been). The degree of reduction in N. A.'s neocortical activity must be too small to reduce his superior verbal intelligence, but great enough to affect his verbal memory, which is impaired. These studies are still at a very early stage, however, and more measures need to be taken in patients and controls who are engaged in memory tasks before any confident conclusions can be drawn. Even so, they do weakly imply that in normal people, the structures that are implicated in amnesia modulate the activity of association neocortex in a way that has little effect on the encoding and retrieval of semantic information, but facilitates the storage of semantic and episodic information. In amnesics, this storage facilitation would not occur.

Varieties of organic amnesia?

The fact that organic amnesia can be caused by lesions of several distinct, although strongly interconnected, brain structures raises the possibility that more than one kind of memory deficit is covered by the rubric of 'organic amnesia'. This possibility has been explored mainly by comparing amnesics with different aetiologies on memory tasks, rather than directly comparing patients with distinct focal lesions. Even though different aetiologies are associated with distinct kinds of lesions, there are problems with this approach. First, differences in memory may not be related to the separate aetiological groups having lesions in distinct limbic, diencephalic, or basal forebrain sites, but to incidental damage to other brain structures, unconnected with organic amnesia. For example, alcoholic amnesics may differ from post-encephalitic amnesics not because they have diencephalic lesions rather than medial temporal limbic system lesions, but because they have a particular kind of incidental impairment of frontal lobe function. Second, there may be very considerable heterogeneity within an aetiological group. This is particularly striking in the two aetiological groups just mentioned. For example, some alcoholic amnesics show no signs of frontal lobe atrophy, whereas others appear to have not only frontal cortex atrophy, but also PTO association cortex atrophy. These problems must be borne in mind in analysing available data so as to identify the elementary memory deficits that constitute amnesia. The risks can be minimized by seeing whether the components of a memory disorder ever occur in isolation and, if they do, whether the brain damage is still present in the 'core' region, but extends less into other areas. If part of the amnesic syndrome is found in isolation, but is caused by a lesion to a brain region not affected in other amnesics, then it may still be an elementary memory disorder, but be quite unrelated to the usual amnesic syndrome because it could be caused by a quite distinct functional deficit.

What, then, is the evidence that organic amnesia caused by limbic system, diencephalic, and basal forebrain lesions is a compound of more basic elementary deficits? Two broad kinds of heterogeneity have been proposed. The first is that the basic amnesic syndrome can be material specific to certain kinds of information; the second is that even the more global amnesic syndrome itself can be fractionated and that it takes more than one form. The existence of isolated verbal and non-verbal material-specific amnesias has been alluded to earlier in this book and is well supported (Milner, 1971). Lesions that affect the left medial temporal lobe cause serious difficulty with the acquisition and retention of verbal materials, but have little or no effect on memory for material that is hard to verbalize, such as abstract pictures or randomly constructed wire shapes that have to be palpated. Equivalent right hemisphere lesions have the reverse effects. More contentiously, it has also been claimed that left hemisphere lesions are associated with poor gustatory memory, whereas right hemisphere lesions are associated with poor olfactory memory (see Mayes & Meudell, 1983). There has been little investigation of whether the anterograde amnesia in these material-specific amnesias is accompanied by material-specific retrograde amnesia. The famous case N. A., whose mainly left-sided diencephalic lesion is associated with an amnesia that affects primarily verbal material, does, however, seem to show retrograde amnesia on some tests (Squire & Cohen, 1982). Clearly, much depends on the extent to which old memories rely on verbal or non-verbal information (such as visual imagery).

If the material-specific amnesias are to count as sub-varieties of amnesia, then they should be characterized by normal intelligence and short-term memory and be caused by a smaller version of the kinds of lesion that normally produce the full syndrome. These conditions appear to be met by the selective verbal and non-verbal amnesias studied by Milner (1971). It has been argued, however, that lesions in PTO association cortex can cause even more specific amnesias for faces, colours, or spatial locations. The most obvious interpretation of these disorders is the one offered in chapter 4 – that they are caused by problems in the storage or retrieval of well-established semantic memories and have no close link to organic amnesia. This interpretation certainly fits facial amnesia, as patients cannot remember massively overlearnt material, such as the faces of close relatives, whereas organic amnesics would have no such difficulty. Even so, there may be some selective memory failures, caused by PTO cortex lesions, that may be sub-varieties of organic amnesia. In these cases, the lesion may have disconnected a cortical region that processes and stores information about, for example, spatial location, from the limbic or diencephalic structures important for memory. The result should be an anterograde and retrograde amnesia that is selective for the relevant information.

This possibility has been supported by Ross (1982), who has described two cases of selective visual amnesia associated with bilateral posterior cortex lesions. One patient had some blind fields, but the sighted fields appeared normal. Despite this, he had loss of memory for all recent visual events. He was, for example, unable to draw a plan of the apartment into which he had moved following his stroke, although he could draw accurately his parents' house, where he had lived for years before his stroke. There was, therefore, an anterograde amnesia accompanied by a milder retrograde amnesia of a kind sometimes seen in amnesics with an organic amnesia associated with limbic–diencephalic lesions. The location of the lesion was consistent with the proposal that the visual cortex had been disconnected from the limbic memory structures in the medial temporal lobe. Ross also described three further patients with unilateral lesions of the tempero-occipital cortex, two of whom showed recent memory deficits for right-sided tactile stimuli and verbal information, but not non-verbal auditory information, and the third of whom showed recent memory deficits for left-sided tactile stimuli and non-verbal auditory information. As would be expected, the first two patients had left hemisphere lesions, whereas the third had a right hemisphere lesion. Ross argued that the sensory inputs to the damaged hemispheres were disconnected from their ipsilateral limbic memory structures and that some recovery might occur if these inputs were transferred via the corpus callosum to the contralateral hemisphere.

The notion that a cortical lesion may cause a material-specific amnesia by disconnecting particular cortical processing and storage areas from the limbic memory structures has, then, received some support from the work of Ross (1982). Whether there are material-specific amnesias for faces, colours, and spatial locations as well as visual information in general is, however, much more polemical. The evidence favouring topographical amnesia (amnesia for spatial location) is the best. Posterior cortical lesions sometimes seem to disturb a patient's ability to learn routes in new environments and the location of objects, as well as affecting memory for routes and geographical knowledge that was acquired pretraumatically. At the same time, these patients show good memory for all other kinds of information, do not seem to suffer from perceptual and attentional problems in processing spatial information, and even show normal short-term memory for the spatial location of a set of blocks. Although spatial memory is disturbed by right hemisphere limbic system lesions, topographical amnesia is caused by lesions of the parietal association cortex. The key question that still needs more investigation is whether patients with this syndrome have spatial retrograde amnesias that are no worse than would be expected in global organic amnesics. Only if the deficits are comparable can it confidently be concluded that topographical amnesia is a material-specific form of organic amnesia rather than a disorder of a specific kind of well-established memory.

If there are material-specific organic amnesias caused by lesions that disconnect PTO association cortex from limbic–diencephalic memory structures, their number is still unknown. It is, however, known that processed sensory information is sent from many PTO association cortex areas to the hippocampus and amygdala, and it seems reasonable that lesions to cortical white matter may sometimes disconnect this input in a highly selective way. In addition to such disconnection syndromes, there is no doubt that material-specific amnesias can be caused by unilateral lesions of the limbic system or diencephalic memory structures. Earlier in this section, mention was made of the possibility that direct bilateral lesions to different parts of these structures might cause distinct forms of global amnesia. *Three* relevant proposals have been made. First, some researchers believe that it may be possible to dissociate anterograde and retrograde amnesia from each other. Second, it has been argued that lesions of the limbic system of the medial temporal lobes and lesions of the diencephalon cause distinct amnesias. Third, it has been argued that severe, permanent amnesia results only if both limbic–diencephalic circuits are damaged. Lesions to either alone cause only mild and probably transient amnesia. Damage to the two circuits is supposed to disturb separate functions that, together, are sufficient for normal memory. This is, of course, the developed form of Mishkin's (1982) hypothesis. The evidence for these three positions will now be considered.

It is a question of great theoretical importance whether limbic–diencephalic lesions inevitably cause retrograde amnesia if they cause anterograde amnesia, and vice versa. If this is not the case, then one must argue that amnesia comprises two disorders, one that affects pre-traumatic memories and one that affects post-traumatic acquisition of memories. In contrast, if no dissociation is found, then a single deficit most probably underlies both pre- and post-traumatic memory deficits. A strong demonstration of the dissociation would require that small lesions in the same locations that normally cause global amnesia produce each kind of deficit in isolation, and that each isolated deficit take the same form that it does in the full syndrome. Less stringently, the dissociation might be supported if the two deficits turn out to be poorly correlated with each other. Strictly speaking, these questions should be asked separately for patients with limbic system and diencephalic lesions because dissociations may occur with lesions in one area but not in the other.

What is the evidence? There have been several reports of retrograde amnesia occurring without anterograde amnesia when the aetiologies included vascular accidents, tuberculous meningitis, and closed head injury. One patient has been described with an isolated and very dense retrograde amnesia, which affected even old, much rehearsed memories (see Goldberg, Hughes, Mattis, & Antin, 1982). For example, he could not remember that Paris is the capital of France. This finding is atypical of organic amnesia, as such long-available and overlearnt information is usually unaffected. There was no evidence, however, of relevant cortical damage that might have disturbed such well-established semantic memories. A similar case was reported by Andrews, Poser, and Kessler (1982); the patient had a retrograde amnesia extending back over 40 years, without an accompanying problem with new learning. Goldberg et al. have, in fact, argued that cases like these two may constitute a new syndrome, caused by an activational failure triggered by a lesion to cholinergic and noradrenergic neurons in the midbrain reticular formation. This view is in accord with the atypical severity of the retrograde amnesia in these cases, and if it is correct, then such cases do not constitute evidence that the global syndrome can be subdivided. They may form a new kind of elementary memory disorder. The possibility that they are caused by a functional memory deficit does, however, need to be excluded. Although an isolated loss of pre-traumatic memories could be caused by storage degradation or state-dependent forgetting, these explanations are problematic, whereas motivated forgetting is usually specific to pre-traumatic events and can be very severe.

Other cases of isolated retrograde amnesia have not been as severe as the two cases just discussed, and seem more typical of the organic syndrome. Furthermore, one such case had a diencephalic lesion, which suggests quite strongly that retrograde amnesia may be a separable deficit within the global amnesic syndrome. One ingenious recent study also suggests that motivated forgetting can be excluded as an explanation of some cases of relatively isolated retrograde amnesia (Kapur, Heath, Meudell, & Kennedy, 1986). The patient had emerged from a series of attacks of transient global amnesia with a retrograde amnesia that seemed to be relatively specific to verbal material and a very mild anterograde amnesia (his WMS score, which measures new learning ability, was an above-average 114). The severity of the patient's retrograde amnesia was comparable with that of a group of alcoholic amnesics, but older memories were more spared in the patient. Kapur and his colleagues compared the ability of the patient and a group of control subjects at learning a list of paired associates, which included items like *John Newcombe–singing* and *Telly Savalas–athletics*. The patient learnt this list faster than the controls. The most obvious explanation is that he had forgotten the occupations associated with the famous names in the task, whereas the controls had not and their memory interfered with their ability to learn the new counterfactual associations. If the patient had been a motivated forgetter rather than the genuine organic article, it seems very likely that he would have been 'fooled' and learnt no better than the controls. Given this probability, it is interesting that the authors argued that the patient's lesion was probably in the medial temporal limbic structures. If correct, he provides strong support for the idea that the amnesic syndrome is subdivisible.

Although there are some early reports of isolated anterograde amnesia (see Mayes, 1987) and Regard and Landis (1984) have described a case of transient global amnesia in which the retrograde amnesia seemed largely to disappear before there was recovery from a severe anterograde amnesia, there have been no recent reports of patients with long-standing isolated anterograde amnesias. It seems likely that the earlier cases might have been shown also to have had mild retrograde amnesias if more sensitive measures had been used. But there is much evidence that indicates that the severity of anterograde amnesia does not predict the severity of retrograde amnesia and vice versa. Butters, Miliotis, Albert, and Sax (1984) have illustrated this point with two patients. One, known as S. S., suffered an attack of herpes simplex encephalitis, which rendered him grossly amnesic, although he retained a post-traumatic IQ of 130 (as measured on the WAIS). The other, R. B., a computer designer, developed amnesia after the clipping of an anterior communicating artery aneurysm. His post-traumatic IQ was 141. These two patients were closely comparable in the severity of their anterograde amnesia. On objective tests of retrograde amnesia, however, S. S. was dramatically impaired and equally so, regardless of how old the memories were, whereas R. B. was not impaired at all on one of the tests and on the other was mildly impaired, but only for memories drawn from the previous decade. Unlike S. S.'s retrograde amnesia, therefore, R. B.'s was mild and steeply graded; that is, only memories acquired in the few years preceding trauma were disturbed.

In addition to these cases, a number of reports exist of patients who have suffered strokes, causing damage to medial thalamic structures, and who showed a retrograde amnesia that was mild relative to their anterograde amnesia. Does the great variation in the severity of retrograde amnesia, despite the relatively similar anterograde amnesias, prove that the two symptoms are caused by distinct functional deficits resulting from different limbic–diencephalic lesions? Unfortunately, the answer is negative because some, or all, of the differences could result from the effects of non-limbic–diencephalic lesions found in some amnesics but not in others. Thus although certain lesions of the diencephalon or limbic system may cause relatively mild and steeply graded retrograde amnesias, the occurrence of severe retrograde amnesias that extend over many decades could be the result of superimposed additional lesions. For example, patient S. S. had a post-encephalitic aetiology, and many, but not all, such patients have very severe retrograde amnesias. When this occurs, it is believed that damage is to not only the limbic system of the medial temporal lobe, but also parts of PTO association cortex. Alzheimer patients also have PTO association cortex atrophy as well as limbic system and basal forebrain damage, and have extremely dense retrograde amnesias that include overlearnt semantic material. In contrast, patient R. B. probably has a lesion that affects his basal forebrain, but leaves his PTO cortex intact.

The frequency of incidental brain damage is particularly high in alcoholic amnesics, so it is interesting that Shimamura and Squire (1986a) recently found no correlation between the severity of such patients' anterograde amnesia and the severity of their memory impairment for events of the 1940s and 1950s. There was, however, a significant correlation between the severity of their anterograde amnesia and their memory impairment for events of the 1960s and 1970s. As there is a correlation between the extent of memory impairment for very remote events and the degree of cortical atrophy, as measured by the CAT scan, and alcoholic amnesics often suffer from frontal cortex atrophy as well as diencephalic damage, it seems probable that the remote memory loss was caused by incidental frontal atrophy in these patients. This view is supported by evidence that frontal lesions do affect remote memory, as discussed in chapter 5. Shimamura and Squire's finding does, however, need to be confirmed because Parkin and Leng (1987) have reported a reliable correlation in a group of alcoholic amnesics between performance on a retrograde amnesia test and a measure of forgetting rate with new memories. In contrast, they found that post-encephalitic and stroke patients with putative limbic system lesions did not show a correlation between these two measures of retrograde and anterograde amnesia. The failure to find a correlation in these latter patients may arise because some of them suffer from extensive PTO association cortex damage.

Although this evidence indicates that cases of isolated anterograde amnesia caused by small limbic system or diencephalic lesions have not yet been clearly identified, there is further evidence compatible with the possibility that anterograde and retrograde amnesias may exist as separate deficits, together constituting organic amnesia. Penfield and Mathieson (1974) described some limbic system amnesics in whom the duration of retrograde amnesia might have been a function of the degree to which the lesion extended into the posterior hippocampus. They argued that posterior regions of the medial temporal cortex may be concerned specifically with the retrieval of remote memories. This idea receives indirect corroboration from the work of Fedio and Van Buren (1974). They found that electrical stimulation of the anterior temporal cortex of conscious patients caused a selective anterograde amnesia, whereas more posterior stimulation caused a selective retrograde amnesia. The support is indirect because it involves a slightly different, although adjacent, brain region, and Fedio and Van Buren were looking at memory over a period of a few seconds, whereas Penfield and Mathieson were concerned with a time scale of years. Nevertheless, the idea that disruption of the anterior medial temporal lobe causes anterograde amnesia, whereas disruption of the posterior medial temporal lobe causes retrograde amnesia warrants further study both with patients and, perhaps more fruitfully, with animal models. The extent to which anterograde and retrograde amnesia are dissociable remains an open question.

The second kind of distinction that has been proposed between the forms of global amnesia is that between the syndromes caused by limbic system lesions and by diencephalic lesions, respectively. Comparisons of the retrograde amnesias associated with each syndrome have proved hard to assess because of the difficulty in differentiating the effects of the 'core' lesions from those of additional cortical damage that frequently accompanies them. The main argument focuses on the claim that lesions of the limbic system structures of the medial temporal lobes cause not only poor learning, but also faster forgetting, whereas diencephalic lesions are associated with poor learning, but normal forgetting. In order to compare rate of forgetting between amnesics and normal subjects, memory at the initial test interval has been equated between amnesics and normal subjects by allowing amnesics longer to study the test items during the learning presentation. Huppert and Piercy (1978a), in the first study of this kind, showed 120 complex pictures to controls for 1 sec each, and to a group of alcoholic amnesics for a mean of 8 sec each. Under these conditions, the groups recognized the same number of pictures at a 10-min delay, and showed similar amounts of forgetting after delays of 1 day and 1 week. As alcoholic amnesics are believed to have diencephalic lesions, this finding, which has been replicated several times, seems to support the claim that such damage is associated with normal forgetting. In contrast, Huppert and Piercy (1979) reported that the patient H. M., who has had bilateral medial temporal lobe removal, forgot at a pathologically fast rate. Using a similar technique, Squire (1981) confirmed that alcoholic amnesics seem to forget at a normal rate under these conditions, as did the patient N. A. In contrast, other patients, who had received a multiple course of ECTs, forgot pathologically fast. As there is some evidence that ECT causes electrical disturbances in the temporal lobes, Squire argued that faster forgetting is caused by dysfunction of the limbic system structures of the medial temporal lobe. Butters et al. (1984) compared forgetting rates in alcoholic amnesics and the patients S. S. and R. B., who probably have limbic system lesions. Although S. S. and R. B. seemed to forget faster than the alcoholic amnesics, they were not matched at the shortest delay; so the conclusion is very tentative.

Most more recent studies have not favoured the view that limbic system lesions cause pathologically fast forgetting. The patient H. M. has been re-examined by Freed, Corkin, and Cohen (1984), who gave him 20 sec to examine each picture, in comparison with the 1 sec allowed to a group of controls. Recognition was tested using both a Yes–No format (in which new and old items are shown separately and subjects judge whether each item is familiar) and a forced-choice recognition format (in which one old and one or more new items are shown together and the subject has to judge which is familiar). H. M. did not forget faster than controls overall with either testing procedure, although with Yes–No recognition, he did show a decrement after a delay of 3 days and a rebound after 1 week.

In a further well-controlled study, Kopelman (1985) compared rate of forgetting in controls with that in a group of 16 alcoholic amnesics and a group of 16 Alzheimer's patients, using Huppert and Piercy's (1978a) original pictures. There were no group differences in forgetting rate, a finding that was particularly impressive because both patient groups had received closely similar learning exposures of around 8 sec. As Alzheimer patients do have limbic system atrophy, this finding is inconsistent with the claim that such lesions are associated with pathologically fast forgetting. Other studies by Corkin's group also suggest that Alzheimer patients do not forget faster than alcoholic amnesics. The notion of faster forgetting after some limbic system lesions, however, has not yet been clearly refuted, as three pieces of evidence support it. First, as will be discussed in chapter 7, several animal studies have found faster forgetting after limbic system lesions. Second, Levin, High, and Eisenberg (1987), using the Huppert and Piercy procedure, have found that closed head injury patients, who probably have damage in the medial temporal lobes, show pathologically fast forgetting when matched to controls at an initial delay of 10 min. Third, Leng and Parkin (see Parkin & Leng, 1987) have found evidence that post-encephalitic amnesics and other amnesics with damage mainly to the limbic system forget faster than alcoholic amnesics. They kept presenting subjects four target pictures until they were perfect at immediate recall and could recognize the target pictures in an array of 16 at a 1-min delay. The two patient groups may have had comparably severe amnesia because their WAIS–WMS discrepancy scores and Rivermead Behavioural Memory Test scores were equivalent, and they achieved criterion on Leng and Parkin's task in the same number of trials. The number of learning trials was repeated exactly with different pictures, and recognition was tested with delays up to 1 hour. It was found that the alcoholic amnesics forgot the pictures less rapidly than the other patients, who had limbic system damage, despite the evidence that both groups had equivalently severe amnesia.

Huppert and Piercy's procedure for studying rate of forgetting is appropriate for comparisons among different groups of amnesics who receive roughly matched learning exposures, but is open to objection when amnesics are compared with normal subjects, who need much shorter learning exposures. This means that doubt can be cast on the conclusion that some or all amnesics forget at a normal rate. The objection arises in the following way: As patients always spend longer learning than do control subjects and the first recognition test is usually given 10 min after the last item is presented, this inevitably means that the delay is longer for the patients. Typically, the average item-to-test delay may be around 11 min for controls and about twice as long for patients. This strongly suggests that if the average delay had been properly equated, the patients' recognition might have been significantly better than that of the controls. It therefore also implies that the procedure underestimates the rate of forgetting for the patients, particularly those who received long learning exposures.

This point clearly applies to Freed et al.'s (1984) reanalysis of H. M.'s forgetting rate because he received 20-sec exposures to each item, compared with the 1 sec allowed to his controls. If the first interval had been adjusted so that H. M. had been tested at the same average delay as his controls, then he might well have shown a faster forgetting rate. The result was that H. M.'s recognition was matched to that of controls who were tested after an average item-to-item delay that was 40 min *less* than the one that was used with him. A further observation of Kopelman's (1985) is supportive of this possibility. He found a correlation between patients' ages and their forgetting rate, indicating that forgetting rate may increase with age. As older patients did not receive longer exposures than younger ones, average item-to-test delay should have been similar in all patients. In other words, when item-to-item delay is matched, then older subjects seem to forget faster. A comparable procedure with amnesics and their controls might produce a similar results. This finding of faster forgetting in older subjects has been corroborated in healthy people, in a study where all subjects were given exposures of 1 sec or less (Huppert & Kopelman, personal communication). In order to check whether amnesic patients forget normally or pathologically fast, future studies will have to match all subjects on average item-to-test delay. This can be done by determining the exposure needed to give something like 75% correct recognition for the worst subject and then ensuring that all subjects have the same delay between item presentations, divided between item presentation proper and a period filled with irrelevant distractor activity. Under these conditions, it may be found that all kinds of amnesic forget faster than normal people, but that some kinds of amnesic forget faster than others. These possibilities remain to be examined fully, although in my laboratory, we have found preliminary evidence that when appropriate procedures are used, even alcoholic amnesics show pathologically fast forgetting. If generally faster forgetting is found in amnesics when the above procedure is used, it could be argued that this is due to a different kind of artefact, as their controls will have received spaced, rather than massed, learning, which may cause slower forgetting. There is, however, no evidence for any such effect. Indeed, there are few, if any, variables that affect rate of forgetting in normal people. It has been asserted that high arousal during learning slows forgetting and that proactive interference speeds it (although little discussed, one would also expect variations in the amount of retroactive interference to affect forgetting rate), but these claims need further support. If faster forgetting is found in a specific group, it could be caused by their low levels of arousal, raised sensitivity to proactive interference (or raised sensitivity to retroactive interference, as this kind of interference increases as the retention interval increases), or some ill-understood storage deficit.

Whether or not all amnesics forget faster than normal people, one problem should be mentioned. It concerns the proposal that limbic system lesions cause faster forgetting than diencephalic lesions. The damaged structures may be serially connected. If they are, then lesions to them may be expected to have similar effects. But each structure receives its own unique pattern of inputs, has some distinct outputs, and, at each stage, there is feedback to structures earlier in the circuit, so it is possible that different lesions would have different effects.

The third proposed kind of distinction between forms of global amnesia relates to Mishkin's (1982) serial-processing view of amnesia, which assumes that medial temporal lobe limbic system and diencephalic structures are linked to form circuits that perform the same functions. This view states that severe, permanent amnesia results only from damage to both circuits. One circuit runs from PTO association cortex to hippocampus, from there via the fornix to the mammillary bodies, to the anterior thalamus, and to the cingulate cortex. The other runs from PTO association cortex to the amygdala, from there via the bed nucleus of the stria terminalis to the dorsomedial and, perhaps, other midline thalamic nuclei, and thence to the orbitofrontal cortex. Each of these circuits probably has its own specific functions relevant to complex memory. As most of the support for Mishkin's view is based on animal models of amnesia, it will be discussed in chapter 7.

Several possible subdivisions of organic amnesia have been considered in this section. There is no question that material-specific kinds of amnesia exist. Some of them are caused by unilateral limbic system or diencephalic lesions, but others may be caused by lesions that disconnect overlying cortical processing and storage areas from underlying limbic–diencephalic memory structures. In both cases, the selectivity of the amnesia is a reflection of the specificity of the cortical region that cannot interact with the underlying structures so vital for memory. The other three subdivisions of organic amnesia are less well established, but their existence would have more profound implications for theories of the functional deficits that cause amnesia. First, atypically severe and isolated retrograde amnesia may be caused by lesions that are not directly involved with the global syndrome, but if they occur, cases of isolated and more typical retrograde amnesia may perhaps be caused by smaller lesions within the regions where lesions do cause global amnesia. If so, the functional deficits underlying these problems are unknown. Second, limbic system lesions may cause faster forgetting than diencephalic ones, although they do not necessarily cause a more 'severe' amnesia. If this is the case, and if all amnesics forget faster than normal people, it is critical to find out what factors influence forgetting rate, something of which we are currently rather ignorant. Third, lesions of hippocampal and amygdalar circuits may affect distinct processes that play a role in recognition and recall. At present, it must be said that all three of these proposed subdivisions of global amnesia need considerable buttressing before they can be regarded as proved.

What is the pattern of breakdown seen in organic amnesia?

Introduction

The pattern of memory deficits seen in organic amnesics constrains the theories that give tenable accounts of the functional deficits that underlie the disorder. But the kind of deficit that has been looked for has been guided by the nature of the currently popular theories. Before discussing the amnesic deficits, it is therefore appropriate to make some general observations about the types of theory that have been advanced to characterize the functional deficit that causes the memory problem. The theories have varied on two dimensions. First, they have postulated specific deficits in encoding, storage, or retrieval of the kinds of information that can be recalled or recognized for which amnesics have poor memory, although some theorists have proposed less specific deficits that include both encoding and retrieval. Second, some theories postulate an impairment that applies equally to all the aspects of complex information for which memory is bad in amnesics. Others postulate that the deficit directly affects only one aspect of the complex information for which amnesic memory is bad. They argue that because memory for this aspect is bad, patients cannot retrieve any other aspect of complex information. In other words, remembering the impaired aspect of information is very important if the other aspects are to be remembered. If, however, some other way of retrieving these other aspects of complex information could be found, then they would be normally remembered by amnesics.

Theories may be classified on both dimensions. For example, Butters and Cermak (1975) proposed that amnesics do not spontaneously encode semantic features to the same degree as normal subjects and that this poor encoding leads to their bad recognition of complex information. The hypothesis therefore proposes that there is a deficit specific to semantic information, caused by an encoding failure. Relatedly, Warrington and Weiskrantz (1982) proposed that amnesia is caused by a failure to store and/or retrieve the kinds of information that require effortful and elaborative encoding because a frontal 'planning' system has been subcortically disconnected from a semantic memory system in PTO association cortex. This hypothesis is similar to that of Butters and Cermak on one dimension because elaborative encoding is particularly directed at semantic information, but differs from it on the other dimension because it denies that amnesics have an encoding impairment with semantic information. This difference still persists even with a more recent version of Butters and Cermak's hypothesis, which proposes that amnesics also do not spontaneously use semantic cueing strategies at retrieval (see Butters, 1985).

A third kind of specific deficit hypothesis is the view that amnesics cannot remember background contextual events (for a review, see Mayes et al., 1985). Like the semantic-deficit hypotheses, which presume that retrieving semantic information is critical for retrieving other aspects of complex information, the context-memory-deficit hypothesis presumes that retrieving background spatio-temporal and other contextual features such as format context (collectively known as extrinsic context) is important for retrieving the remaining aspects of complex information. Different versions of the theory postulate that the failure is one of storage or of encoding and perhaps retrieval (see Cermak, 1982). A fourth and related hypothesis, of Kinsbourne and Wood (see Cermak, 1982), seems to propose that amnesics cannot encode or retrieve either background contextual information or the kind of semantic information that is processed with attentional effort. In their view, when an amnesic sees a doctor, he encodes this fact, but none of the other contextual and semantic details that mark the event as a unique episode. Thus he may remember meeting white-coated, stethoscoped personnel, but not specific individuals because he has not encoded sufficient background contextual and semantic details.

There is a fifth kind of specific-deficit hypothesis, akin in some ways to the context-memory-deficit views, which proposes that amnesics have a specific problem in remembering specific links among components that were not previously related in a memory (see Teyler & DiScenna, 1986; Wickelgren, 1979). This view can be illustrated by an analogy with the way in which normal people have been claimed to process information implicitly. It has been argued that although implicitly processed information is analysed to the level of meaning, only explicitly processed information is synthesized in the sense that previously unrelated elements are linked to one another (Marcel, 1983). Whether or not this is true of implicit processing, it can be argued that amnesics may be able to encode information in this synthesized way, but that their later poor memory suggests that they fail either to consolidate the newly integrated material properly or to retrieve it or both. This kind of deficit is specific because it is proposed that only the links among encoded attributes are disrupted, whereas the attributes themselves may be normally stored but not retrievable because the memory is not an integrated whole. Several theorists have proposed that features encoded in the neocortex may be associated with one another in the hippocampus (see, e.g., Teyler & DiScenna, 1986). If these theorists are correct, then the lesions found in organic amnesics may specifically disrupt the storage and/or retrieval of the integrating links among previously unrelated attributes. Indeed, it would be expected that such lesions would also disrupt the encoding of integrative links.

All five hypotheses postulate that the amnesic deficit(s) are specific to a subset of recognizable and recallable information, and that poor recognition and recall of other kinds of information are a secondary result of such specific deficits. In other words, specific-deficit hypotheses propose that memory for a specific subset of recallable and recognizable information is directly disrupted by brain damage, whereas memory for other kinds of recallable and recognizable information is not so disrupted, but may be poorly remembered because of the memory deficit for the first kind of information. Hypotheses of this kind should therefore make different predictions about the pattern of deficits to be found in amnesics than any hypothesis that postulates that a non-specific deficit causes amnesia. A non-specific hypothesis postulates an equivalent impairment in memory for all those kinds of information that can be recalled or recognized. For example, Butters and Cermak (1975) should predict that as amnesics do not spontaneously encode semantic information to the same extent as normal people, their memory for highly meaningful material will be little different from the memory of meaningless material, whereas normal people's memory will be much superior for more meaningful material. Warrington and Weiskrantz (1982) should make a similar prediction, but in addition, they should predict that amnesics will encode semantic information as well as normal people. For example, both hypotheses predict that normal people will show a bigger memory advantage than amnesics for a word list that is categorizable into semantic groups relative to an uncategorizable list. Distinctive predictions are harder to glean from the context-memory-deficit hypothesis, but one that will be further discussed in this and the next section is that amnesics should be disproportionately bad at remembering contextual features.

This means that they will be worse than their controls at remembering contextual features of target items, such as words or pictures, even when their recognition of the targets is matched to that of the controls by testing the controls either after a longer delay or after they have been given less opportunity to learn.

The oldest kind of non-specific-deficit hypothesis of amnesia is the view that patients fail to consolidate memories of complex information properly. A more recent version of this non-specific storage-deficit account is the hypothesis of Squire, Cohen, and Nadel (1984), which proposes that medial temporal lobe lesions disturb consolidation so that forgetting is faster for post-traumatically acquired information, and graded retrograde amnesia occurs because the damaged system is essential for a consolidation process that continues for several years after memories are initially acquired. The suggestion that amnesics have a deficit in a consolidation process that goes on for years will be discussed in the next section, but it raises an interesting point about retrograde amnesia. If anterograde and retrograde amnesia are seen as a single deficit caused by one kind of functional failure, then there is a problem for selective encoding and storage-deficit accounts of the syndrome. They fail to predict that retrograde amnesia will occur unless special assumptions are made. A retrieval deficit does make this prediction. It should be noted, however, that Squire et al. argue that there may be storage-deficit accounts that do so as well. Nevertheless, they do so only if one assumes that storage changes continue for years after the original acquisition of information.

One other non-specific-deficit hypothesis that has been influential in guiding research postulates a failure of retrieval and not of encoding or storage. This hypothesis proposes that amnesics are excessively sensitive to interference operating at the time of retrieval (Warrington & Weiskrantz, 1974). Its initial protagonists have now rejected this hypothesis, which predicts retrograde as well as anterograde amnesia and is non-specific because it claims that any kind of memory exposed to high levels of interference will be poor in amnesics. The hypothesis does not, however, clearly explain why patients should be so sensitive to interference operating at the time of retrieval. This issue will be further discussed after the relevant evidence has been considered.

The hypotheses make different predictions, and most research effort has been directed at discovering which ones fare best. Several kinds of evidence have been particularly relevant. First, it is important to know the types of task at which amnesics show normal memory. Second, it is vital to know whether amnesics are disproportionately bad at any memory tasks, as such deficits might be expected if any of the specific-deficit accounts were correct. Third, any evidence about treatments that disproportionately improve the memory of amnesics are important for similar reasons. Fourth, evidence about the form taken by retrograde amnesia and its possible relationship to anterograde amnesia is central to distinguishing whether there are deficits of encoding, storage, or retrieval.

Two precautions must be borne in mind in assessing relevant evidence. The first is to make sure that effects are not results of incidental damage to non-limbic–diencephalic structures (or the basal forebrain), particularly the frontal lobes. As already indicated, many amnesics have such incidental damage, so that superimposed on their basic deficit may be further cognitive-mnemonic losses. Although of interest in their own right, these disorders will probably be distinct from the deficits that underlie organic amnesia. The first precaution applies mainly to studies of alcoholic amnesics, or Korsakoff patients, because much research into amnesia has involved these patients, the majority of whom are believed to have incidental frontal lobe damage. This belief is based on evidence that Korsakoff patients often perform poorly on tests sensitive to frontal lobe lesions, whereas other amnesics do not, and on evidence from CAT scans and post-mortem analyses that up to 80% of Korsakoff patients show some frontal cortex atrophy (see Moscovitch, 1982; Parkin & Leng, 1987). There is independent evidence for frontal lobe atrophy in chronic alcoholics who do not have severe memory problems, as do Korsakoff patients (see Parkin & Leng, 1987). Korsakoff patients therefore are at particular risk of this form of brain damage. Its extent in them seems, however, to be highly variable, as patients have been described with intact frontal lobes (see, e.g., Mair et al., 1979). Future work should use MRI to measure frontal atrophy more sensitively in Korsakoff patients and other amnesics, such as those who have had aneurysms of the anterior communicating artery, so that the influence of this kind of incidental damage can be more accurately assessed.

The second precaution arises out of the fact that most evidence has been based on comparing poor amnesic memory with good control memory. This issue has been discussed at length by Mayes et al. (1985). Such comparisons are very prone to floor and ceiling effects, in which amnesics perform at chance or controls perform perfectly. If this happens, it is pointless to look at the effects of different conditions on amnesic and control performance. Much relevant evidence takes this form, as investigators wish to know whether amnesics are normal on task A, bad at task B, and very bad at task C. Even if obvious floor and ceiling effects are avoided, problems remain. Thus amnesics may seem to perform normally on a task, simply because the test involved is very insensitive. Also, if they do badly on two tasks, it is more or less meaningless to say that they are worse at one of them unless the tests are matched for sensitivity (see chapter 2).

Until recently, research on amnesia has not taken this second type of problem seriously, with the result that much work is uninterpretable. As it is extremely hard to develop tests of equivalent sensitivity, researchers have preferred to match amnesics and controls on one memory test, and then under precisely the same conditions to examine performance on another test (see chapter 2). For example, amnesic and control recognition of a list of words could be equated by testing the controls at a much longer interval or following reduced learning opportunity, and under the same conditions, subjects could be asked whether the words were presented visually or auditorily (a question relevant to the context-memory-deficit hypothesis). This kind of procedure makes it unlikely that any deficit could be a result of amnesics' poor memory rather than indicative of its cause. It is also conservative because it need make no assumptions about normal forgetting. For example, it could be that normal forgetting over time is caused by a selective

loss of background contextual information, somewhat similar to what has been proposed for amnesics. If so, amnesics would not show impaired contextual memory when their recognition of target material is matched to that of controls by testing the latter after a long delay. This would not refute the context-memory-deficit hypothesis, but merely provide it with no positive support. In contrast, if a context-memory deficit was found, the hypothesis would be strongly supported. The hypothesis could also be double-checked by lowering control recognition to amnesic levels by giving the controls reduced learning opportunity, which may not have detrimental effects on memory for context.

Preserved memory in anterograde amnesia

As well as normal intelligence and short-term memory, amnesics have been reported to show normal acquisition and retention of certain kinds of information despite their great impairment at learning new kinds of episodic and semantic information when recognition or recall tests are used. They have been reported to show normal classical conditioning of an eye-blink response (Weiskrantz & Warrington, 1979), to learn and retain normally a wide range of motor, perceptual, and cognitive skills (see Cohen, 1984), and to show normal priming; that is, they process items differently as a result of having seen them recently (see Cohen, 1984). Although these tasks differ from one another in many respects, theorists have argued that they must all lack one or more properties that depend on the integrity of the structures that are damaged in amnesics. For example, it has been suggested by Squire (1986) that amnesics show preserved procedural memory. It is proposed that this form of memory knowledge can be indicated only indirectly. Interestingly, this is Schacter's (1987b) definition of implicit memory, which he contrasts with explicit memory, a form of memory that can be indicated directly either verbally or by pointing. Schacter posits that only implicit memory is preserved in amnesics. This argument is plausible because there is reason to believe that those kinds of memory that are unaffected in anterograde amnesia are also unaffected in retrograde amnesia. For example, Squire and his co-workers (see Squire, 1986) showed that the skill of reading mirror-reversed words, acquired before patients received a course of ECT, is retained normally, although the patients show poor recall and recognition for other information acquired pre-traumatically. Previous work, to be discussed, had shown that this skill is acquired normally in amnesics of several aetiologies. Identification of the properties of memories that are spared in amnesics requires a fuller analysis of the preserved kinds of memory.

Unfortunately, not all studies of preserved memory in amnesics have included controls. For example, although one can say that amnesics learn a classically conditioned eye-blink response well, it is uncertain whether they are completely normal because controls were not included in the relevant study. The patients in this study did, however, show effective conditioning whilst showing little or no recognition of the apparatus that had been used to train them. This indication that one kind of memory but not another is present is usually referred to as the Claparède effect, after the French neurologist who first described it early in the twentieth century. After shaking hands a few times with Claparède when he had a pin in his hand, his patient became reluctant to be so greeted by him, even though she was apparently unaware that she had met him before.

Studies of amnesic skill learning have generally incorporated controls in recent years, and it is well established that many amnesics can learn pursuit rotors normally. This task requires subjects to keep a stylus in contact with a small rotating area for as long as possible. When patients do appear below normal on this task, it is probably because they have additional impairments that slow their rate of responding (see Cohen, 1984). Without these extra deficits, amnesics would probably learn a range of motor skills normally. Perceptual-skill acquisition and retention may also be normal in patients. For example, Cohen and Squire (1980) required ECT patients, alcoholic amnesics, and the patient N. A. to read low-frequency mirror-reversed words on 3 consecutive days. Both new and previously seen words were presented on the second and third days and on a fourth day, over 13 weeks later. The amnesics became quicker at reading new words at the same rate as controls and retained the ability normally over the 13 weeks. Their ability to read the repeated words did not improve quite as fast as in the controls. As the amnesics had very poor recognition for repeated words, it seems likely that the superior control performance depended not only on the use of the skill of reading mirror-reversed words, but also on the recognition of the pattern of repeated words. This explanation is likely because the words were shown in triads, so that normal subjects could infer what the second two words were after reading the first. This study shows that amnesics can learn and retain a general perceptual skill normally. When that skill is exercised on material that was used in practice, however, amnesics may not perform quite normally because control subjects can sometimes rely on direct recognition as well as the skill, whereas the patients can use only their normally acquired skill. Amnesics not only show poor recognition for the items that were used to train their skill, but also, like normal subjects, will probably not be able to describe what they are doing when they perform. This is a feature of what was referred to as procedural memory in chapter 1.

In the absence of any theory of skill as a procedural form of memory, it is very hard to know whether a 'skill' task is a pure test of skill or whether it also depends on recognition and recall, which are impaired in amnesics. Tasks cannot be specified in advance as pure measures of specific memory processes, but only after careful analysis of the processes on which they depend. One task that illustrates this point is currently the source of some controversy. It has been reported that a group of alcoholic amnesics and the patient H. M. learn and retain the Tower of Hanoi problem as well as their control subjects (Cohen, 1984). This problem uses five wooden blocks, graded in size, and three pegs. At the start of the problem, the five wooden blocks are placed on the left-hand peg, with the smallest on top and the largest at the bottom. Subjects are asked to move the blocks so that they are in the same position on the right-hand peg, moving one block at a time and never putting a larger block on a smaller one. The optimal solution takes 31 steps. Cohen found that amnesics improved on this task at a normal rate over 4 consecutive days of practice. In support of the view that the task was procedural for the amnesics at least, he found that the patients were unable to discriminate intermediate positions that were on the optimal-solution path from others that were not, despite being able to solve the task as well as controls. This suggests that they could demonstrate the skill only in action rather than by recognition of the knowledge that it incorporates – a feature of procedural memory. Cohen also found that patients had no trouble solving a modified form of the puzzle in which blocks had to be moved to the middle, not the right-hand, peg. This suggests that they had acquired normally a set of skills that generalize to similar problems.

Although another study of learning in amnesics that used the Tower of Hanoi problem has found normal performance (Saint-Cyr, Taylor, & Lang, 1987), it has not always been found, so more studies are needed to see how general preserved performance in this task actually is. In one respect, it is surprising to see normal amnesic performance because control subjects should show good recognition of the various moves necessary to solve the task, and their ability to recall such information should put them at an advantage with respect to the patients. In other words, unless the task is entirely dependent on a cognitive skill that subjects are unable easily to analyse or describe, the control subjects should have the advantage of being able to recall the most effective strategies. If such an advantage is not found, this can only be because normal subjects are not helped by using such strategies, which seems implausible. It is particularly surprising because frontal lesions impair performance on a task similar to the Tower of Hanoi, which suggests that its solution depends on the planned recall of strategically relevant information. Any task that depends on solving a problem with one set of material offers normal subjects a chance to use their superior recall ability to retrieve item-specific strategic information. This may explain why amnesics do not learn jigsaw puzzles quite as well as normal people. If performance on a task depends on both acquiring a skill and recalling strategically relevant information, more or less normal performance might be found in mildly impaired amnesics, but not in severely impaired ones. Thus although some amnesics are able to learn and retain the application of a simple mathematical rule for up to 17 weeks and to learn cognitive problems for which normal subjects show poor awareness on questionnaires of the solution strategies, the severely amnesic patient H. M. shows little sign of being able to learn either task (Gabrieli, Haimowitz, & Corkin, 1985).

Skills are acquired procedures for achieving certain goals with a given class of materials. They may be indicated by better achievement of those goals with the exact materials on which they were practised or with new materials of the same general type. The tentative proposal made here is that amnesics will show normal learning and retention on tasks where performance depends entirely on the use of procedures not accessible to consciousness; that is, performance does not depend on recalling strategies and information relevant to the solution. When performance also depends in part on strategy recall, amnesics should not be completely normal. This is most likely to occur when the skill is being applied to material on which it was practised, but may also occur if it is possible consciously to monitor the components of the skill in question and to recall when each component is appropriate. Amnesics should therefore be more likely to perform normally when exercising skills on new material or when the skills are ones that normal subjects have difficulty in articulating verbally. Although appealing, this proposal needs to be rigorously checked with tasks that have been carefully analysed to determine whether normal people's solution of them benefits from the recall of relevant strategic information. Such analyses face several problems. First, it has to be ascertained not only whether subjects can verbally describe relevant strategies, but also whether this helps them solve the task. Second, it has to be ensured that the questions that are aimed to tap subjects' verbal knowledge of the task do not require a higher level of knowledge than is evident from the level of skill that has been achieved.

Whereas skills can be applied to new material, priming is specific to items or material that was perceived recently. In the late 1960s, Warrington and Weiskrantz showed that under certain test conditions, amnesics can display normal or nearly normal memory for words or pictorial material (see Shimamura, 1986). Similar, but less rigorous demonstrations had been made in long-overlooked German studies at the beginning of the century. These demonstrations of preserved amnesic priming were made in two ways. In the first, subjects were shown progressively more complete fragments of words or pictures of common objects and had to say what they were as soon as possible. Subjects could identify pictures and words sooner if they had already seen the progressive series of fragments, and amnesics did very well, despite having appalling recognition for the words and pictures. The fact that amnesics were not completely normal could have been because they cannot use recognition to mediate identification of the object and word fragments, but normal people can. Amnesics have to rely solely on priming. The second way of testing involved presenting subjects with a list of words to learn and then giving them the first three letters of each word as a cue. Amnesics sometimes do as well as controls at this task, despite being unable to recognize most of the words that they correctly generate from the cues.

The fact that amnesics failed to recognize the words that they correctly generated from the cues was inconsistent with suggestions that the test was simply one of cued recall. This point was reinforced by the finding that when subjects are given explicit instructions to use cues to help them retrieve items that were shown them recently, controls do far better than amnesics (see Shimamura, 1986). In contrast, when subjects are given instructions to complete the opening three letters with the first word that comes to mind and are generally encouraged not to treat the test as one of memory, amnesics perform as well as controls. Under these word-completion instructions, amnesics are as likely as controls to produce a recently presented word as a response, despite being unable to recognize that word as one they have recently seen. This tendency returns to chance within 2 hours under some conditions, so it cannot plausibly be argued that the word-completion test is markedly less sensitive than a recognition test. Spared amnesic performance is, then, unlikely to be an artefact of test insensitivity, and word completion can be regarded as a form of priming because items are processed differently as a result of having been recently perceived.

As with skilled performance, it has been argued that amnesic priming will not be completely normal if control subjects can augment their performance by using monitoring strategies and recalling specific information. It seems that the use of such strategies by control subjects can often be eliminated by giving non-memory instructions. This point is further illustrated by a second area in which preserved amnesic priming has been claimed. Amnesics have been reported to learn and remember lists of related paired-associate words as well as controls (see Shimamura, 1986). These lists comprised either semantically related words, such as *soldier–army*, or rhyming word pairs, such as *burner–learner*. Although this result has been repeated several times, we have never been able to obtain normal amnesic performance in my laboratory with memory instructions. The explanation became apparent when Shimamura and Squire (see Shimamura, 1986) found that their alcoholic amnesics remembered as well as controls when they were given non-memory 'free association' instructions (subjects were asked to give the first word that came to mind associated with the first word of each pair), but that controls did much better when memory instructions were given. With the 'free association' instructions, subjects were also told to rate the degree of relatedness of the word pairs at presentation, so that they would not treat the task as one of memory. One must assume that in the earlier studies that found normal amnesic performance, subjects must have interpreted the task so that they did not use strategies dependent on recalling specific information. It is notable that when control subjects do perform better than amnesics, it is because the performance is significantly improved relative to its level with non-memory instructions. This improvement is not found with amnesics.

The idea that priming is tapped most cleanly when a task does not appear to involve memory is also supported by a third kind of priming test at which amnesics perform normally (Jacoby & Witherspoon, 1982). The test depends on the selection of homophone pairs containing a rare and a common member, such as *reed* (rare) and *read* (common). If asked to spell the spoken homophone, the most common response is to spell the common form. The test required subjects to answer questions about the rare form of the homophone and then later spell items in a list of spoken words that included the homophones about which they had answered the questions. Both amnesics and control subjects showed a significant shift towards spelling the rare form of the homophone, and, if anything, the amnesics showed a bigger shift than the controls. Despite the evidence for normal memory, tested by the indirect means, another test revealed that the amnesics had far worse recognition of the rare forms of the homophones about which they had answered questions than did the controls.

Word completion, free association, and changes in spelling performance may be kinds of priming, but they are superficially rather different from priming as traditionally conceived. Traditionally, priming has been associated with tasks in which subjects have to name a string of letters or decide whether a string of letters is a word or a non-word (a lexical decision task). The speed with which subjects can make lexical decisions is faster if they have recently perceived an item (the repetition priming effect). Cermak and his colleagues have shown that alcoholic amnesics show a normal repetition priming effect for recently seen words, but, unlike controls, they do not show a repetition priming effect for recently presented non-word strings (see Shimamura, 1986). It has been argued that normal amnesic priming was found for only the words because priming in amnesics depends on the temporary activation of information that is already present in memory. Non-words have no such representation, and so amnesics do not show priming to them. This view and possible exceptions to it will be considered in more detail shortly. No one has yet tested to see whether amnesics show normal semantic priming, where seeing a semantically related item, such as *nurse,* speeds the lexical decision about a later item, such as *doctor*. It has been shown, however, that when alcoholic amnesics were told to expect a word corresponding to a body part after three *x*s were presented, they made faster lexical decisions (see Shimamura, 1986).

One feature shared by the forms of spared amnesic priming so far discussed is that of being relatively short-lived. The effects of priming on both word completion and free association have been reported to last about 2 hours (see Shimamura, 1986). Most word-completion priming has used opening three-letter stems that begin at least 10 words, such as *mot——*as a cue for *motel,* but cues can be unique to the correct word. These cues can be the opening letters, such as *oni——*as a cue for *onion,* or assorted letters, such as *a——a——in* as a cue for *assassin*. In normal people, priming facilitates these kinds of word completion for at least 1 week, but in amnesics, there is evidence that priming does not match that of controls even at immediate testing and disappears after 2 hours (see Shimamura, 1986). The reason for this deficit is still uncertain, but control subjects may, for some reason, be more likely to use recall strategies with these tasks, even though non-memory instructions are given. It should not be assumed that all forms of amnesic priming fade within 2 hours. For example, Meudell and Mayes (1981) found that alcoholic amnesics displayed good (but not quite normal) learning and normal retention of the ability to find shapes hidden in cartoon pictures over a delay of about 1 month, despite having very poor recognition for the pictures. Subjects did not get better at finding the shapes in new pictures, so skill acquisition was not involved, and this finding makes it plausible to propose that performance depended on a kind of pictorial priming. The fact that amnesic learning of the task was not quite normal is probably a reflection of the controls' ability to recall where shapes were hidden in the pictures, which the amnesics could not do.

One feature of the last task is that if it involves priming, it cannot be regarded as dependent on the temporary activation of an already existing semantic representation in memory because the subjects had never seen the pictures before.

All the other kinds of priming mentioned above could be interpreted as involving the activation of pre-existing memories. If priming can occur to items that prior to their presentation had no semantic memory representation, then this is probably a different kind of priming because it is very hard to explain in terms of the activation of pre-existing memories. It is important to determine whether amnesics show preservation of this kind of priming as well as that involving the activation of established memories. There is, in fact, evidence that priming does not occur in amnesics, at least sometimes, if novel material is presented. For example, amnesics do not show free association priming when unrelated word pairs, such as *dog–wall,* are used and they do not show word-completion priming when non-words, such as *numdy,* are cued by their first three letters.

There are, however, a number of reports that spared amnesic priming sometimes occurs in situations where there can be no existing semantic representation to activate. First, Johnson, Kim, and Risse (1985) have shown that amnesics and controls displayed an equivalent enhancement in preference for recently heard Korean melodies (previously totally unfamiliar) in spite of the amnesics' impaired recognition of the tunes. In the amnesics, therefore, this priming-like evidence of memory for the novel material occurred in the absence of recognition. Second, Moscovitch and colleagues (see Schacter, 1987b) have shown that amnesics speed up their reading of lists of unrelated and degraded word pairs as much as their controls and that this effect is not due simply to their reading the individual words faster. Third, Nissen and Bullemer (1987) presented subjects with a serial reaction-time task comprising a repeated 10-trial stimulus sequence. Alcoholic amnesics became faster at reacting to such repeated sequences, even though they failed to recognize that they had seen them before. These patients were therefore showing implicit memory for the temporal order in which events were presented, although it was not possible to show whether such memory was completely normal. Fourth, McAndrews, Glisky, and Schacter (see Schacter, 1987b) showed subjects difficult-to-comprehend sentences, such as 'The haystack was important because the cloth ripped', and required them to generate cues that made the sentences intelligible (for example, the word *parachute* for the sentence just given). Amnesics were able to generate the correct cues on the basis of a single prior exposure to sentence-cue pairs, but failed to recognize either sentences or cues. Fifth, Graf and Schacter (1985) presented amnesics and controls with unrelated word pairs, such as *house–sheep,* using an incidental learning task, and then asked for word completion either in the context of the same stimulus word (for example, *house–she——*) or in the context of a different stimulus word (for example, *town–she——*). Both groups performed equally well and did better when tested in the same context as that in which the word pairs had initially been presented.

Another recent line of evidence is relevant to the problem of the kinds of novel material that amnesics may prime to normally. The evidence involves measuring subjects' skin resistance whilst they are performing a recognition test with stimuli that they have just been shown. For example, Tranel and Damasio (1985) showed a series of novel face pictures to an amnesic, and later gave her a recognition test in which the recently shown pictures were intermixed with completely novel ones. Although the patient showed markedly impaired recognition of the faces she had just seen, her skin-resistance responses appeared to discriminate between recently shown and new faces about as well as did the controls'. As the faces had not been seen before the experiment, the patient displayed indirect evidence of memory despite her very poor recognition. Similar results have been reported with stimuli that are already in semantic memory. For example, although amnesics do not recognize recently shown words, there is some evidence that their skin-resistance responses can discriminate such words from ones that have not been shown recently (see Moscovitch, 1985). These findings suggest that amnesics maintain a kind of unconscious memory for recently shown material, whether or not there was a pre-existing representation of that material in long-term memory. The findings need to be replicated, and it will be particularly important to see whether these 'autonomic' indices of memory are normal in amnesics rather than merely more sensitive than recognition measures. This will be a difficult goal to achieve because there is evidence that skin-resistance responses are themselves not normal in amnesics.

Glisky, Schacter, and Tulving (1986) have recently shown that some amnesics are capable of learning the domain-specific knowledge needed for operating and interacting with a microcomputer. The patients were taught by an adaptation of the method of vanishing cues, in which a target is cued by a decreasing number of letters as the subject improves, until no cues at all are used. For example, patients were required to complete the following incomplete sentence 'A sequence of characters enclosed in quotation marks is called a ———'. In order to help them, one or more letters of the word string could be provided to guide them. Under these conditions, the patients learned much more slowly than their controls, and the knowledge they acquired seemed to be qualitatively different. The major difference was that the patients could access their memories only under a narrow range of conditions. The most amnesic patients were particularly dependent on the wording of the instructions being precisely the same as it had been during learning with the vanishing cues. If the wording was changed, even though the meaning was not, they frequently were unable to produce the proper response. They were also unable to answer general questions about what they had learnt and showed no ability to generalize their knowledge. Although the patients may have learnt to recall and recognize the computer definitions and operations at a much slower rate than their controls, this seems relatively unlikely, given the qualitatively distinct nature of their memories. What they may have slowly developed is a kind of priming to novel material, which would be of considerable interest because some of the patients who showed such learning were severely amnesic. The patients' retrieval of correct responses may therefore have depended on priming, even if they had some ability to recognize the responses.

If these recent studies are correct in their implication, then amnesics may show two kinds of preserved priming. The first kind involves reactivation of already established memories, whereas the second seems to involve implicit memory for new semantic and, possibly, episodic information. It is currently uncertain whether these are two radically different kinds of priming or whether they lie at different ends of a continuum of priming processes, each of which may have unique features. There are, however, several pieces of evidence relevant to this issue. First, Graf and Schacter (1985) argued that the priming of new associations occurred in their task only if subjects processed the unrelated word pairs using a semantic strategy, whereas the priming of already established associations (for example, *sour–grapes*) occurred equally well, regardless of whether subjects processed the pairs semantically or merely compared the number of vowels each word contains. If correct, this would suggest that the priming of new associations depends on the effortful, semantic processing of the novel material, whereas the priming of already established memories does not. In my laboratory, however, we have twice found that free association priming of related word pairs (for example, *soldier–rifle*) is markedly better in normal people if subjects process the pairs semantically rather than compare how many vowels they contain. In the second study, we excluded any subjects who did not strictly obey the free association instructions to ensure that performance was unaffected by the mediation of explicit memory (i.e., recall of the pairs). In contrast, we have found little evidence that word-completion priming is greater when words are processed semantically rather than in terms of their vowel structure. It would seem likely, therefore, that semantic processing is important for some kinds of priming of already established memories as well as for the priming of new information.

Graf and Schacter (1985) have also highlighted a second possible distinction between priming of new associations and that of established memories. They argue that priming of new associations occurs only if the test cue includes parts of both words in the pairs, whereas priming of already established associations does not require this. For example, priming of *house–sheep* occurs only if subjects are given the cue *house–she*——with word-completion instructions, whereas priming of *sour–grapes* can be shown when subjects are given merely the cue *sour* – with free association instructions. This distinction seems compatible with most of what is currently known about the various kinds of new information priming preserved in amnesics. McAndrews and his colleagues (see Schacter, 1987b) did find, however, that amnesics were able to produce disambiguating cue words when shown difficult-to-comprehend sentences that had been inspected on only a single occasion. This form of new association priming therefore seems to occur without the need for test cues comprising parts of both related items (sentence and cue in McAndrews's task).

A third possible difference between the two putatively distinct kinds of priming concerns the extent of their preservation in amnesics. It has become clear recently that not all amnesics show the kind of priming to new associations reported by Graf and Schacter (1985). These researchers have re-examined the data from the 12 amnesics that they originally tested, divided them into moderately and severely amnesic subgroups, and found that only the mildly amnesic subgroup showed any priming of new associations (see Shimamura, 1986). This, of course, raises the critical question of whether all priming with new material occurs normally only in mildly impaired amnesics. Currently, the evidence would seem to be against this possibility because Moscovitch and his colleagues (see Schacter, 1987b), Nissen and Bullemer (1987), and McAndrews et al. (see Schacter, 1987b) found that even severely amnesic patients showed 'speeded reading' priming, serial reaction-time priming, and cue-generation priming, respectively. Furthermore, Cermak, Blackford, O'Connor, and Bleich (in press) have shown that, unlike Korsakoff patients, the severely amnesic post-encephalitic patient S. S., displays not only repetition priming to non-words, but also the kind of unrelated word-pair priming reported by Graf and Schacter (1985). Although much more research is necessary, it seems likely that some forms of priming that depend on the formation of new representations in memory occur, even in severely amnesic patients. As priming of previously established memories is also often preserved in severe amnesics, the extent of preservation in amnesics may not be a function of amnesic severity. It may, instead, depend on the absence of incidental damage to the frontal lobes because such damage occurs in Korsakoff patients, who sometimes fail to show priming of previously novel information.

A fourth point that has been the focus of some recent discussion concerns the longevity of priming effects. There is evidence that several forms of word-completion and free association priming for already established memories typically last for only a few hours (see Shimamura, 1986), whereas the kind of new association priming demonstrated by McAndrews et al. was robust in severe amnesics even after a 1-week delay. It remains to be determined whether durability is a reliable difference between the two putatively different distinct forms of priming.

The fifth point concerns the relationship between priming and contextual information. It has been suggested that new association priming may occur with novel semantic *and* episodic information. If it occurs with the latter, then such priming may depend on the storage of the background spatiotemporal and format contexts that specify an episode. This has not yet been investigated systematically. It has been shown, however, that priming for already established memories is affected by changes of the sensory modality in which information is presented (a kind of format context). Thus amnesics show normal word-completion priming whether words are presented auditorily or visually, but, like normal subjects, when words are presented auditorily and tested visually, they show less priming than when words are also presented visually (see Shimamura, 1986). In my laboratory, we have tested free association priming under conditions in which both format context and background context were changed between presentation and test. We found that both kinds of change had an equivalent detrimental effect on this kind of priming, so priming for well-established memories may be affected by stored information about both format and background context. Nissen and Bullemer's (1987) study also suggests that it is possible to show priming directly for a newly acquired memory about the temporal order of events. This further supports the idea that contextual information can be stored normally in amnesics in a form that is suitable to mediate priming.

Although many aspects of preserved amnesic priming remain obscure, it is clear that even severely amnesic patients can show normal, or near normal, implicit memory for both novel and well-established information for which they show no recognition. It has not yet been demonstrated that these two forms of priming depend on radically distinct mechanisms. The fact that both are preserved in patients must be relevant to the problem of what deficits cause the poor recognition shown by amnesics for recently presented information, whether novel or previously familiar. One argument that is difficult to maintain in the light of good amnesic priming and poor recognition is that the processes of priming are sufficient to support recognition under any circumstances. There is, in fact, evidence that priming is more or less unaffected whether recognition is good or bad. In normal subjects, it seems to be difficult to predict whether an item will be recognized because there is priming to it, and whether or not an item is recognized has little bearing on whether there will be priming to it later. It has been reported by Squire and his colleagues that ECT patients performed normally on a word-completion task 45 min after their last treatment, but that their recognition was around chance at this time and improved gradually over 9 hours following treatment (see Shimamura, 1986). The occurrence of normal priming when recognition is at chance indicates that some or all of the processes underlying recognition are independent of those underlying priming. If priming and recognition depend on distinct memory processes, then problems are raised for the view, discussed in chapter 1, that recognition can sometimes be mediated by a familiarity mechanism. As familiarity is believed to be attributed to items that are processed with above-average speed, and some forms of priming preserved in amnesics are manifested in this way, it becomes difficult to argue that increased processing speed is *sufficient* for good recognition. Recognition may, however, sometimes depend on an increased speed of processing familiar items (dependent on priming), together with the judgement that processing speed has been increased. Amnesics would have a selective inability to make this kind of judgement. If the processes underlying priming are sometimes necessary for recognition, however, one would expect to see *some degree* of dependence between the two. This dependence has been denied by some workers. If they are correct and the processes underlying priming never contribute to recognition, then it should be possible to find patients in whom recognition is normal and priming is impaired. As no such patients have been convincingly tested yet, it remains possible to argue that some of the processes underlying priming do contribute to recognition. If so, amnesia must disrupt some other component of recognition, possibly the hypothetical judgmental ability just mentioned.

Priming is the most theoretically interesting of the three kinds of implicit memory for which amnesics show sparing. This is because, unlike conditioning and skill learning, it is a form of item-specific memory at which patients perform normally, despite their appalling recognition and recall of the same items. The theorist's attention is therefore focused on the differences between the two forms of memory because it is there that the amnesic impairment must lie. These differences will be discussed in the final section of this chapter, when theories of amnesia are considered.

Disproportionately poor or qualitatively different memory?

Much of the evidence discussed in the first part of this section is relevant to the context-memory-deficit hypothesis, as it purports to show either that background contextual information is remembered worse by amnesics than target information that was the focus of attention during learning or that contextual information is remembered in a qualitatively different way in patients and control subjects. Most of the studies discussed equate amnesic and control recognition or recall of targets by testing controls after a longer delay or with reduced opportunity for learning.

First, Squire (1982) has reported that alcoholic amnesics were disproportionately bad at discriminating in which of two lists simple sentences were presented. The amnesics were tested with 3 min between lists, and then 10 sec after the second list had been shown, their recognition of the sentences was tested. If sentences were correctly recognized, then patients were asked from which of the two lists they had been drawn. Controls were tested at a longer delay after the second list, so that their recognition was matched to that of the amnesics. Despite being matched on sentence recognition, controls could discriminate from which lists the sentences came far better than the amnesics, who performed around chance. In an earlier study, Squire and his colleagues (see Squire, 1982) found that the patient N. A. and some ECT patients did not have disproportionate deficits for list discrimination under similar conditions. It has also been found that H. M. does not have specific problems with either recency or frequency judgements with different tasks from those used by Squire (Sagar, personal communication). As there is no evidence that ECT patients or the patients N. A. and H. M. have extensive frontal lobe damage, whereas alcoholic amnesics often do, these findings suggest that amnesics may show disproportionately bad temporal discrimination only if they have incidental brain damage that affects the frontal lobes. This suggestion is consistent with Squire's observation that his alcoholic amnesics did poorly on tests sensitive to lesions of the frontal lobes, and that their performance on these tests correlated with a combined measure of their performance on the list discrimination and degree of release from proactive interference (using the test procedure discussed in chapter 5). However, the contribution of the list-discrimination scores to this correlation is unclear because the alcoholic amnesics performed near chance on this test. Even so, the suggestion is also consistent with Kohl's (1984) finding that patients with frontal lobe lesions are impaired at a list-discrimination task, even though their recognition of targets is normal. Furthermore, in my laboratory, we have found a significant correlation between performance on tests sensitive to frontal lobe lesions and list discrimination when patients' and controls' recognition was matched by giving the latter briefer learning exposures to words (Pickering, 1987).

An alternative to the view that the disproportionate amnesic memory deficit for temporal order is caused by incidental frontal lobe damage has been advanced by Parkin and Leng (1987). These workers compared a mixed group of amnesics with limbic system lesions with a group of alcoholic amnesics, who have diencephalic lesions, on a recognition task that required patients to make increasingly difficult judgements about which 4 of 16 pictures they had seen most recently. In other words, task performance implicitly depended on the patients' ability to judge item recency. The alcoholic amnesics performed much worse at this task than the patients with limbic system lesions. Parkin and Leng argued that diencephalic lesions, but not limbic system lesions, impair directly the ability to encode temporal information and, indeed, contextual information in general. To support their view, they would have to show, however, that patients with focal diencephalic lesions perform as badly on their task as did their alcoholic amnesic subjects, who may well have had incidental frontal lobe damage. It should also be noted that they failed to show that their patients with limbic system lesions did not have excessive temporal memory deficits, although this would be expected by both their view and the incidental frontal lobe damage hypothesis.

Congruent with Squire's (1982) findings, Huppert and Piercy (1978b) reported that another group of alcoholic amnesics made judgements about item recency and frequency in a qualitatively different way from control subjects. They showed subjects two long lists of pictures 1 day apart. Half the pictures in each list were shown once, and the other half were shown three times. Ten minutes after seeing the second list, subjects were required to indicate, with half the pictures, the list from which they came; then, with the other half, they had to judge whether the pictures had been shown once or three times. The amnesics confused item frequency and recency in making these judgements. For example, they were more likely to judge erroneously that an item was recent if it had been presented frequently, and more likely to judge erroneously that an item had been shown frequently if it had been shown recently. In contrast, controls made the opposite pattern of errors, being more likely to judge incorrectly that an item was recent if it had been shown only once, and more likely to judge incorrectly that it had been shown frequently if it had not been shown recently. These results might have reflected the fact that amnesics remembered the pictures far worse than the controls. The study has, however, been repeated with additional control groups, in which recognition was brought down to amnesic levels by using either short exposures or long retention intervals (Meudell, Mayes, Ostergaard, & Pickering, 1985). This did not affect the controls' pattern of performance with recency and frequency judgements, so the amnesic performance pattern cannot be a simple result of their poor memory.

Not only do alcoholic amnesics seem to be disproportionately bad at recency judgements, but Kohl (1984) has some evidence that they are similarly impaired with frequency judgements. Although her patients' recognition of rare words improved when the words were shown more often, they were very poor at judging how often the words had been shown. Control subjects' frequency judgements were far better, even when their recognition of words was roughly equated to that of the amnesics by showing them a list of common words for which recognition is harder. It is not therefore surprising that Huppert and Piercy's (1978b) results suggest that alcoholic amnesics base their judgements of frequency and recency on how familiar a memory feels rather than on specific information about temporal cues, which are presumably unavailable to them. Although it has been reported that at least 80% of alcoholic amnesics show signs of frontal lobe atrophy (see Moscovitch, 1982), not all workers believe that their qualitatively distinct and very poor performance with recency and frequency judgements is a result of such incidental damage. Thus Hirst and Volpe (1982) reported that a mixed group of amnesics were insignificantly worse than controls at recognizing words previously shown in two lists, but were much worse at identifying the list from which the words came. Similarly, they reported that patients recognized relatively recent news items about as well as controls, but were far worse at dating the news items. Furthermore, they claimed that their patients did not seem to be impaired on tests sensitive to frontal lobe lesions. It has, however, been argued that it is very unusual for patients not to show a recognition deficit for target words, although Volpe, Holtzman, and Hirst (1986) have reported that patients with lesions of the CA1 field of the hippocampus show very poor recall, but only very mild recognition deficits, and some of Hirst and Volpe's patients had lesions of this kind. A small deficit in recognition might well have been concealed by a ceiling effect. The amnesics' performance also fell below chance on some of the temporal judgement conditions, on which they did worse than controls. The evidence that amnesics without frontal lobe pathology are disproportionately bad at temporal discriminations is therefore not yet compelling. It needs to be examined in amnesics with selective limbic system and diencephalic lesions, who have clear recognition deficits.

The issue of whether amnesics have a disproportionate problem with recency and frequency judgements that is not caused by incidental frontal lobe damage should be kept open. It may be that frontal lobe lesions impair such judgements for reasons different from those that underlie the amnesic deficit, as has been argued by Kohl (1984). She found that frontal patients making list-discrimination judgements tended to judge items as coming from the first list and that their ability to recognize list words was not affected by instructions to remember the list from which the words came. In contrast, alcoholic amnesics showed no judgement bias towards the first list, and did show impaired recognition when told to remember the list from which the words came. Finally, the evidence that some amnesics do not show disproportionate deficits needs to be carefully examined. For example, in Squire's (1982) study, the control subjects may have had a harder discrimination to make than the patients. If N. A. and the ECT patients were less impaired than the alcoholic amnesics, then their deficit may have been hidden. The argument for this view is that discrimination difficulty is a negative function of the ratio of the interval between lists to the interval between the second list and test. In Squire's study, this ratio was far greater for the patients than for the controls. Future studies should keep this ratio constant whilst reducing control recognition to amnesic levels. They should also examine whether there is a correlation between patients' recognition scores and their performance with temporal discrimination tasks, using easier discrimination tasks so that patients can score better than chance on them.

The second type of contextual memory for which some amnesics have been reported to have a disproportionate problem is memory for the source of target information (Schacter, Harbluk, and McLachlan, 1984). It has been found that relative to a group of controls, a mixed group of amnesics displayed more amnesia for the source of target information than loss of recall of the targets. All subjects were given obscure and trivial facts about well-known people, such as 'Jane Fonda hates milk'. The facts which the subjects were to learn were presented by either of two experimenters. The subjects were later asked to recall the facts one at a time and, if successful, had to indicate whether they had been told them in the experimental situation and, if so, by which of the experimenters. The test session included other easier facts as foils, so that it was sometimes appropriate to say that a fact had been learnt extra-experimentally. It was found that the amnesics, but not the controls, made a large number of extra-experimental errors; that is, they claimed that they had heard about facts elsewhere when they could have heard them only in the experiment. This difference held even though control recall was reduced to amnesic levels by testing them at a much longer delay (1 week as opposed to the few seconds or minutes used with the amnesics). Schacter and his colleagues found that there was a correlation between the degree of patients' source amnesia and how badly they performed on tests that are sensitive to frontal lobe lesions. Although this suggests that the deficit is secondary to the patients' incidental frontal lobe damage, it was also found that four patients with probable frontal lobe damage, but no amnesia, did not show source amnesia. This could mean that source amnesia results only when poor memory, caused by limbic–diencephalic lesions, is accompanied by frontal lobe damage. If frontal lobe damage does contribute to the deficit, it could be either because such damage limits the use of attentional resources or because it affects temporal discrimination. It is also possible that source memory is largely independent of target memory. Certainly, Squire (1982) reported that temporal discrimination did not predict sentence recognition, and recently Shimamura and Squire (1987) found that, although some alcoholic amnesics are disproportionately poor at source memory, the extent of source amnesia does indeed seem to be independent of target memory.

The third and fourth claims that amnesics have disproportionate problems with contextual memory are related to each other and also indirect. They involve the use of an A–B, A–C interference paradigm. The learning lists are constructed either from words cued by their first three letters at test, such as *stamp* cued by *sta——* for A–B and *station* similarly cued for A–C, or from related paired associates, such as *soldier–rifle* for A–B and *soldier–army* for A–C. In experiments that used these specific interference paradigms, although subjects do not appear to have been given the non-memory instructions appropriate for tapping priming in a selective fashion, amnesics were reported to learn the first list as well as controls. They were, however, far worse at learning the second list and produced many first-list responses as intrusion errors (for a review, see Mayes & Meudell, 1983). With paired associates, the deficit was apparent from the first trial with the A–C list, but with the cued word lists, it became apparent only after the first trial. In both cases, the amnesics made an excessive number of A–B intrusion errors in trying to learn the second list. These results have been interpreted to mean that amnesics fail to discriminate the contextual markers of the two lists and hence find it almost impossible to decide whether a B or a C response is appropriate, although the absence of a deficit on the first A–C trial is hard to explain on this view. The interpretation indicates that amnesics have a *disproportionate* deficit in remembering the background contextual markers that distinguish the lists. If correct, it would mean that amnesics are more susceptible to interference at retrieval and show poor memory because they cannot retrieve contextual information. In other words, amnesic sensitivity to interference would be explained in terms of a context-memory deficit.

There are, however, serious problems with the interpretation of the evidence said to support this claim, although in a modified form, it may eventually prove to be correct. First, it has been suggested by Kinsbourne and Winocur (see Mayes & Meudell, 1983) that some of the interference effect may be caused by a generalized problem with encoding the A–C list rather than with retrieving contextual markers. In their experiment, the A–B pairs were used as the stimuli for the A–C list. For example, if *soldier–battle* was an A–B pair, then its matching A–C pair would be *soldier + battle–army*. Under these conditions, alcoholic amnesics, not surprisingly, made few intrusion errors, but were nevertheless slow to learn list A–C. Some of this difficulty might, however, relate to incidental frontal lobe atrophy common in such patients because such atrophy is likely to impair the ability to switch to new and more appropriate hypotheses about how to process information.

A second problem with the interpretation is that the studies used to support it utilized memory instructions. It is therefore possible that amnesic performance was based mainly on priming, whereas controls could rely to a much greater extent on their ability to recall specific item information. A recent study clearly supports this interpretation (Mayes, Pickering, & Fairbairn, 1987). Alcoholic amnesics and controls were given A–B, A–C lists of related word pairs to learn. In the first condition, amnesics were given five trials on the A–B list before being tested on it with memory instructions after a 2-min delay. Controls were tested in the same way, except that they received only one trial. This was necessary in order to match amnesic and control recall of the A–B list. The A–C list was learnt and tested in precisely the same way immediately after the A–B list had been tested. Whereas the controls remembered the second list as well as the first one, the amnesics were markedly impaired and made many intrusions from the first list. This replicated the usual amnesic interference effect. In the second condition, the procedure was repeated with a different pair of lists, except that memory instructions were avoided. Both groups of subjects were presented the lists five times and were told to rate the relatedness of the pairs rather than learn them. Then, after the 2-min delay, they were shown the first word in each pair and asked to produce the first associate that came to mind. Under these free association conditions, the two groups performed very similarly. Their memory for both lists was the same, and both groups showed an interference effect on the A–C list, comparable with that displayed by the amnesics in the first condition.

These results suggest that interference occurs in this paradigm when performance is based on priming without the help of the ability to recall specific information from the two lists. Although performance was matched on the A–B list in the first condition, it was based on different memory processes in the two groups. In amnesics, it depended almost entirely on priming, whereas in controls, it depended largely on recall of the response terms. If item recall is not used by subjects when free association instructions are given, it is much less likely that the correct response will be selected for the A–C list. Further support for the view that with memory instructions different mechanisms are at play in the two groups was found in a third condition, in which the only change from the first condition was that a 2-hour, rather than a 2-min, delay was used before testing the A–B list. Although matched at 2 min, the amnesics did worse than controls at the longer delay, performing very close to chance. As it is known that free association priming of this kind decays in about 2 hours, control performance must have depended largely on recall of the response terms.

In other words, these results mean that the amnesic interference effect in this paradigm is a result of the patients' poor recall ability rather than a direct indication of why their recall is so bad. It remains possible that recall and recognition are bad because of a selective failure of contextual memory, but that interference occurs in this paradigm because of the overall failure of recall. If so, the patients' context-memory deficit would mean that they recognized neither the A–B nor the A–C responses, and showed intrusion errors and interference because priming works in that way when operating in isolation. If amnesics do have a selective context-memory deficit, one would still predict that they should suffer more from interference than controls even when all subjects are matched on A–B recognition by appropriate manipulations, such as giving amnesics more learning trials, on a task where performance cannot depend on priming. At present, no convincing demonstration exists showing that when amnesics without frontal lobe damage are matched to their controls on A–B recognition with a memory task that does not depend on priming, they suffer from more interference when they learn an A–C list. In my laboratory, Ratcliffe and I have shown, however, that Korsakoff patients still show more proactive interference than controls even when conditions are arranged so that the groups are matched to each other on A–B recognition with a task (memory for stories) that does not depend on priming. Nevertheless, we could not conclusively exclude the possibility that frontal lobe atrophy caused the patients' increased sensitivity to interference.

The fourth claim that there is disproportionately poor amnesic memory for context, which also involves the interference paradigm, was reported by Winocur and Kinsbourne (1978). They found that when they made amnesics learn the A–C list in a very different context from the one used for A–B learning, the amount of interference was greatly reduced. Control subjects were not affected by this manipulation, which involved changing the learning room so that it was either standard or illuminated with a red light, with music playing and incense burning. These results were interpreted as showing that the manipulation helps amnesics to make the contextual discrimination between the A–B and A–C lists, so that they are less likely to confuse B and C responses. Why controls were not helped is not explained, but the implication is clearly that amnesics are disproportionately bad at contextual memory. The interpretation seems to imply that the manipulation does not affect recall of the A–B list, but simply makes it more discriminable. This is implausible because the procedure is a minor modification of one that is used to demonstrate context-dependent forgetting, so that one would expect an impairment of A–B recall. Such an impairment would clearly aid A–C recall. This second interpretation of the data implies that amnesics have difficulty re-trieving context only when the relevant contextual features are no longer present. This implication is not one that follows from the context-memory-deficit hypothe-sis because according to this, amnesics have special problems with contextual memory even when the relevant features are still present – that is, when there has been no change of context. Contextual memory should be less available even un-der these circumstances, and it is unclear whether one should expect less, more, or a normal amount of forgetting when context is changed at the time of test. Fortunately, detailed consideration of this issue may be unnecessary, as the next paragraph makes plain.

There is evidence that the Winocur and Kinsbourne (1978) effect is an artefact of testing poor memory. Mayes, Meudell, and Som (1981) reported that memory for strongly associated word pairs is very little affected by a testing delay of 1 week. At that delay, however, there is a considerable amount of context-dependent forgetting when normal subjects are tested in a radically different room. This effect is absent when memory is tested after a 1-min delay. Context-dependent forgetting therefore seems to be more likely to occur if recall is relatively weak. It might be predicted that normal subjects will show context-dependent forget-ting, like that shown by Winocur and Kinsbourne's amnesics, at short retention delays, provided they are presented with related A–B, A–C word pairs with free association instructions, as this seems to prevent the use of recall memory. In other words, context-dependent forgetting may be found with priming in A–B, A–C paradigms, but not with cued recall instructions. This prediction has not yet been tested, although we have found a reduction in A–B priming when context was shifted between presentation and test, which is certainly consistent with a context-dependent forgetting effect in the A–B, A–C paradigm.

The above discussion makes it clear that it is not proved that disproportionate amnesic problems with temporal discriminations and memory for the source of information are the inevitable results of limbic and diencephalic damage. It is equally plausible that they are caused by incidental frontal lobe damage. Also, amnesic problems with interference and context-dependent forgetting, of the kind that has been shown so far, may actually be caused by poor recall and recognition. This does not mean that the context-memory hypothesis is false, but merely that the evidence so far described does not unequivocally support it. There is, however, more evidence. Winocur and Kinsbourne (1978) also reported that their alcoholic amnesics showed a marked improvement in memory for related word pairs if learning and testing took place in an unusual and distinctive setting. This improvement was not found in control subjects, even when a retention interval of 1 week was used (Mayes et al., 1981). It is not therefore a result of testing poor memory. Alcoholic amnesics have also been reported to benefit differentially when words are presented in a new and striking manner, such as being printed in red on a green background, instead of in black on a white background.

What do these results mean? It has been suggested that the patients benefit from striking contextual cues mainly at encoding, but that there is some benefit at retrieval as well. The results seem to suggest that amnesics do, in some circumstances, process context to relatively greater effect than control subjects, and do so voluntarily rather than automatically. If so, the findings are hard to reconcile with most versions of the context-memory-deficit view, which predict that amnesics will not process context in a mnemonically effective way and that it is usually processed automatically. There seem to be two possible routes to a reconciliation between Winocur and Kinsbourne's findings and the usual versions of the context-memory-deficit hypothesis. First, the beneficial effect of a striking context has been shown only in alcoholic amnesics. It has not been shown in amnesics of other aetiologies. If it occurs only in alcoholic amnesics, it may be a result of the incidental frontal lobe damage commonly found in these patients. This would indicate that the beneficial effect of a striking context in these patients is probably causally unrelated to the deficit underlying their amnesia, which could be caused by a selective failure to remember extrinsic context. Second, the selectively impaired amnesic processing of contextual information, whether it is essential to the syndrome or an incidental result of frontal lobe damage, could be improved when particularly impressive material is presented to amnesics, and this beneficial effect might not be found in normal people. Processing and hence memory might benefit because contextual features may be processed by voluntarily deploying attentional resources when the features are striking enough, even if such processing is normally carried out using minimal attentional resources. Amnesics might differentially benefit from effortful processing of context because their primary deficit is either in the processing of information that involves minimal attentional effort or in remembering the products of such processing. There is, indeed, some evidence that alcoholic amnesics show better memory for the temporal order, frequency, and spatial position of items when their attention is focused on these features, in circumstances where controls show no such benefit

(Kohl, 1984). This attentional focus seems to impair target memory rather than benefit it, but other kinds of effortful contextual encoding possibly do improve target memory.

Recently, in my laboratory, we have obtained preliminary support for the view that amnesics have disproportionately poor memory for items' modality of presentation and spatial location. Two experiments related to memory for modality of presentation. In one experiment, alcoholic amnesics and their controls were presented with lists of words to learn. Half the words were visually presented on cards, and half were spoken – that is, auditorily presented. Recognition was tested immediately after presentation of short lists to the amnesics. Controls were tested after a longer delay and were also given longer lists to learn. Recognition was good and the same in both groups. Immediately after recognition of each word had been tested, subjects were asked what modality it had been presented in during learning. The controls did significantly better than the amnesics at this task (Pickering, Mayes, & Fairbairn, in preparation). Memory for modality of presentation of words did not improve in controls, even when they knew it would be tested, suggesting that this kind of format context is automatically encoded, as other evidence indicates. There was also a significant positive correlation between patients' scores on tests sensitive to frontal lobe lesions and their memory for recognized words' modality of presentation, and between these scores and patients' general recognition ability. The possibility that disproportionately poor memory for modality was caused by incidental frontal lobe damage was, however, weakened by the finding that a patient with selective bilateral frontal lobe damage was not disproportionately poor at modality memory. In the second experiment, Bateman and I showed a group of alcoholic amnesics and their controls a series of objects (visual presentation) and later tested memory for half the objects by two-choice forced-choice *visual* recognition and for the other half by two-choice forced-choice *tactual* recognition (cross-modal recognition condition). Although patients and controls were matched on visual recognition by presenting longer lists of objects to the latter, with briefer presentation times and longer retention intervals, the amnesics were significantly worse in the cross-modal recognition condition. We are currently exploring this disproportionate deficit further, but it could well be related to the patients' poor memory for sensory modality of item presentation.

Spatial memory was also investigated in two experiments. In the first, subjects had to learn a list of words, in which each word was presented in a different position on a large file card. The controls were then tested at a longer delay than the alcoholic amnesic patients, so as to match word recognition in the two groups. After recognition was tested, subjects were asked to place cut-out copies of the correct words in the places where they had originally been on the file card. Although recognition in the two groups was closely matched, the patients were far worse than the controls at correctly locating the test words. In the second experiment, subjects were asked to estimate the cost of the real objects represented by 16 toys and to remember the toys. During this presentation phase of the experiment, the subjects saw the toys laid out in different positions on a grid. After a brief delay for the patients and a long delay for the controls, subjects were asked to recall as many toys as they could. Performance was matched in the two groups. Immediately after this test was completed, subjects were given the toys and told to place them on the grid in the positions they had occupied during the learning stage of the experiment. The patients were less accurate at the spatial memory task than were the controls (Pickering, Mayes, & Fairbairn, in preparation). Performance on these spatial tasks does not correlate with signs of frontal dysfunction in the patients, and there is also evidence that patients with frontal lobe lesions, even if they are bilateral, are not impaired on similar spatial tasks (see Kohl, 1984).

The above evidence is preliminary and tentative. It is, however, supported by studies from other laboratories, although these studies did not directly attempt to match patients and their controls on recognition or recall of target material. Even so, Kohl (1984) found greater deficits in spatial memory than target memory in a group of alcoholic amnesics. Indeed, in one condition with incidental learning of the spatial positions of verbal material, the patients were not worse than their controls at word recognition, but were markedly worse at locating the words. Hirst and Volpe (1984) have also found evidence that memory for spatial location is more impaired than memory for targets in amnesics. They compared the performance of a mixed group of amnesics with that of a control group on a task that required subjects to walk down a New York street and try to remember both the buildings and their positions. The amnesics showed a larger deficit with their spatial memory than with their memory for the buildings. Hirst and Volpe have argued that amnesics are unable to encode spatial features automatically, but have some ability to do so if they apply attentional effort to the encoding. They have reported that amnesics' memory for the spatial position of target items improves when their attention is directed towards encoding such information, and that control subjects do not show a similar improvement under these conditions. Kohl has found similar results. It is not certain, however, that normal people would not show similar results if tested when their memory was reduced to amnesic levels. In studies in my laboratory, we have found some evidence that this occurs. If this is so, Hasher and Zacks's (1979) claim that spatial features are automatically encoded must be wrong, because this implies that the application of effort will not improve memory for the automatically encoded feature. Nevertheless, it remains true that spatial and other contextual features are normally encoded with minimal attentional effort.

The anterograde amnesic deficits that have been described so far relate specifically to memory for context. Recently, Hirst et al. (1986) reported a kind of disproportionate amnesic deficit that may relate to contextual memory, but that could also have implications for memory that depends on elaborative encoding strategies. These workers found that recall was more impaired than recognition in a large group of amnesics that included alcoholic amnesics and patients with other aetiologies. Subjects were shown lists of 40 words that were either unrelated or were divided into a number of semantic categories. After learning, they were asked to recall as many words from a list as possible; when this was done, they were given a recognition test for the words in the list. Amnesic recognition was matched to that of the controls by allowing them to study the words for 8 sec each, compared with the controls' 0.5 sec. Although they were as good as the controls at recognition, the amnesics were significantly worse at recall. The amnesics who did not have an aetiology of chronic alcoholism did not show any impairments on tests sensitive to frontal lobe lesions, so it is difficult to argue that the recall deficit is caused by incidental lesions of the frontal lobes. The possible implications of this deficit will be discussed in the final section of this chapter. It is, however, worth stating here that although recall may be more impaired in amnesics than recognition, the extent of this differential impairment is not as great as in some other brain-damaged patients. For example, as discussed in chapter 5, frontal lobe lesions often impair recall, but leave recognition unaffected. As Huntington's choreics are believed to suffer from frontal lobe atrophy, it is interesting that their recognition is better than that of alcoholic amnesics, whereas recall in the two groups is often equally bad (see Butters, 1985).

Some of the other deficits in anterograde amnesia that have been reported may, however, result from incidental frontal lobe damage suffered by patients. For example, Shimamura and Squire (1986b) have looked at an aspect of meta-memory, known as feeling-of-knowing, in controls and amnesics with mixed aetiologies. Feeling-of-knowing refers to a subject's ability to predict whether an unrecalled item will later be recognized. It is counted as metamemory because it requires the making of a judgement about a person's memory. Shimamura and Squire gave their subjects general-knowledge questions until a total of 24 incorrect responses had been accumulated. They then assessed feeling-of-knowing by getting subjects to rank unrecalled items in terms of how likely it was that they would recognize the correct answer if given several choices. A recognition test for the unrecalled items was then given to determine the validity of these rankings. The judgements of ECT patients, the patient N. A., and two patients with aetiologies involving hypoxia and hypotension, respectively, were as accurate as those of control subjects. In contrast, alcoholic amnesics were poor at making feeling-of-knowing predictions. Although the authors argued plausibly that the alcoholic amnesics' disturbed metamemory was not a result of testing weak memory, they did suggest that it might be caused by incidental damage and not be essentially connected to the amnesia. Evidence reviewed in chapter 5 makes it likely that frontal lobe lesions would cause this kind of metamemory deficit, which probably results from a poor ability to make inferences from information that is in memory. If this is so, metamemory deficits in amnesics provide no support for the view that limbic–diencephalic lesions impair the ability to access a particular kind of information.

Alcoholic amnesics have also been reported to do poorly on a task sensitive to the processing of semantic information, at which patients with frontal lobe lesions are also impaired, as was described in chapter 5 (see, e.g., Squire, 1982). Subjects were shown several items in a given category, and after a brief distraction interval, their recall of these items was tested. The procedure was then repeated with more items from the same category. On the fifth trial, items from a different category were presented. With normal subjects, recall got progressively worse from trial one to trial four, a process that is ascribed to proactive interference. On the fifth trial, there was release from proactive interference, and recall significantly improved. The same release was seen in alcoholic amnesics when there was a change from presenting letters to presenting numbers, but the patients showed little, if any, release when there was a shift from one semantic category to another (for example, from plant words to animal words). Butters and Cermak (1975) argued that this finding supported their view that amnesia is caused by a habitual tendency not to process semantic information. But as discussed in chapter 5, Moscovitch (1982) has reported that a similar deficit occurs in patients with frontal lobe lesions, whereas patients with left temporal lobe lesions, who have bad verbal memory, performed normally. Alcoholic amnesics who fail to show release generally perform poorly on tests, such as the Wisconsin Card-Sort, that are sensitive to the effects of frontal lobe lesions. Furthermore, amnesics with non-alcoholic aetiologies show normal release after semantic shifts, although this has not always been found. It remains possible that the deficit underlying the failure to show release is different after frontal lobe lesions than it is in the amnesic patients who fail to show release. Freedman and Cermak (1986) have reported, for example, that some frontal patients fail to show release even when the procedure is repeated five times, whereas alcoholic amnesics fail to show release on only the first occasion. The final resolution of the problem will require further experiments, but it is clear that failure to show release is not found in all amnesics.

The release from proactive interference paradigm uses a modification of the Brown-Peterson task that was described in chapter 5, which involves testing subjects' short-term memory for a series of word triplets drawn from the same semantic category before presenting a word triplet from another semantic category to see whether memory improves. The basic task tests subjects' ability to remember items over a few seconds whilst performing a distracting activity. Although there is no doubt that some amnesics remember normally in this task with delays of 30 sec or more, others are impaired even at very short delays. Butters (1984) has argued that alcoholic amnesics are always impaired at this task, although Kopelman (1985) found normal performance in a group of 16 such patients with delays of up to 20 sec. At the longest delay, however, the patients did appear to be deteriorating faster than controls. Kopelman found that there was a just significant ranked scores' correlation between patients' recall and a measure of cortical atrophy. He also found that Alzheimer patients, who have far more cortical atrophy than alcoholic amnesics, performed much worse on the Brown-Peterson task. Recently, Parkin and Leng (1987) reported that alcoholic amnesics are impaired at the task, whereas amnesics with limbic system lesions are not. The deficit is almost certainly incidental to the core amnesia, and is probably at least partially caused in Korsakoff patients by the kind of frontal lobe lesion problem already discussed; that is, it is caused by a difficulty in switching rapidly between two actions (rehearsing and doing the distractor task). In patients with Alzheimer's disease, this kind of lesion may also contribute to their poor performance, but their more extensive PTO association cortex damage probably also plays a role.

Alcoholic amnesics also show more intrusion errors in the Brown-Peterson task than do patients with Huntington's chorea, although recall is equally bad in the two groups (see Butters, 1985). In other words, the alcoholic amnesics are more likely to recall items from previous lists inappropriately. Kopelman (1985) has made a similar observation in comparing groups of alcoholic amnesics and patients with Alzheimer's dementia. Although the dementing patients made fewer intrusions, their recall was also worse in this study, so items from earlier lists might have been beyond recall for them. This suggestion is compatible with the results of another study, described by Butters (1985), in which alcoholic amnesics, patients with Huntington's chorea and Alzheimer's disease, and controls were given four short stories to remember. Recall in all groups except the controls was equally poor, but the alcoholic amnesics and Alzheimer patients showed an equivalent number of prior story intrusions and more than the patients with Huntington's chorea. The tendency to produce intrusions could be caused by frontal lobe damage, which impairs temporal discrimination and perhaps increases impulsiveness. This needs to be proved, however, because Huntington's chorea is also associated with frontal lobe atrophy. In other words, when Alzheimer and Korsakoff patients show equally poor recall, both make excessive intrusion errors. This may occur because both groups have frontal lobe damage (although PTO association cortex damage is more prominent in Alzheimer patients and may play a role in their case). But patients with Huntington's chorea, who show equivalent recall, do not make excessive intrusions and are believed to have frontal lobe atrophy. If frontal lobe lesions cause excessive intrusion errors, then either Huntington's choreics must have very small frontal lobe lesions or the lesions must be differently placed than in Korsakoff patients.

The evidence reviewed above suggests that amnesics may be disproportionately bad at remembering various kinds of contextual information, and all these deficits cannot be easily attributed to incidental frontal lobe lesions. Amnesics may also be disproportionately bad at recall relative to recognition, and this deficit may also be an essential feature of their memory deficit. This seems much less likely with the other deficits that have been discussed, as they are usually not found in all amnesics and are very similar to deficits caused by frontal lobe lesions. Some further experiments have directly tested the view that amnesics do not either encode or remember elaborated semantic information. As these experiments relate closely to two of the theories already mentioned, they will be discussed in the final, theoretical, section of this chapter.

Retrograde amnesia

The best known generalization about retrograde amnesia is that memories of events happening shortly before the brain trauma are impaired, whereas older memories are spared. This generalization is often made in relation to the amnesias that are caused by the closed head injuries, common in road accidents. Unless the injury is very severe, durations of retrograde amnesia of over 30 min are unusual, and recovery tends to occur with time so that the amnesia shrinks to cover only the seconds or minutes before trauma (Russell, 1971). The initial extent of retrograde amnesia seems to be related to how long severe anterograde amnesia persists after trauma. Care should be taken in interpreting these observations, however, as they are usually based on clinical impression. In a recent study, Maring, Deelman, and Brouwer (1984) compared 32 unselected patients with closed head injury with the same number of controls. Subjects were given a multiple-choice test of public events that occurred between 1971 and 1982. This recognition test was given with a similar recall test. The patients' memory was impaired, and there was no sign that their deficit was reduced for the older events. The impairment was also greater for recall. As closed head injury often causes frontal lobe damage, it is possible that frontal cortex lesions may explain the observed memory performance (to a greater extent than in amnesia, these lesions impair recall more than recognition). This study indicates that objective tests of remote memory yield results that may be different from clinical impression. It should not be concluded, however, that closed head injury does not cause a temporally graded retrograde amnesia. Patients may have a steeply graded amnesia, affecting both recognition and recall, combined with a variable, but usually mild, recall failure that extends equally to all pre-traumatic memories. Another possibility is suggested by a study of Levin et al. (1985). These workers found that closed head injury patients showed a flat retrograde amnesia with a test of old television shows that had lasted only one season, whereas on autobiographical events, they showed a temporally graded retrograde amnesia. As autobiographical events would have received far more rehearsal than the television shows, and more rehearsal the older they were, these results could indicate that rehearsal protects memories from the deficit underlying amnesia. Older autobiographical memories will be more rehearsed, but not older memories about briefly shown television shows, so there will only be temporally graded retrograde amnesia for the former.

Objective tests of remote memory have been given to amnesics of several aetiologies and have often revealed sparing of older memories. Squire and Cohen (1984) have argued that limbic system lesions cause a temporally limited retrograde amnesia, whereas diencephalic lesions may cause an extended retrograde amnesia with less obvious sparing of old memories. In support of the first part of the claim, the famous patient H. M., who has limbic system damage, showed impaired recall of events that occurred 1 to 3 years before his surgery in 1953, but normal recall of earlier events, under some test conditions. Thus Marslen-Wilson and Teuber (1975) gave H. M. a test of faces of people who had been famous either before or after his operation. They found that his memory for the pre-morbidly famous faces was as good as that of controls, whereas he had terrible memory for those famous in the 1950s and 1960s. However, Corkin and her colleagues (see Corkin, 1984) have recently given H. M. some formal tests of remote memory and found that for some material, his amnesia extends back to 1942, the date at which he developed temporal lobe epilepsy. These tests may have given an exaggerated impression of the temporal extent of his retrograde amnesia for two reasons. First, they were given nearly 30 years after he became densely amnesic, and this condition may have prevented him from rehearsing the affected memories like normal people. His retrograde amnesia might therefore have been less extensive if Corkin et al. had tested him shortly after his operation, as did Milner. Second, he became severely epileptic in 1942, and this disorder disturbs the ability to acquire new information so some of his memory loss for remote events may have been anterograde.

The findings with H. M. indicate that his retrograde amnesia is probably graded. Indeed, Corkin et al.'s (1983) results may give the impression that his disorder is more temporally extensive than it really is. The findings are also consistent with the suggestion that the apparent extent of amnesia is a function of the tests used. Corkin et al.'s tests are more sensitive than clinical interview or the famous-faces test. Is there evidence that other patients with limbic system lesions have temporally graded retrograde amnesias when sensitive tests are used? Milner (1971) described such amnesias in temporal lobectomy cases in her early work, but generally there is very little evidence because locus of damage has been confirmed in very few cases. Formal tests of post-encephalitic amnesics, who very probably have limbic system damage, have generally shown a very severe and extensive retrograde amnesia with little sign of sparing of memories, even when they are several decades old (for a review, see Mayes & Meudell, 1983). There are indications that retrograde amnesia in post-encephalitic patients is variable, and steeply graded memory losses have been reported in some patients. Most of these reports were, however, based on clinical impression, although more recently, they have been confirmed with sensitive formal tests (Parkin & Leng, 1987).

Like H. M., post-encephalitic patients (for more detail, see the second section of this chapter) have an amnesia with an acute onset; unlike him, there is no reason to suppose they had pre-existent problems with learning that could have caused poor memory for remote events. The reason that their retrograde amnesia is usually so extensive is probably that their brain damage is more widespread. Butters et al. (1984) speculated that the lesions of post-encephalitics may extend further posterior in the temporal lobes than in the case of H. M. and that more posterior lesions particularly affect older memories. Warrington and Shallice (1984) have found, however, that some post-encephalitics have impaired memory for very well-established semantic information, probably first acquired in childhood. Such deficits are not usually found after selective limbic–diencephalic lesions, but are after PTO association cortex lesions. This would suggest that these patients' extensive retrograde amnesias are results of such cortical degeneration. At present, neither possibility can be eliminated, and both may apply. Whatever turns out to be the case, brain damage in post-encephalitic amnesics is variable, as is the severity of their retrograde amnesia.

Other cases who do show temporally limited retrograde amnesia have been reported. Thus Butters et al. (1984) have described the case of R. B., who developed amnesia following the clipping of an anterior communicating artery aneurysm. This patient had a post-morbid IQ of 141 and very severe anterograde amnesia, but performed normally on the famous-faces test when the faces belonged to people who had been famous in R. B.'s pre-morbid period. He was mildly impaired on a recall test for public events that had occurred in the 1970s, but was normal for events that had occurred between 1930 and 1970. Although anatomical confirmation is needed, R. B.'s lesion probably involved the structures of the basal forebrain that project to the hippocampus and amygdala, and if so, he is likely to be suffering from a dysfunction of the limbic structures of the medial temporal lobes, like H. M. and post-encephalitic patients.

The largest group of amnesics that have been reported to have temporally graded retrograde amnesia are bilateral ECT patients. These patients have been studied extensively by Squire and his colleagues with a variety of formal tests, including one that taps knowledge of television programmes that were screened for 1 year only (for a review, see Squire & Cohen, 1984). On this test, amnesia was observed for programmes broadcast between 1 and 2 years prior to the ECT, but not for programmes that were broadcast 3 to 8 years previously. Other studies have given convergent results. The deficit is transient and usually disappears within 6 months. Although the memory of control subjects became progressively worse for older public events or TV programmes, that of the ECT patients was actually worse for TV programmes screened in the 2 previous years than it was for programmes screened 4 to 6 years previously. Squire and Cohen (1979) have also reported that ECT affects equally what they describe as detailed and salient information. Detailed information comprises highly specific facts that are rapidly forgotten, whereas salient information comprises centrally important facts that are slowly forgotten. ECT was reported to affect both kinds of information in the few years before treatment and neither kind for older memories.

There are some interpretive problems with the ECT studies, although they give clear evidence of temporally graded amnesia. First, it is largely speculative to argue that the treatment causes a limbic system dysfunction in the medial temporal lobe rather than in the diencephalon or elsewhere. Second, the patients are being treated for depression and also receive a general anaesthetic, both of which are known to affect memory. Furthermore, ECT should improve depression, and it has been shown that during depressed moods, unpleasant experiences are more readily recalled than pleasant experiences (see chapter 2). As the Squire studies compared patients' memory before they received ECT with their memory after a course of five ECTs, the patients may have experienced an improvement in mood. This mood change could produce state-dependent forgetting for events that occurred during the severely depressed period, which might extend back for several years prior to treatment. In other words, the patients might have difficulty remembering things that happened during the time when they were most depressed. Although Squire used recognition tests, which are not supposed to be susceptible to state-dependent forgetting, as well as recall tests, it is difficult to be sure what combination of factors gives rise to the graded retrograde amnesia seen in his patients. This feeling is supported by a unique study that controlled for depression and compared ECT with a sham condition in which patients received anaesthetic only (Frith et al., 1983). On one test, patients had to indicate whether names shown to them belonged to famous people from the past 40 years or were fictitious. Patients given sham ECT were impaired on this remote memory test, whereas ECT patients actually showed improved performance! Frith and his colleagues suggested that ECT may activate established memories and so make their recognition easier.

The above discussion indicates that anaesthesia, ECT, and changes in depressed state may all influence remote memory and in different ways, so that several independent factors may be contributing to graded retrograde amnesia. Graded retrograde amnesia is not, however, always seen after ECT (see Squire & Cohen, 1984). When no sparing of older memories occurred, it was noted that control subjects remembered equally well across all the time periods tested; that is, they showed no signs of forgetting. The patients showed temporally graded amnesia only when control subjects showed forgetting of the test items drawn from the earlier time periods. Squire and Cohen argued that as memories are forgotten, then, paradoxically, they become increasingly resistant to the kind of disruption that causes organic amnesia, but Butters and Albert (1982) have found graded retrograde amnesias (albeit long ones) in patients using tests on which controls remembered old items as well as newer ones (so that old memories did not seem to be forgotten relative to new ones). When old items are remembered as well as newer ones, this suggests that they have been better learnt and have perhaps received more subsequent rehearsal. This seems to imply that ECT patients are impaired at remembering older items only when they have been well learnt. This directly contradicts what was argued above in connection with the retrograde amnesia shown by patients with closed head injuries. It was argued there that the more a memory has been rehearsed, the less disrupted it will be by amnesia. This seems to be a far more plausible principle than its opposite. There may have been other, as yet undiscovered differences between the Squire tests that showed graded amnesia and those that did not. The factors in tests that determine the temporal extent of amnesia are still poorly understood. For example, although ECT patients showed an amnesia extending back only 2 years before treatment for the names of TV programmes, the amnesia extended to 7 years when they were asked to date programmes (see Squire & Cohen, 1984).

The case that limbic system lesions of the medial temporal lobe cause a retrograde amnesia confined to events experienced only a few years before trauma is still based on a very small number of patients. Other patients with lesions that include the limbic system, such as post-encephalitics, often show temporally extensive amnesias, with no sparing of older memories. Even if one accepts that selective limbic system lesions produce a temporally graded amnesia, this finding has to be interpreted. One suggestion, made above, is that older memories are relatively spared because they have been rehearsed and perhaps reorganized to a greater extent than newer memories. Formal tests of retrograde amnesia have tried to control this factor to some degree. They try to sample public events, which can be given a fairly precise date, and ideally, they also try to provide equivalence; that is, events from the different periods should have been initially learnt to the same extent and forgotten at similar rates. If this requirement is met, then older events should be less well remembered by control subjects, and subjects too young to have experienced the events at first hand should not remember them. Not all tests meet this strict requirement [for example, those of Butters & Albert (1982), where older items are as well remembered as newer ones], but even if it is met (as it is by the TV tests), one cannot assume that the older events have not been more rehearsed than the newer ones. It may well be that 'normal' forgetting would be much faster if memories were not frequently rehearsed, however indirect such rehearsals might be.

This speculation about the role of rehearsal in normal forgetting may be relevant to the findings of Sanders and Warrington (1971). They gave a public-events questionnaire to a mixed group of amnesics, including patients with probable limbic system and diencephalic lesions, and found retrograde amnesias with no sparing of older memories. Their test was carefully devised to satisfy the equivalence criterion and contained items that were selected so that there was a minimum likelihood that they would be subsequently rehearsed. The older test items therefore may have received little, if any, more rehearsal than the newer ones. The absence of sparing for the older items may, however, have been an artefact caused by the amnesic patients performing at floor level. This possibility receives some support from results obtained with Albert's tests. On these tests, alcoholic amnesics showed retrograde amnesias that extended back for decades, but with partial sparing of the oldest items, whereas patients with Huntington's chorea and Alzheimer's disease showed no sparing of memory for the oldest items (Butters & Albert, 1982). Indeed, the Huntington's patients were less impaired than the alcoholic amnesics with the newer items and more impaired with the older items. This strongly suggests that the remote memory impairment has different causes in these patients and that whatever sometimes protects the remote memories of alcoholic amnesics is ineffective against the deficit found in patients with Huntington's chorea.

This conclusion is theoretically important with respect to the causes of organic amnesia, but may be unjustified if one interpretation of the retrograde amnesia found in patients with an aetiology of chronic alcoholism is correct. Although all studies of alcoholic amnesics, apart from that of Sanders and Warrington (1971), have found the patients to show a remote memory deficit that extends back for decades, but with sparing of the oldest memories (for reviews, see Mayes & Meudell, 1983; Squire & Cohen, 1984), this temporally graded remote memory impairment has sometimes been interpreted as a consequence of the slow development of amnesia that may occur in these patients. In other words, the patients may have become gradually amnesic over many years because of their alcohol addiction, and the effect of this would be that they became progressively unable to remember new information. The patients could therefore have a progressively worsening anterograde amnesia that is superimposed on a genuine retrograde amnesia that shows no sparing of even the oldest memories (just like the patients with Huntington's chorea). This interpretation receives some support from observations that non-amnesic alcoholics have mild learning problems and show some deficits on remote memory tests that are confined to the most recent time periods (see Butters, 1985). The impairment on the remote memory test affects only recall, however, and might be caused by a genuine retrograde amnesia rather than being secondary to a slowly developing anterograde amnesia. Given that the remote memory impairment in alcoholic amnesics may extend back 40 years, it is hard to imagine how a progressive memory disorder could affect 30-year-old memories more than 40-year-old ones unless the patients began heavy drinking whilst still in the pram.

A recent case report by Butters (see Butters, 1985) also fits most easily with the view that the remote memory impairment shown by alcoholic amnesics is a genuine result of a retrograde amnesia, not appreciably contaminated by a gradually progressive anterograde amnesia. The patient was an eminent scientist who developed alcoholic amnesia at the age of 65, just after he had written his autobiography. On a detailed test of information available in his autobiography, Butters was able to show a severe amnesia that became milder as the date of origin of the information became older; that is, there was a temporally graded amnesia that extended back over several decades. As well as showing amnesia for personal episodes, this patient was very impaired at recalling definitions of terms that must have been very familiar to him during his scientific career. Now, the patient is known to have had an acute breakdown, known as a Wernicke-Korsakoff episode, after writing his autobiography. Wernicke-Korsakoff episodes are characteristic harbingers of many alcoholic amnesic states and are associated with confusion, a variety of motor symptoms, and delirium. If patients survive and recover from this episode with the aid of thiamin therapy, they emerge with a severe amnesia, which seems to have an acute onset. It is therefore tempting to argue that the scientist's graded retrograde amnesia was genuine and not caused by gradually worsening learning ability. This view is clearly supported by the evidence that the lost memories had been readily available to him in the years before the Wernicke-Korsakoff episode. Although his learning ability was undoubtedly deteriorating during this time, it probably did not appreciably affect the form taken by his subsequent retrograde amnesia.

Although alcoholic amnesics do have diencephalic lesions, it has been argued that their extensive retrograde amnesias are caused by incidental lesions, probably of their frontal lobes. This view is supported by the finding of Shimamura and Squire (1986a) that there was no correlation between the severity of patients' anterograde amnesia and the severity of their memory impairment for the remote past, although a correlation was found between the severity of their anterograde amnesia and the severity of their memory loss for the recent past. This strongly suggests that patients' poor memory for events that occurred decades before has a different origin from their new learning deficits and poor memory for the recent past. The poor memory for the recent past can be interpreted in two ways. First, it may be that it is a steeply graded genuine retrograde amnesia of the same kind that Squire has argued exists in ECT patients. Second, it could result from an anterograde amnesia that progressively worsened over the previous few years (the same argument as before). The first interpretation is supported by evidence from patients who have focal diencephalic lesions of sudden onset. One such case has been reported by Winocur, Oxbury, Roberts, Agnetti, and Davis (1984). Their patient had suffered a vascular accident that affected the blood supply to the thalamus bilaterally. Although his anterograde amnesia was moderately severe, his retrograde amnesia was much less extensive than that seen in alcoholic amnesics.

It is clearly important to give remote memory tests to other amnesic patients with lesions confined to the diencephalon and to compare their performance on the same tests with that of amnesics who have focal limbic system lesions. At present, there is no convincing evidence that diencephalic and limbic system lesions cause different kinds of retrograde amnesia. Both kinds of lesion are associated with temporally graded retrograde amnesia on some formal tests. Not all tests show sparing of older memories, and it has been suggested that those that do not have been devised so that older items will have received little more rehearsal than newer ones. If so, both limbic system and diencephalic lesions cause a functional deficit that results in poor memory for things acquired pre-traumatically, but less so to the extent that those memories have been rehearsed. In contrast, the deficit in memory for pre-traumatically acquired information caused by Huntington's chorea and, probably, by frontal lesions is just as great whether or not memories have been well rehearsed. Alcoholic amnesics have been a difficult group to study because their amnesia may have a gradual onset (although there is a surprising lack of direct evidence for this widely held view) and because they often have damage to the frontal lobes.

The formal tests of retrograde amnesia have tapped publicly available information. Subjects might be asked, for example, to identify Ronan Point (a high-rise block of flats in London part of which collapsed after a gas explosion in the late 1960s). Thus the memories that are tapped are semantic, rather than episodic. Clinical interviews have established that amnesics also often have very poor memory for pre-traumatically acquired autobiographical information. Some people have argued that such episodic memories are far more seriously affected than semantic ones. Zola-Morgan, Cohen, and Squire (1983) have shown, however, that amnesics are capable of recalling personal episodes when given appropriate encouragement. They required subjects to recall personal memories associated with concrete cue words, such as *book,* and found that amnesics could do this, contrary to some other reports, when they were pressed to do so. It was noted that the personal memories tended to be drawn from their early lives. They therefore came from a period for which public-events questionnaires indicated patients' semantic memory was also good. This suggests that episodic and semantic memories that have been rehearsed to about the same degree are equally affected in amnesics.

Before turning to the theoretical discussion, one final feature of retrograde amnesia will be considered. This is simply whether the disorder is a failure of retrieval or of storage.

The view, advanced in this book, that storage occurs within the brain regions where processing occurs would suggest that retrograde amnesia is caused by a disruption of storage as well as retrieval. It has been argued, however, that retrograde amnesia is caused by a selective impairment in retrieval. This argument has been based on two kinds of empirical evidence. First, patients can show recovery from retrograde amnesia, and this recovery can be rapid even when the disorder has been relatively long-lasting. Thus Victor et al. (1971) reported that 21% of their alcoholic amnesics recovered completely, and 25% recovered partially. Similarly, some post-encephalitic amnesics have shown total recovery after suffering from severe retrograde as well as anterograde amnesia (see Weiskrantz, 1985). Victims of transient global amnesia sometimes have amnesias that extend back for decades, but they usually disappear very quickly when the patient recovers. Retrograde amnesia has also been induced experimentally by stimulating the limbic system structures of the medial temporal lobes (see Weiskrantz, 1985). Interestingly, the amnesia became more temporally extensive the longer the stimulation was maintained. In all cases, it recovered within a maximum period of 2 hours, taking longer when the amnesia was more temporally extensive. The longest stimulation used was 10 sec, and that resulted in an amnesia that extended back several weeks. If one supposes that longer stimulations cause a greater amnesic disruption, then it is possible that very long stimulations might have produced an amnesia that extended back for years. This is quite consistent with what has been argued here – that older, more rehearsed memories are more immune to the deficit underlying amnesia. Even the most extreme form of this deficit may not affect very well-rehearsed memories.

The second kind of evidence that has been used to support the argument that retrograde amnesia is caused by a selective retrieval failure relates to Shallice's (1986) criteria for distinguishing between storage and retrieval deficits, discussed in chapter 4. One of these criteria is that success or failure of recall of particular items should not be consistent from one occasion to another if the deficit is one of retrieval. Cermak and O'Connor (1983) have tested the remote memory of the post-encephalitic amnesic S. S. on two occasions, well apart in time, and found that although the patient's memory was very poor on both occasions, he failed different items on the two tests. In Shallice's view, this is what would be expected with a retrieval failure. Clearly, it is important to repeat this procedure with other patients to determine whether it applies to all amnesics. There is preliminary evidence that it does not apply to alcoholic amnesics, as these patients tend to make stereotyped recalls from one occasion to another (Pickering, personal communication). There has been no attempt to apply Shallice's other criteria to the problem of retrograde amnesia. This would be interesting to do. Cueing has, however, been shown to improve remote memory in amnesics, and this perhaps corresponds to Shallice's second criterion for a retrieval failure – that item retrieval can be improved by priming. More relevantly, it needs to be determined whether amnesics can demonstrate normal implicit memory for pre-traumatically acquired information for which they show no explicit memory. No one has examined whether patients are equally bad at recalling what corresponds to superordinate features and attribute information in remote memories. If they are, then, for example, they should find it no more difficult to recall that there was an explosion at Ronan Point, given that they knew it was a building, than to recall that it was a building.

Do these two kinds of evidence prove that retrograde amnesia is caused by a selective retrieval deficit? The answer is surely no. It has already been argued in chapter 4 that Shallice's criteria are open to question. Even if the features of retrograde amnesia satisfied all five of Shallice's (1986) retrieval criteria (and they may well not), it would still be quite possible that the disorder involves a storage failure. Most people believe that the strongest evidence favouring a retrieval deficit view is that indicating that recovery can occur from retrograde amnesia. If the store has been destroyed, how can the memory return? This argument is based on an overly simple view about recovery of function. The true view must surely run as follows: Trauma causes dysfunction in limbic–diencephalic structures. This either causes the disruption of a retrieval mechanism or disrupts a store. If the neurons that provide the retrieval mechanism or the store have been destroyed, then there is no recovery. In contrast, if the function has merely been put out of action temporarily, then memory will recover. Recovery in no way discriminates between the deficit being one of retrieval or one of storage. In my view, there are still no criteria that can reliably distinguish between storage and retrieval failures. It is worth making one further comment about such deficits. The comment relates to what is meant by retrieval. A retrieval mechanism might perform a systematic search for cues that were encoded during learning. It is possible that such a systematic search mechanism could be damaged without destroying the store. Once this search mechanism has activated enough cues that were encoded during learning, then the rest of the memory will be activated automatically. This is also a retrieval mechanism, but it will involve the activation of the same neurons that are storing the memory. Any lesion that affects this type of retrieval mechanism must also disrupt the store. Unless retrograde amnesia is shown to be caused by a failure to plan memory retrieval, it is most likely to result from a simultaneous breakdown of storage and retrieval.

What functional deficit causes organic amnesia?

Any account of the functional deficit(s) underlying amnesia must be consistent with the pattern of preserved memory and disproportionate memory deficit found in anterograde amnesia, as well as the form taken by retrograde amnesia. If it is assumed that the underlying deficit causes both anterograde and retrograde amnesia, then it becomes hard to argue that an encoding or even a storage failure produces the memory disorder. Even if this were not assumed, however, there is evidence against the view that anterograde amnesia is caused solely by an encoding deficit. Halgren, Wilson, and Stapleton (1985) simultaneously electrically stimulated the hippocampus and amygdala of epileptic patients for periods of less than 1 sec whilst they were viewing pictures of complex scenes or when their recognition of these scenes was being tested or on both occasions. Memory was not affected when recognition was tested immediately, which suggests that the patients' short-term memories were probably intact and that their processing of the stimuli was not grossly impaired. Stimulation during both encoding and retrieval did, however, disrupt recognition about equally when this was tested after a delay, and the disruption was far greater when stimulation was given during both encoding and retrieval than when it was given during either alone. Halgren and his colleagues argued that the stimulation must disturb encoding and retrieval processes engaged in by the limbic structures of the medial temporal lobes. Other work, described in the last section, also indicates that more intense stimulation in the delay before retrieval can disturb memories that were acquired up to at least weeks beforehand. As the effects of stimulation resemble those of a reversible lesion, it seems probable that amnesics must at least show disturbed encoding and retrieval of certain kinds of information.

Two of the theories mentioned earlier in the chapter propose that amnesics either do not habitually encode (and possibly do not habitually retrieve) semantic information when this requires the use of planned and effortful processing (the view of Butters & Cermak, 1975) or cannot retrieve and/or store the semantic products of the kinds of effortful processing controlled by the frontal cortex (the view of Warrington & Weiskrantz, 1982). These views are consistent with several pieces of evidence.

First, there is some electrophysiological evidence that amnesics show reduction in an electrical component generated by the brain, which some have argued is a correlate of semantic processing. Greenwood, Volpe, and Gazzaniga (see Gazzaniga, 1984) recorded EEG activity from patients' scalps and looked particularly at an electrical component, found by averaging many responses to similar stimuli, that occurs 300 msec or later after attended events happen. This positive, scalp-recorded component is known as P300. It was found that this component was absent in a patient who was very poor at recognition, reduced in one with a mild recognition impairment, and normal in a patient without a recognition loss. These findings are intriguing because the amplitude of P300 has been related to the kind of attentional effort that is associated with semantic processing, has been found to be larger in response to words that are later recognized, and is believed by some to be generated by the limbic system structures of the medial temporal lobes. This last claim has, however, been challenged, and it is also very unlikely that P300 is a specific correlate of semantic processing. Finally, it has been reported by Donchin (1984) that P300 is absent in certain elderly subjects with apparently normal memory. The absence of P300 in certain amnesics is interesting and warrants further study, but it cannot be regarded at present as strong support for the view that these patients fail to encode or retrieve semantic information.

The second piece of evidence with which an amnesic semantic encoding and retrieval deficit is consistent is the report of Hirst and his colleagues (1986) that recall is more affected than recognition in amnesics. There is considerable evidence that recall of a list of items depends more than recognition on the encoding and, presumably, retrieval of elaborative semantic links among the items. If these semantic links were not encoded and/or retrieved normally, then recall would be more affected than recognition.

Third, Butters and Cermak (1975) have assembled an extensive body of data that suggest that alcoholic amnesics may have problems in processing semantic information. There are, however, several serious problems with these data. Other amnesics do not appear to suffer from the deficits shown by alcoholic amnesics. There is reason to suppose that some or all of the deficits are caused by incidental frontal lobe lesions that do not relate to the core amnesic problem. Also, if the semantic-processing deficits were genuine features of amnesia, then one would expect to see, contrary to fact, that amnesics show marked reductions in intelligence.

Butters and Cermak's hypothesis predicts that if amnesics are encouraged to process meaningful aspects of stimuli, then they will be quite capable of doing so, and this will improve their memory differentially with respect to normal people who are given the same encouragement. The strongest form of this prediction is that the procedure will actually make the amnesics' memory normal. If the meaningful information has to be elaboratively processed, then Warrington and Weiskrantz (1982) make an opposite kind of prediction. As their hypothesis states that amnesics cannot remember elaboratively encoded information, orienting tasks that encourage the encoding of meaningful features of items should not improve memory as much as they do in normal people. We have tested these predictions with alcoholic amnesics using a variety of materials, including words, pictures of faces, nonsense shapes, and complex cartoon pictures (for a review, see Mayes & Meudell, 1983). Subjects learned the material in their own way or their attention was directed towards low-level features of the stimuli in order to impair their memory or it was directed towards meaningful features of stimuli in order to improve their memory. Control subjects were tested at a longer delay in order to match their memory in the spontaneous learning condition with that of the amnesics. Our results are easy to describe. Amnesics and controls were affected in exactly the same way. Their memory was improved when their attention was directed towards meaningful aspects of stimuli and made worse when attention was directed at mnemonically irrelevant aspects of stimuli, and the size of these effects was the same in both groups. There was also some evidence that the groups performed the orienting tasks in the same way. In addition, Warrington and Weiskrantz should predict that amnesics will not benefit from using visual mediating imagery to link together unrelated words in tasks that require the learning of lists of word pairs. There is, however, good evidence that amnesics with both limbic system and diencephalic lesions show much improved learning of word pairs if they use linking imagery (see Parkin & Leng, 1987).

If valid, these results must mean that neither the Butters and Cermak (1975) nor the Warrington and Weiskrantz (1982) hypothesis is correct. There have, however, been some reports that alcoholic amnesics benefit differentially from having their attention directed towards meaningful aspects of stimuli, and others that they do not benefit at all. In one study, McDowall (1979) found that alcoholic amnesics improved differentially when asked to say during learning what semantic category words belonged to. This effect was relative to the level of memory found after a spontaneous learning condition. It disappeared when semantic cues were given at retrieval, because this greatly improved the patients' memory in the spontaneous learning condition. The patients were, however, significantly worse than the controls on the similarities subtest of the WAIS, and poor performance on this subtest has been linked to poor semantic processing and is probably caused by incidental cortical atrophy in these patients. My interpretation of the overall pattern of results is that amnesics respond in the same way as normal people to having their attention directed to meaningful features of stimuli during learning and retrieval, indicating that their spontaneous processing of such features is normal. If they do show differential improvement, this is because of incidental cortical damage. This damage will probably include lesions of the frontal lobes, as some evidence, discussed in chapter 5, shows that these lesions cause poor spontaneous processing, but memory improves dramatically if encoding is carefully guided by the experimenter. This interpretation accords with the impression that the memory failures of highly intelligent amnesics cannot be explained in terms of disturbances in the elaborative processing of semantic information. Less convincingly, it also accords with the evidence that indicates that some of the kinds of priming at which amnesics seem to be normal depend on semantic processing.

If the evidence that amnesics have a selective processing deficit for semantic information is weak, there is perhaps better support for the view that they have a selective problem with memory for extrinsic context, comprising format and background contextual information. First, a deficit in processing such features of stimuli is compatible with preservation of normal intelligence in amnesics. Second, it is also compatible with normal short-term memory in the patients if one assumes that immediate recall of information does not depend on the initial retrieval of items' contextual markers. It is only after a delay or a distraction that such markers are likely to prove necessary for identifying retrieved items. A nice illustration of this point is provided by Yarnell and Lynch's (1973) observations of concussed and temporarily amnesic American football players. Immediately after regaining consciousness, the players *could* recall the move in which they had just been engaged, but on removal to the different context of the touch-line, they were no longer able to do so. The third feature of amnesia presents more serious problems for the context-memory-deficit view. It is plausible to argue that conditioning, skill learning, and priming, the kinds of implicit memory that are preserved in amnesics, depend on a form of retrieval that does not require the accessing of contextual information. In contrast, the kind of explicit memory disturbed in amnesics is more likely to do so. There is, in fact, direct evidence that classical conditioning is unaffected by changes in background context between learning and test (Mackintosh, 1985), which suggests that conditioning does not usually depend on the retrieval of contextual features. No similar evidence exists for skill learning, but, in my laboratory, Hargreaves and I have recently found evidence that free association priming may also show context-dependent forgetting. This result needs confirmation, and it remains to be determined whether the effect is identical to that found with explicit memory because, under the conditions of our experiment, there seemed to be little relationship between the effect of a context shift on free recall of the word pairs and the effect of such a shift on free association priming. It also seems to be confined to free association priming because we have not found context-dependent forgetting with word-completion priming.

If our finding proves reliable, it indicates that at least one kind of priming preserved in amnesics may depend on a kind of retrieval of contextual information, despite the fact that with priming there is no obvious requirement to retrieve an item's contextual markers. In this respect, priming resembles recall and recognition of semantic information and differs from recall and recognition of episodic information. This is because recall and recognition of semantic information make no explicit reference to the context in which information was acquired, whereas recall and recognition of episodic information do and may occur only if an event's contextual markers are also retrieved. It is, therefore, clearly dangerous to argue that because it makes no explicit reference to contextual markers, a particular form of memory does not partially depend on the retrieval of context. The occurrence of context-dependent forgetting with free association priming presents a serious problem for the context-memory-deficit hypothesis of amnesia because amnesics are normal at this kind of priming, and yet the hypothesis argues that they have a specific deficit in processing (encoding and retrieving) extrinsic contextual features. There are two responses to this problem. The first is to reject the hypothesis, and the second is to argue that contextual and target information are represented in radically different ways in implicit memory (preserved in amnesics) and explicit memory (i.e., recall and recognition, at which amnesics are impaired). There is currently little direct evidence to distinguish between these possibilities (although the study in my laboratory is weakly consistent with the idea that context-dependent forgetting may depend on different mechanisms with explicit and implicit memory), but there is other, related evidence that supports the context-memory-deficit view, so the second possibility will be discussed further. Before doing this, however, it is worth highlighting one possible implication of accepting the first possibility and rejecting the context-memory-deficit hypothesis. As discussed earlier in the chapter, amnesics may show preserved priming not only for items already established in memory, but also for novel target information. Context-dependent forgetting effects and the study of Nissen and Bullemer (1987) further suggest that patients' implicit memory for format and background context may also be normal. If so, they may store novel target and contextual information normally, and their poor recall and recognition for it result possibly from a deficit in judging that their processing of such information has become faster [as suggested by Jacoby's (in press) hypothesis about recognition]. This suggestion that amnesics have a kind of judgemental deficit that applies to all recognizable and recallable information is an interesting one that will need to be pursued if the context-memory-deficit view turns out to be false. Even if the view is true, amnesics may, of course, also have a familiarity-judging deficit. Indeed, if Jacoby's extension of Mandler's (1980) hypothesis that recognition sometimes depends on a judgement of increased speed of processing and sometimes on contextual retrieval is correct, then amnesics might need to have deficits in both contextual memory and a judgemental process. This implication becomes otiose if a minor modification is made to the hypothesis so that it claims that recognition always depends on a judgement about whether there has been an increase in item-processing speed, but that this increased processing speed sometimes depends on retrieving contextual features and sometimes not (Downes, personal communication). Alternatively, sometimes the increased speed of item processing is insufficient for the making of a confident judgement, so this attribution based on processing speed for the target is supplemented by the processing of related contextual features about which judgements are also made, with the recognition decision being based on the integral of all these judgements. On these views, impaired judgemental ability must disrupt recognition under all circumstances. The predictions of the judgemental-deficit view need to be worked out, but one is that, at least in some cases, priming and recognition should decline in parallel. In broad terms, there should be some kinds of priming that reflect changed speeds of item processing (e.g., perceptual identification priming, which reflects the rate of processing a complete item rather than a fragment), and they should decline at the same rate as recognition under some circumstances.

The idea that the memory representations underlying priming (particularly of novel associations) differ from those underlying recall and recognition has been developed by Schacter (1985). He has argued that the memory representations of new associations that amnesics are able to create are quite distinct from those that underlie recall and recognition. He distinguishes between 'unitized' structures, which underlie priming, and nested structures, which underlie recall and recognition. His distinction seems to incorporate a modified form of the context-memory-deficit hypothesis. 'Unitized' structures comprise integrated information, such as familiar words, idioms, and associates. The presence of part of a 'unitized' structure is sufficient to activate the whole. More important, the 'unitized' structures can be modified by what Schacter calls the encoding of information in the 'local context' in which they are used. Local context includes the semantic information that is encoded when the structure is activated (this could be another unrelated word), the modality in which the structure is presented, and the form in which it is presented. In other words, local context includes all those kinds of information that the priming of novel associations might suggest can be remembered by amnesics. In contrast, nested structures incorporate and can be retrieved only by accessing the 'global context' in which they were acquired. Global context comprises the spatial and temporal features of the episode in which the nested structures were formed. The global context is the same for each item in a list, whereas local context is unique to each item.

Schacter seems to argue that 'unitized' structures do not contain information about global context and that recall and recognition can be achieved only by accessing the latter kind of information. Amnesics' ability to develop 'unitized' structures for newly presented faces may explain why they may show discriminating skin-resistance responses to these stimuli, whereas their recognition failure may occur because they cannot develop nested structures for the faces. He also proposes that whereas normal people can acquire nested structures from a single episode, 'unitized' structures are modified only gradually. Although local context can be incorporated in one trial into a 'unitized' structure, the structure cannot be activated directly by this new component. This, Schacter argues, is why part of the pre-existing structure has to be present for priming to occur. For example, in a task when unrelated word pairs have been presented under semantic-processing conditions, priming occurs when cues like *window–rea* are presented with word-completion instructions (subjects having earlier seen *window–reason*), but not when *window–* is presented alone with free association instructions, if the novel pair was seen only once. He does, however, allow that with a great deal of repetition, local context can modify 'unitized' structures, so that it can act as a cue in isolation, which is sufficient to activate the structure. This is perhaps what happened in the study where patients learnt computer definitions and operations. Similarly, when amnesics were trained by the method of vanishing cues with un-related word pairs, such as *tobacco–boulder,* after a very large number of trials, they had some success in cueing the second word from the first word alone, without any of the letters from the second word to help (see Schacter, 1985). If this is like the amnesic learning of computer definitions, then it, too, should be very sensitive to local context, unlike the memory of normal people, which is much less constrained.

Schacter's (1985) hypothesis requires proper assessment, but is currently the only explanation of priming that tries to account for priming of new associations as well as priming of previously well-established memories. His hypothesis does, however, seem to imply that the representations underlying priming do not involve background contextual information because this is the same as what Schacter terms 'global context', and he argued that this form of context is not involved in 'unitized' structures. If so, priming should not be affected by changes in this kind of context between presentation and test. Our recent results, showing context-dependent forgetting of free association priming, imply that this is not the case. Furthermore, Schacter's view suggests that amnesics should not have a problem remembering items' format context, as this is part of the local context, which, according to his hypothesis, is involved in 'unitized' structures. Such information would include sensory modality of item presentation and mode of presentation within a sensory modality. This implication of Schacter's view seems to conflict with the most direct kind of evidence for the context-memory-deficit view, which suggests that amnesics are disproportionately bad at remembering various kinds of extrinsic contextual information, including memory for the sensory modality by which information is presented as well as spatiotemporal context ('global context', in Schacter's terms). There does not have to be a conflict, however, if one assumes that amnesics can create memory representations of items' sensory modality and background context in 'unitized' structures, but not in nested structures. Whether or not this assumption is correct is currently unknown. It must be admitted that it is entirely ad hoc and that, at present, evidence about priming presents a challenge to the context-memory-deficit hypothesis. There is, nevertheless, growing evidence that amnesics are particularly bad at remembering contextual information and that these deficits cannot always be explained as results of incidental frontal lobe damage. There is also some evidence for kinds of memory deficit that might be expected to be caused by context-memory failures. Thus Hirst and his colleagues (1986) have found recall to be more impaired than recognition in amnesics, and we have preliminary evidence that alcoholic amnesics are more sensitive to interference even when matched to their controls on initial learning, as would be expected if they cannot contextually tag competing memories. It is worth noting that greater amnesic sensitivity to interference would be consistent with faster forgetting in all amnesics (for which we have preliminary evidence), provided the amount of interference increases with retention interval. The role of frontal lobe damage in amnesic sensitivity to interference still cannot be discounted, however. Nevertheless, even when frontal lobe lesions cause similar context-memory deficits, as with poor temporal discrimination ability between items, some evidence to be discussed in chapter 7 suggests that the disorders may be distinct.

Amnesics may, then, be disproportionately bad at remembering the kind of background contextual information that normal people process with minimal attentional effort. Whether this deficit is specific to contextual features, or represents a general problem with processing that normally requires minimal attentional effort, is unresolved. Hirst and his colleagues have argued that amnesics cannot process information automatically, as can normal people, and have to process everything with attentional effort. This might occur because of an overall reduction in processing capacity in amnesics. If so, one would expect that normal people, given a second task to perform whilst learning, would suffer a disproportionate disruption of their contextual memory. It is difficult to see, however, how such a reduction in processing capacity could leave intelligence unaffected. These issues remain to be completely resolved, but in my laboratory, we have found that performance of a secondary task by normal people does not disproportionately disrupt their memory for modality of item presentation, although it seems to impair word-completion priming. If these findings are valid, the amnesic deficit cannot be caused by reduced central processing capacity.

More central to the context-memory-deficit hypothesis is the assumption that retrieving contextual markers is critical for normal recall and recognition. If this assumption is correct, then there should be a correlation between amnesics' recall and recognition of target items and their memory for contextual markers of those targets. This prediction has not yet been systematically tested. It is quite possible to find no correlations, or small ones, between target memory and memory for individual contextual features in amnesics and normal people, despite the truth of the assumption. One should expect only a correlation between target memory and some composite measure of contextual memory, although a significant correlation was reported in the previous section between target recognition and memory for presentation modality. Recent work in Manchester has confirmed this correlation between target recognition and modality memory in normal people, and found a similar one between target recognition and spatial memory. Memory for list of presentation and target recognition do not appear to correlate, however, in normal people. Even so, it has to be admitted that we do not really know which, if any, contextual features play an important role in target recall and recognition. For example, patients with left temporal lobe lesions have poor verbal memory, but their spatial memory appears to be normal (see Milner, Petrides, & Smith, 1985). Although these patients are likely to have other, as yet unidentified contextual memory problems, it is clear that poor spatial memory cannot cause their verbal memory problem. Evidence from state- and context-dependent forgetting in normal people might suggest that the hypothesis is wrong because these forms of forgetting mainly, if not solely, affect recall.

Three comments should be noted about this failure to disrupt recognition by removing items' contextual markers between learning and test. First, some kinds of contextual change do seem to affect recognition. These include the order in which items are presented during learning and test, and variations in speaker's voice, modality of presentation, and type font (see Morton, Hammersley, & Bekerian, 1985). Other kinds of contextual change may also affect recognition, but have not yet been examined. Second, shifts of state or context between learning and memory testing do not prevent contextual markers from being retrieved, but merely make it less likely that they will be. Not only do subjects still probably retrieve some contextual markers, but if they are encouraged to imagine the original learning situation, their recall deficit is largely eliminated. This suggests that both state- and context-dependent forgetting depend on fairly small reductions in the retrieval of contextual information. The third point is related to the second. If amnesics become less able to retrieve the kinds of contextual markers that become less available in state- and context-dependent forgetting, and this deficit becomes more severe as the amnesia worsens, then one might expect that mild amnesics would be relatively worse at recall than they are at recognition. In other words, mild amnesics may be chronically in a state that resembles the condition of normal people who are displaying context-dependent forgetting. Their recall should therefore be more impaired than their recognition. This is exactly what has been reported by Hirst and his colleagues (1986). More severely impaired amnesics might not show this pattern because when access to contextual markers becomes drastically affected, recall and recognition may be equally disrupted. In chapter 1, evidence was cited that suggests that recall may depend on accessing target material from contextual cues, whereas recognition depends on the strength of the links between the target and its contextual markers. It may also be the case that recall and recognition depend on slightly different contextual cues. This remains to be explored.

It is possible that amnesics suffer not so much from a processing failure with contextual information *per se,* as from an inability to integrate this information with target material. Although both contextual and target information might be stored in memory, the latter would be largely unavailable because its recognition and recall would be very difficult without the links to contextual markers. This view is very similar to the hypothesis, mentioned in the last section, that proposes that amnesics are unable to store or retrieve newly integrated material. Halgren (1984) has suggested that the subcortical structures damaged in amnesics initially unify the stored representations of previously unrelated semantic and episodic material by linking them to common contextual markers that they also store. This suggestion is an attractive amalgam of the context-memory-deficit and integrated-memory-deficit hypotheses. In effect, the proposal is that amnesia is caused by a processing and storage failure for contextual information that links together target material attributes. A slightly different view has been advanced by Teyler and DiScenna (1986), who propose that the hippocampus stores an index of the presumably thousands of neocortical modules that are activated by particular events and that, initially at least, no storage changes occur in these neocortical modules. Their view is based on the anatomical links between neocortex and hippocampus (discussed in chapter 7) and on the phenomenon of LTP (see chapters 1 and 7). The hypothesized memory changes, which are initially confined to the hippocampus and which index the activated neocortical modules, are proposed to be LTP-like modifications. Teyler and DiScenna's view is in some ways very similar to Halgren's and the context-memory-deficit hypothesis in that it claims that the structures damaged in amnesia normally integrate the complex information represented in the cortex. Like the context-memory-deficit hypothesis, it also states that with rehearsal, complex memories eventually come to be stored entirely in the cortex and their retrieval becomes independent of limbic and diencephalic structures. The major difference is that it postulates no initial neocortical storage. This seems to be an extreme and unlikely assumption, as LTP-like changes also occur neocortically. It is also focused solely on the hippocampus, giving no heed to the role of the other structures that may be damaged in amnesics.

Can the context-memory-deficit hypothesis account for retrograde as well as anterograde amnesia? If the two forms of amnesia have a single explanation, then the hypothesis postulates that this is a failure to process and store contextual information. If retrograde amnesia can occur in isolation, then the hypothesis must postulate that there can be a selective deficit in retrieving and storing contextual information. It has been argued that although temporally graded amnesia has often been observed, it occurs only when older memories have been more rehearsed than younger ones. In other words, the temporal gradient is an artefact of how well rehearsed and organized are memories of different ages. If recent memories were repeatedly rehearsed, then they, too, might be immune to the deficit found in amnesics. As memories are rehearsed and reorganized with the passage of time, their retrieval may become 'decontextualized' and therefore increasingly independent of the structures that are damaged in amnesics. This is presumably what has happened to very overlearnt semantic information. Although the amnesic lesion may destroy the storage of the contextual markers that used to unify well-rehearsed memories, the markers will be no longer necessary to retrieve them. It is proposed that this decontextualization occurs with highly rehearsed semantic and episodic memories. Clearly, this suggestion is currently speculative and needs more direct support. It is interesting to note, however, that older autobiographical memories tend to be described from the perspective of an observer, whereas more recent ones are more likely to be described from the point of view of the actor. This may indicate that older episodic memories are more decontextualized.

To account for the amnesia caused by limbic system lesions, Squire et al. (1984) have advanced a proposal similar in certain respects to that just discussed. Whereas that proposal suggests that the structures damaged in amnesics are important for the encoding, storage, and retrieval of the contextual markers that integrate newly associated target attributes, but less important in the processes that decontextualize memories, Squire and his colleagues argued that the limbic system lesions basically impair whatever process it is that changes the organization of memories through time as a result of rehearsal. They also argue that this reorganizational deficit underlies the faster forgetting of newly learnt material, which they believe characterizes limbic system amnesia. This second assumption is, however, implausible. It does not follow from their view that limbic system lesions disrupt the reorganizational process because the faster forgetting that has been reported in amnesics with limbic system lesions occurs before reorganizational processes are likely to have had any effect. With respect to their first assumption, it does indeed seem to be possible that amnesics fail to rehearse and reorganize their old memories, as there is some reason to suspect that retrograde amnesia gets worse with time; but the evidence that has been reviewed in this chapter makes it probable that this happens because amnesics cannot retrieve memories that have not been reorganized.

It is therefore tentatively concluded that amnesics' memory problems arise from a failure to process and store contextual markers that serve to integrate the memory representations of new facts and experiences. This hypothesis needs far more rigorous testing and may well prove to be wrong in many of its details. The problems it faces in explaining the phenomena of priming are particularly severe, and it is possible that, in the end, the context-memory-deficit hypothesis will be rejected and a familiarity-judgement deficit view advanced. Nevertheless, it fits available evidence better than other accounts. Whether amnesia should be regarded as a unitary disorder remains a moot point. There are certainly material-specific subforms of amnesia, and there is quite good evidence that retrograde amnesia can occur in isolation, although it needs to be convincingly shown that this syndrome is caused by a smaller version of the kind of lesion that normally produces global amnesia. The evidence for distinct forms of limbic and diencephalic amnesia is less good, but should be taken seriously. Finally, it is possible that damage to hippocampal and amygdalar circuits produces distinct deficits, both of which contribute to amnesia. As will be discussed in chapter 7, it is possible that these deficits involve different aspects of contextual memory.

7   Animal and biochemical models of amnesia

It has proved difficult through the study of human amnesics to elucidate several matters critical to understanding the disorder. First, human cases are not usually appropriate for identifying the critical lesions that cause the core memory problems because their lesions often extend into brain regions where damage causes unrelated deficits. Second and relatedly, it is hard to determine from human amnesics the extent to which their memory deficits result from damage to neurons that release specific transmitters, such as acetylcholine or noradrenalin. Third, despite developments with electrophysiological recording techniques and the emergence of the PET scan, study of human amnesics and healthy people is not an effective means of exploring the anatomical connections and physiology of the brain regions lesioned in amnesics in order to gain a clearer idea of precisely what functions are disrupted in patients. These three issues have been more effectively examined through physiological studies with animals and pharmacological studies with animals and humans. The next section discusses animal models of the amnesic state. The third section briefly reviews what light pharmacological studies have thrown on amnesia, and the last section considers animal work involving lesions, electrophysiological recordings, and manipulations of long-term potentiation (LTP). As indicated in chapter 1, LTP is an increase in neural responsiveness, particularly striking in hippocampal neurons, that occurs when brief bursts of high-frequency stimulation are given to the inputs of the relevant neurons. It may persist for weeks and is believed by many to be based on a memory-like change. LTP is of interest here because it has been used to examine the functions of the structures whose damage is believed to be critical in amnesia.

Animal modelling has been used in one other way that will be referred to cursorily here – to elucidate precisely what aetiological factors underlie different forms of amnesia as well as what damage and what effects on memory such factors have. Most such work has focused on the aetiology of alcoholic amnesia. It has long been generally believed that this syndrome is caused by thiamin deficiency, which is secondary to chronic alcoholism. Nicotinic acid deficiency has also been implicated by some. The complexity of the aetiology is apparent from attempts to model the syndrome in animals. For example, De Witt and Goldman-Rakic (1983) studied the effects on monkeys of one to four episodes of thiamin deprivation and failed to find any signs of mammillary body or dorsomedial thalamic damage. They did, however, observe lesions in other brain regions, such as the striatum, in the basal ganglia, and the cerebellum. Their monkeys were also impaired at various learning tasks, including one that was designed to be analogous to recognition. The animals were not bad at this task, however, when unique items were used on each trial, whereas human amnesics probably would have been. Although the authors argued that more prolonged deprivation might have caused appropriate diencephalic lesions, there is no evidence to support this view. There may, of course, be species differences, as is perhaps suggested by Irle and Markowitsch's finding (see Markowitsch & Pritzel, 1985) that thiamin deprivation in the cat consistently affects the mammillary bodies. It has even been found that such deprivation in rats may cause specific reductions in acetylcholine turnover (see Mayes & Meudell, 1983).

Although the effects of thiamin deprivation may differ in humans and monkeys because of a species difference, other factors may be involved. Thus cultured cells from alcoholic amnesics have been reported to be deficient in the thiamin-dependent enzyme transketolase, although this has not always been found (see Mayes & Meudell, 1983). Some alcoholics may therefore develop amnesia because of an inherited deficit in transketolase, which makes them abnormally vulnerable to the effects of the thiamin deprivation often associated with alcoholism. The syndrome may also be exacerbated by the direct effects of repeated intakes of alcohol. Studies of rodents given vitamin-fortified diets and regular intakes of alcohol have found learning disturbances and evidence of neuronal loss from the hippocampus (see Mayes & Meudell, 1983). Similar damage has been noted in some alcoholic amnesics. This work indicates that the causes of alcoholic amnesia are still far from being properly understood, but it seems likely that in different patients, the role of hereditary factors (such as transketolase deficiency, which is found in some alcoholic amnesics), thiamin deprivation, nicotinic acid deprivation, the direct effects of alcohol, and other as yet unidentified factors is likely to vary, and such variation may be associated with overlapping, but not identical neuroanatomical damage and memory deficits (Mayes & Meudell, 1983).

Amnesia has sometimes been found in people who have suffered cardiac arrest or temporary periods when there is vascular insufficiency in the brain. In order to gain greater understanding of this syndrome, Volpe, Pulsineli, Tribuna, and Davis (1984) temporarily occluded four major blood vessels supplying the brain in rats. The animals survived the insult, but showed an impairment on a spatial learning task likely to be affected by hippocampal lesions. On histological examination, they were found to have suffered severe loss of neurons in the CA1 region of the hippocampus and in the striatum of the basal ganglia. This damage is similar to that Volpe and his colleagues have noted in some human cases of cardiac arrest, and it should be remembered that the patient studied by Squire and his colleagues (see Squire, 1986), who suffered a hypotensive episode whilst undergoing open-heart surgery, was also reported to have had very similar damage. Lesions that are confined to the CA1 field of the hippocampus are particularly interesting; Volpe, Holtzman, and Hirst (1986) have reported that patients with predominantly CA1 lesions show very poor recall in the face of much more normal recognition. They have also reported that forgetting, tested by recall, is lost pathologically fast in such patients, whereas this does not apply to recognition. The animal model may be a means of checking and extending this work.

Animal models of organic amnesia

Early attempts to model organic amnesia in animals were not successful. As interest was focused at the time on the case of H. M. and it was believed that his syndrome was probably caused by hippocampal resection, the animal studies concentrated on the effects of this lesion. Some of the monkey studies were, however, deliberately modelled on H. M.'s surgery, so their apparent failure to demonstrate amnesia cannot be explained simply in terms of the lesion being inadequate. There are three major possible reasons why animal and human studies might appear incongruent. First, there have been evolutionary changes in limbic–diencephalic structures, which would mean that this system has a unique role in human memory. Second, the tests given to animals were inappropriate ones in the early studies, in the sense that one would have expected human amnesics to perform normally on them as well. Third, the early animal lesions were usually too small or in the wrong structures. All three explanations might, of course, apply to some extent. If, however, the first is too important a factor, there would be little chance to see whether the second two explanations can account for the discrepancies found in the earlier studies.

It is well known that human amnesics perform badly on tests of recognition and recall, but may show normal learning and retention of conditioning, skills, and priming. Thus a minimal requirement of an animal model of amnesia should be that the animals perform poorly on tests that, it is likely, tap recognition or recall, and are unimpaired at most skill learning and conditioning tasks. Despite the failure of early studies to model amnesia by giving hippocampal lesions, Gaffan (1974) reported that when the fornix of juvenile monkeys was transected, the animals were impaired on a recognition task, although they performed normally on a test of associative memory. The former task involved delayed matching-to-sample with trial unique objects. The monkeys were shown objects, which were then removed from sight for a given delay; after the delay, the first object was shown with another object, which had never been seen before. Animals were rewarded for picking the object they had just seen. Test objects were not shown on more than one trial. The monkeys were impaired at delays of longer than a few seconds and when lists of objects were used. For the associative task, monkeys were repeatedly shown some objects that were presented with reward and other objects that were not. The animals learnt to distinguish between rewarded and non-rewarded objects normally.

Gaffan's study suggested that fornix lesions can produce an amnesic-like state with poor recognition and normal performance on a task that might be regarded as akin to conditioning or skill learning. Lack of recognition after delays of more than a few seconds would be expected, as it is also found with human amnesics. Unfortunately, it is impossible to be absolutely sure that animal tasks tap the same processes that are tapped by human tasks, even when the two are formally equivalent, because humans may approach such tasks with strategies based on verbal skills that are unavailable to animals. If the above interpretation of Gaffan's study is correct, then selective lesions of the hippocampus and its Papez circuit connections should be sufficient to cause amnesia. There is, however, considerable controversy about the meaning of Gaffan's findings. First, subsequent work has shown that fornix-transected monkeys are not normal on all associative tasks (Gaffan et al., 1984). When rewards are paired with some objects but not others, the lesioned animals have great difficulty in following the rule of choosing objects not previously associated with reward. This result raises in acute form the questions of what determines normal performance in fornix-lesioned monkeys and, specifically, whether the kinds of associative tasks used by Gaffan can be equated with the memory tasks that human amnesics would perform normally.

Second, and more seriously, there is controversy about the severity of the recognition deficit in fornix-lesioned monkeys. Although other studies have reported such deficits in animals with these lesions, they have not usually been as great as those initially found by Gaffan (see Bachevalier, Saunders, & Mishkin, 1985). In one study by Owen and Butler (1981), an impairment was revealed only if lesioned monkeys had some degree of familiarity with all the stimuli used. In other words, the monkeys could tell whether they had seen stimuli before, but they could not judge which of two familiar stimuli they had seen more recently. This result is consistent with the possibility that the monkeys had a deficit in making temporal judgements, but not in recognition *per se*. Zola-Morgan, Dabrousska, Moss, & Mahut (1983) have also argued that fornix lesions do not cause a recognition impairment. They found that fornix lesions caused a motivational change so that animals showed enhanced preference for novelty. This change might perhaps affect animals' recognition performance.

Bachevalier, Parkinson, and Mishkin (1985) have compared the effects of isolated lesions of the fornix or of the pathways between the amygdala and the thalamus with those of combined lesions. They examined recognition by using a variant of the task employed by Gaffan (1974). In this delayed non-matching-to-sample task, animals have to choose a novel object in preference to one they have just seen, a task that they find easier to learn than delayed matching-to-sample. Sectioning the pathways individually had only a small and unreliable effect, whereas the combined transection caused a severe deficit. In further work, Mishkin and his colleagues have tried to identify why their results and Gaffan's were different. Once again, they found that fornix transections caused only a small recognition impairment and that testing with juvenile monkeys and with a delayed matching-to-sample task (as in Gaffan's experiment) made no difference. As Gaffan has shown that fornix-lesioned animals have difficulty coping with rapidly shifting demands and, in his experiments, different delays and lists were intermixed respectively within sessions and across short blocks of sessions in a way not replicated by Mishkin and his colleagues, this testing procedure may explain the discrepant results. There is also evidence that more prolonged retraining on the task reduces deficits in fornix-lesioned animals. The evidence therefore suggests that these lesions have a minor effect on recognition in monkeys.

This minor effect of fornix lesions on recognition was consistent with an earlier

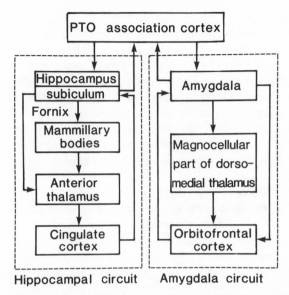

Figure 7.1 A schematic illustration of Mishkin's (1982) two-circuit hypothesis. He postulates that amnesia is far more severe if there is damage to both hippocampal and amygdalar circuits. The circuits process information that they receive from the association neocortex and feed back the results of their processing to the neocortex. As will be apparent from the text, many connections, including those between the two circuits, are not illustrated. The importance of these other connections for recognition is an important issue.

result of Mishkin (1978), who had found that lesions of the hippocampus or amygdala alone had very little effect on delayed non-matching-to-sample performance in monkeys, whereas combined lesions of these two structures had a disproportionately great effect. The results of this initial study triggered Mishkin's (1982) two-circuit hypothesis, which is illustrated in Figure 7.1. More recently, Aggleton (personal communication) has found similar results with rats using an analogue of the delayed non-matching-to-sample task. Whereas hippocampal or amygdalar lesions alone appear not to have affected recognition, combined lesions did. Aggleton has also been able to show that human alcoholic amnesics are impaired at a very similar delayed matching-to-sample task using difficult-to-verbalize pictures.

   One rival to Mishkin's two-circuit hypothesis, as well as to the view that hippocampal lesions alone can cause amnesia, was the temporal stem hypothesis of Horel (1978). In order to discriminate between the temporal stem and the two-circuit hypotheses, Zola-Morgan, Squire, and Mishkin (1982) compared performance of monkeys with temporal stem (see chapter 6) and conjoint hippocampal and amygdalar lesions on two memory tasks. On a delayed non-matching-to-sample task, the animals with conjoint lesions were markedly impaired, with delays of 15 sec or longer, whereas the animals with temporal stem lesions performed at a level almost identical with that of control animals. The second task required the learning of simple pattern discriminations. On this task, the animals with temporal stem lesions were massively impaired, whereas those with conjoint lesions performed practically as well as their controls. The authors argued that the animals with temporal stem lesions performed badly on this task because of disturbed visual information processing, caused by damage to the afferents and efferents of the visual regions of the temporal association cortex. Conjoint lesion animals were not impaired because the pattern discrimination may have tapped the same processes as are involved with skill acquisition. The double dissociation clearly provides strong support for the conjoint lesion hypothesis of amnesia, is consistent with the hippocampal hypothesis, and indicates that the temporal stem view is incorrect.

Squire and Zola-Morgan (1985) have reported that monkeys with conjoint lesions are impaired on three tasks in addition to delayed non-matching-to-sample. These tasks involved delayed retention of object discriminations (monkeys learnt which objects were associated with reward and were tested after a 48-hour delay), the concurrent learning of object discriminations (monkeys had to learn which members of eight pairs of junk objects were associated with reward when the trials with the different pairs were intermingled), and a delayed-response task (the animals saw food placed under one of two wells, which were then withdrawn from view during a delay that could be filled with distraction, after which they could try to retrieve the food from the correct well). It was argued that these tasks were sensitive to the lesions because human amnesics are particularly affected by tests after long delays, especially when the retention interval is filled with distractions. The fact that the impairments were striking with delays that were only a few seconds long when the interval was filled with distraction corresponds well with our knowledge that amnesia in humans affects memory only after attention has been withdrawn from material to be remembered. The impairments also affected memory for all categories of information tested – that is, memory for objects, memory for spatial positions, and memory for associations between objects and rewards – as would be expected from our knowledge of human amnesia. Work from Mishkin's laboratory also indicates that recognition impairments are not confined to visual stimuli, but apply to tactile stimuli as well.

Whereas monkeys with conjoint hippocampal and amygdalar lesions were found to be poor at the tasks just discussed, they have been shown to acquire a couple of motor tasks normally (see Squire & Zola-Morgan, 1985). One of these tasks required the monkeys to reach through a barrier and manipulate a breadstick into a position so that it could be taken back through the barrier unbroken and then eaten. The other task involved moving a sweet with a hole in the middle (Lifesaver, or an American Polo) along a rod with two right-angled bends. The experimenters also confirmed that these animals could learn a relatively difficult pattern discrimination fairly normally, although they were very impaired at learning object discriminations that normal monkeys could learn in a few trials. It was argued that discrimination learning has two components: one procedural, and one declarative (to use their terminology). First, animals must learn how the two stimuli differ and which of these differences are relevant to the task. This ability is acquired gradually over a large number of trials and may be a form of procedural memory preserved in amnesics. Second, animals must identify which stimuli are associated with reward, knowledge that is acquired relatively rapidly, except in amnesics. Object discriminations, which take 20 to 30 trials to learn, presumably depend mainly on the second kind of memory, whereas pattern discriminations, which take 200 to 300 trials to learn, depend mainly on the first kind of memory. Although this argument requires further support, there is good evidence that conjoint hippocampal and amygdalar lesions provide a close model of human amnesia.

Indeed, Saunders, Murray, and Mishkin (1984) have argued that not only is conjoint damage necessary to produce a severe recognition deficit, but the deficit's extent is directly related to the amount of conjoint damage. They compared monkeys' performance on a delayed matching-to-sample task after either bilateral hippocampal and unilateral amygdalar removal or bilateral amygdalar and unilateral hippocampal removal. Over delays that ranged from 10 sec to 2 min, the groups averaged, respectively, 75% and 80% correct. Earlier studies had shown that performance following selective lesions of these structures averaged 91%, whereas after complete conjoint lesions, it fell to 60% correct. The experimenters discussed the human neurosurgical literature and showed that this corresponds well with their own findings with the monkeys; that is, humans with bilateral hippocampal and unilateral amygdalar resections perform on recognition tests at a level intermediate between that of controls and that of the patient H. M., who had a complete conjoint lesion. They therefore argued that at least with respect to recognition, the hippocampal and amygdalar lesions play a more or less equal role.

Although Squire and Zola-Morgan (1985) agree with Mishkin that the conjoint hippocampal and amygdalar lesion produces a good model of amnesia, they are less confident that the two selective lesions have equal effects on recognition and about the kind of damage that is actually critical with the amygdalar lesion. Initially, they argued that conjoint lesions were more likely to damage anterior hippocampus than were isolated lesions of the hippocampus, so that the conjoint lesions' effects might be greater because they involve more hippocampal damage, rather than because they also damage the amygdala. They now accept, however, that this argument cannot be correct, because even in animals in which hippocampal lesions have histologically been confirmed to be complete, recognition impairments were not as great as those in animals with conjoint lesions. More recently, however, Squire, Zola-Morgan, and Amaral have found that when isolated lesions of the amygdala are made by a radio-frequency lesion maker so that any cortical damage is minimized, animals were not impaired on the delayed non-matching-to-sample task, even at a 10-min delay (see Squire & Zola-Morgan, 1985). The usual method of lesioning the amygdala with conjoint lesions involves a frontotemporal surgical approach, which also causes damage to temporal cortex structures overlying the hippocampus and projecting to it, as well as to other brain regions. This lesion does cause a small, but significant impairment on the delayed non-matching-to-sample task. Although this finding suggests that it is cortical rather than amygdalar damage that aggravates the effect on recognition found after hippocampal lesions alone, this idea needs to be directly tested by examining the effects on recognition of conjoint lesions where amygdalar lesions are made with the radio-frequency lesion maker. On the whole, the human evidence suggests that lesions confined to the hippocampus do cause a mild disturbance of memory, whereas amygdalar lesions do not. Further evidence that Mishkin has gathered on the effects of lesions to other parts of the hippocampal and amygdalar circuits does, however, provide some support for a role of the amygdala itself. This evidence will now be considered.

It has already been mentioned that Bachevalier, Parkinson, and Mishkin (1985) reported that separate transections of the fornix and pathways connecting the amygdala to the medial thalamus cause only mild recognition deficits, whereas combined lesions have a very serious effect. Although there is evidence that hippocampal and fornix lesions do not have identical effects, this finding does support Mishkin's view that hippocampal lesions alone will not have a dramatic effect on recognition memory [in agreement with the observations of Volpe and his colleagues (1986), who found only a mild recognition deficit in human patients]. Unlike animals with conjoint hippocampal and amygdalar lesions, those with both tracts cut quickly relearnt what the delayed non-matching-to-sample task involved; that is, they quickly grasped again what they were supposed to be doing in the task. The experimenters suggested that this difference might have been related to the fact that the tract operation was done in two stages rather than because of the difference in lesion location. Despite this mild effect on relearning the task, however, recognition following a delay was almost as bad as that caused by conjoint hippocampal and amygdalar lesions. The experimenters argued that this finding supported their view that amygdalar damage plays a critical role in amnesia caused by medial temporal lobe lesions.

As well as to the mammillary bodies, the fornix sends projections to the anterior nucleus of the thalamus, which it also indirectly influences via the mammillary bodies. It is also known that almost all regions of the amygdala project to the dorsomedial nucleus of the thalamus, with the greatest number of projections being to the most medial, magnocellular part of this nucleus. These projections from the amygdala are either direct or indirect via the bed nucleus of the stria terminals. Human studies had indicated that large thalamic lesions that included the anterior and dorsomedial nuclei caused amnesia, so Aggleton and Mishkin (1983a) tested to see whether similar lesions in monkeys impaired delayed non-matching-to-sample performance. Although the lesioned monkeys relearnt the task with short delays, they were seriously impaired when the length of the delay was increased. There was no effect on the learning of pattern discriminations or of a spatial delayed-response task, which are also not affected by conjoint hippocampal and amygdalar lesions. In a follow-up to this study, Aggleton and Mishkin (1983b) lesioned monkeys medially either in the anterior thalamus or posteriorly in the dorsomedial thalamic nucleus, thus separately compromising the projections of the hippocampal and amygdalar circuits. These lesions produced moderate deficits on the delayed non-matching-to-sample task and on tests of object reward association learning. Comparison with the results from the larger medial thalamic lesion suggested that a severe amnesia was produced only if there was damage to both the thalamic sites that received amygdalar and direct and indirect hippocampal projections.

Aggleton and Mishkin (1983b) argued that the mild amnesic effects of the posterior thalamic lesions were probably caused by the damage to the magnocellular part of the dorsomedial thalamic nucleus rather than to the adjacent nuclei, such as the centre median, which were affected more variably. Evidence suggests that posterior dorsomedial thalamic lesions have more severe effects on recognition than do anterior dorsomedial thalamic lesions. The anterior lesion not only damaged the anterior thalamic nucleus, but also consistently produced degeneration in the mammillary bodies. In a later study, therefore, Aggleton and Mishkin (1985) destroyed the mammillary bodies bilaterally in a group of monkeys that were then tested on the delayed non-matching-to-sample task. Although the lesioned animals were impaired at relearning the task after the post-operative recovery period, they were not significantly impaired at delays up to 2-min long when they had relearnt what the task was about. They did, however, show a consistent trend towards impairment. The experimenters concluded that mammillary body lesions probably do cause a mild recognition deficit, basing this conclusion on their own results and previous work, which found significant deficits in the most difficult conditions of two similar object and picture recognition tests after mammillary body lesions. This conclusion has been more recently strengthened by the finding that conjointly lesioning the mammillary bodies and the bed nucleus of the stria terminalis (both nuclei on the undirect route between limbic system and thalamus) caused a recognition deficit, whereas either lesion alone had a minimal effect (Saunders & Mishkin, 1987).

The anterior thalamus projects to the cingulate cortex, and the magnocellular part of the dorsomedial thalamic nucleus projects to parts of the orbitofrontal cortex and the anterior cingulate. The combined cingulate and orbitofrontal region is sometimes referred to as ventromedial frontal cortex (Figure 7.2). Mishkin and Bachevalier (1983) compared a complete lesion of this region with one of the dorsolateral frontal cortex. Monkeys with the latter lesion were slightly impaired at relearning the delayed non-matching-to-sample task to criterion, with a delay of 10 sec between seeing an object and having memory for it tested. In striking contrast, animals with ventromedial lesions were severely impaired and did not properly succeed in reattaining the criterion. It was concluded that whereas the effects of the dorsolateral frontal lesions on performance in this and other tasks might be partly caused by a problem with spatial relations, the ventromedial frontal lesion had a more direct effect on recognition. Both these suggestions are speculative and require much more support. It has already been indicated that relearning what the delayed non-matching-to-sample task is about may not be a

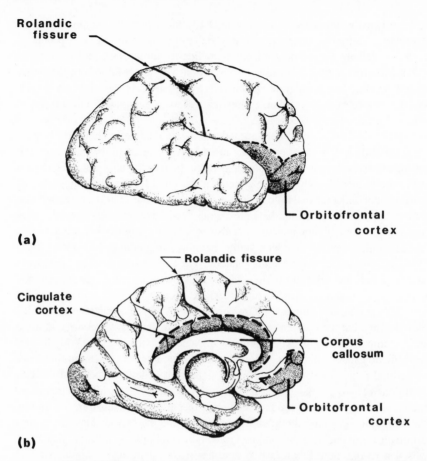

(a)

(b)

Figure 7.2 The location of the ventromedial frontal cortex, comprising cingulate and orbitofrontal cortex. (a) A lateral view of the right hemisphere showing the orbitofrontal cortex, but not the more medial cingulate cortex. (b) A medial view of the left hemisphere showing both structures.

form of learning affected by amnesia. It would be useful to determine whether animals with ventromedial frontal lesions are still impaired when the object to be remembered and the two choice objects are presented at the same time. Under these circumstances, an impairment would probably indicate a learning problem unrelated to recognition because the recognition load would have been reduced to zero. This issue raises in acute form the difficulty of determining whether an animal is showing a recognition deficit or some other problem that does not characterize human amnesics. Evidence from comparable lesions in humans would be valuable, but there are no reliable reports on the effects on recognition of ventromedial frontal cortex lesions, although there are scattered reports of transient, amnesic attacks following cingulate cortex lesions (see Mayes & Meudell, 1983).

It has been shown in one case that difficulty in relearning the delayed non-

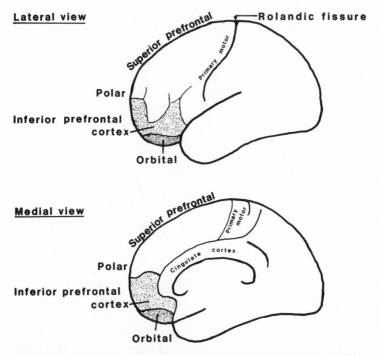

Figure 7.3 The location of inferior frontal cortex is illustrated, particularly in relation to the structures of the ventromedial prefrontal cortex. The upper drawing gives a lateral view of the left hemisphere, and the lower drawing gives a medial view of the right hemisphere.

matching-to-sample task was not caused by a recognition impairment. Kowalska, Bachevalier, and Mishkin (1984) lesioned another frontal lobe region, the inferior prefrontal cortex (Figure 7.3), which receives a projection from the more laterally placed parvocellular division of the dorsomedial thalamic nucleus. Animals were given lesions of the inferior prefrontal cortex, and after a 2-week post-operative recovery period, they were retrained on the non-matching task. They needed a very large number of trials to reattain the criterion with a 10-sec delay, but once they had done so, they performed within the normal range with longer delays and longer lists of objects. It was argued that their slowness in reattaining the criterion was caused by the perseverative tendencies that this lesion produces. This interpretation was supported by the observation that the monkeys had very strong position preferences throughout the period when they were having trouble reattaining the criterion. It is compatible with Mishkin's (1982) view that the magnocellular, but not the parvocellular, division of the dorsomedial thalamic nucleus forms part of the amygdalar circuit, lesions to which cause severe, permanent amnesia. It also agrees with the conclusion reached in chapter 5 that most frontal cortex lesions influence learning only because they disturb planning processes.

The literature reviewed so far suggests that Mishkin's hypothesis warrants serious consideration. There is evidence that combined lesions at a number of points on the hippocampal and amygdalar circuits lead to more severe recognition failures than does damage to either circuit alone. At the level of the hippocampus and amygdala, however, there is still uncertainty about what kinds of damage are responsible for the deficits in recognition. There is some evidence that hippocampal lesions may be more important than amygdalar ones and that lesions of temporal cortex that overlies the hippocampus may also play a role. At the level of the frontal cortex, it has not been convincingly demonstrated that ventromedial frontal lesions seriously impair recognition as opposed to a form of learning that may not be impaired in amnesics. Furthermore, the effects on delayed non-matching-to-sample tasks of isolated cingulate and orbitofrontal lesions also need to be examined, as such lesions might be expected to cause mild recognition deficits if Mishkin is correct. The problems with interpreting the effects of the ventromedial frontal lesions indicate that it is often difficult in non-verbal species to identify the cause of a performance deficit. Certainly, evidence from human patients with a variety of frontal lobe lesions does not support the view that any such lesion seriously compromises recognition.

The non-matching task has also been given to monkeys with damage in the basal forebrain. In an initial study, the neurotoxin ibotenic acid was used to produce lesions in the nucleus basalis of Meynert, the part of the basal forebrain that sends cholinergic projections to both neocortex and amygdala. Although there was no impairment, the animals proved to be more sensitive to the mnemonically disruptive effects of the anticholinergic drug scopolamine. Aigner et al. (1984) compared these animals and their controls with others that had been lesioned in the diagonal band of Broca and the medial septum, the parts of the basal forebrain that send cholinergic projections to the hippocampus. Another group of monkeys were given lesions in all basal forebrain sites. Only the last group was reported to be impaired on the recognition task. This finding supports the idea that basal forebrain atrophy may contribute to the memory problems shown by Alzheimer patients. The presence of such damage in Alzheimer patients is not itself convincing, because they also have damage in many other regions, including the hippocampus. The finding that only lesions to all three cholinergic basal forebrain structures impair recognition also provides support for the dual-circuit hypothesis (Mishkin, 1982) because severe recognition deficits were reported only after lesions that disrupted the input to both hippocampus and amygdala, so that the activity of both structures was disturbed. It does not, however, prove that the critical disruption is of the cholinergic input to these structures because both electrolytic and ibotenic acid lesions destroy not only cholinergic neurons in the basal forebrain, but also neurons that release other transmitters.

In chapter 1, it was noted that both the hippocampus and the amygdala receive inputs of processed sensory information from association neocortex. The striate cortex, which is the primary visual receiving area of the neocortex, sends its outputs that fan out into the more anterior prestriate cortex, where different regions separately encode such visually identified attributes as shape, size, colour, and texture. This information may then be integrated by even more anterior regions of PTO association cortex, such as the inferotemporal cortex, where object perception may be achieved. The prestriate cortex also sends projections to parietal regions of PTO association cortex, which may achieve some kind of spatial representation of the objects identified by the inferotemporal cortex. Mishkin's argument is that a newly perceived object leaves a lasting effect on inferotemporal neurons once they have triggered the dual cortico-limbic-diencephalic-frontal circuit. The result is some kind of strengthening of the prestriate–inferotemporal connections that encode and store a memory of what was perceived. Lesioning studies on the inferotemporal cortex have theoretical significance for Mishkin (see Mishkin, 1982). They also have methodological significance in relation to the non-matching tasks.

Mishkin (1982) lesioned two regions of the inferotemporal cortex in monkeys (see Figure 1.1): the more posterior region, TEO, which perhaps is important in visually based shape perception. This information is sent to other regions, including TE, which integrates shape and other visual information into a representation of a perceived object. After a 2-week recovery period, the animals were retrained. Group TE took many more trials than group TEO and the control groups, and still after 1,500 trials none of its members had fully reattained the criterion of 90% correct performance at 10-sec delay. With delays between 10 sec and 2 min, group TE monkeys deteriorated far faster than control animals as soon as the delays became longer than 10 sec. The TEO animals performed normally with delays up to 2 min. When, however, they were given increasingly long lists of objects to remember, they also showed an impairment of intermediate severity. Mishkin therefore argued that the TEO monkeys' poor performance reflected a failure in shape discrimination. The animals could still distinguish the to-be-remembered object's colour, size, and texture; with normal recognition memory, this was sufficient for them to distinguish the to-be-remembered object from the novel one at test. When lists of objects were presented, however, successful discrimination may depend critically on shape perception, so performance dropped significantly. As the deficit of the TE animals was apparent even when objects were presented and tested one at a time, it was argued that the deficit was probably caused by a severe recognition impairment.

If area TE stores representations of visually presented objects, then lesions to it probably disturb not only storage, but also the final stages of encoding for such representations. Precisely this has been argued by Gaffan et al. (1985). They compared the effects of inferotemporal lesions on the learning of a serial-reversal task, in which the reward associations of two very familiar objects were repeatedly changed, and an object discrimination learning set task, in which animals had to learn to discriminate many pairs of objects. As the monkeys were impaired on only the latter task, the experimenters suggested that the lesion had disrupted the ability to identify visual stimuli. The disruption might have resulted because the lesion restricts the number of visual attributes that animals can access (this is like a generalized version of Mishkin's account of TEO lesions). This restriction does not apply to visuospatial attributes (as would be expected from what has been said above) because another experiment showed that the animals could still discriminate the direction in which a figure was pointing. If this interpretation of the TE lesion is correct, it must be possible for a perceptual deficit to impair performance on the delayed non-matching-to-sample task. This seems particularly likely, given the TE-lesioned animals' great difficulty in relearning the task even with a minimal delay. In processing terms, if a stimulus is poorly encoded, then it may be rapidly forgotten. With a zero delay, however, the monkeys with TE lesions may be able to encode sufficient visual attributes to perform within normal limits. This possibility needs to be tested.

Area TE sends projections to both hippocampus and amygdala within the limbic system of the medial temporal lobe. If storage of information necessary for visual recognition requires the flow of information through the dual circuits, then disconnecting area TE from underlying limbic structures should cause a severe deficit on the non-matching task. In an ingenious experiment, Mishkin (1982) lesioned the hippocampus and amygdala on one side of the brain and area TE on the other side. The animals that were given this crossed lesion were impaired on the recognition task, but performed better than animals with conjoint hippocampal and amygdalar lesions. Mishkin argued that this lesion is less devastating than a bilateral conjoint hippocampal and amygdalar lesion because visual information can still reach the spared hippocampus and amygdala on one hemisphere from the spared area TE on the other hemisphere via the intact anterior commissure (a fibre tract within the temporal lobes that connects parts of the right and left hemispheres). A second group of animals received the same lesion, but also had resections of their anterior commissures. The resection prevented visual information from passing from the intact area TE of one hemisphere to the intact medial temporal limbic structures of the other hemisphere. This group of animals performed very little better than monkeys with conjoint hippocampal and amygdalar lesions. The implication of Mishkin's crossed-lesion and disconnection design study is that the normal function of the limbic system structures in visual recognition memory depends on their receiving processed visual information from area TE. The design is very elegant because it allows one to draw this implication from the cross-hemisphere disconnection when it would be far harder to sever the intrahemispheric links between area TE and the limbic system structures.

The effects of Mishkin's (1982) disconnection experiment are consistent with the interpretation offered in chapter 6 for some cases of material-specific amnesia, in which there appeared to be cortical damage rather than direct damage to the limbic system. Such lesions may disconnect cortical regions concerned with the processing of specific kinds of attributes from the limbic system circuits essential for recognition and recall. How specific are the cortico-limbic connections? There is increasing evidence that the cerebral cortex comprises a large number of vertically organized units, some of which are roughly columnar in shape, identified by their input–output relations and by their internal synaptic connections. It has been suggested that these columns are the basic operating units of the cerebral cortex,

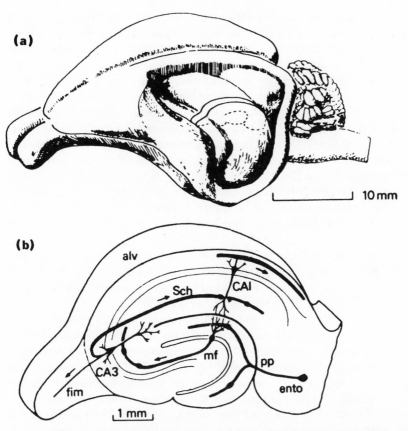

Figure 7.4 The lamellar organization of the hippocampus in the rabbit's brain. (a) A lateral view of the brain with the parietal and temporal cortices removed so as to expose the hippocampal formation. The lamellar slice indicated is presented separately in (b) to show the circuitry involved, alv refers to alveus; ento, entorhinal cortex; fim, fimbria; pp, perforant path; Sch, Schaffer collateral. (From Gray J. A., *The neuropsychology of anxiety*. Oxford University Press. Copyright 1982.)

and, if so, the circuitry of the columnar modules should provide constraints on how information is processed within the association cortex as well as primary sensory cortex (where the columns were first identified). It has been speculated by Phillips, Zeki, and Barlow (1984) that these processing modules may share an abstract function, involving the formation of new associations between the informational components that they process. These basic columnar modules, comprising perhaps 10^3 to 10^4 neurons, may be organized into larger units, corresponding to the kinds of module considered in chapter 1. Each basic columnar module processes and stores a specific kind of informational attribute. It has been speculated that the basic modules themselves consist of smaller components, containing 30 to 100 neurons, within which the neurons are equivalent in that they process and store exactly the same information (see Squire, 1987). Goldman-Rakic (1984) has traced projections from the prefrontal cortex to the hippocampal region and found that cortex overlying the hippocampus is also organized in a columnar fashion. She argued that the pattern of termination may relate to the way the hippocampus is organized into slices, or lamellae, at right angles to its long axis (Figure 7.4). Each lamella has its own input–output relationships and can operate in parallel with other lamellae. On the basis of this and other evidence, Goldman-Rakic proposed that each prefrontal column may be uniquely connected with a hippocampal lamella, and speculated that this relationship may also apply to all cortical inputs to the hippocampus. If different hippocampal lamellae are specifically linked to particular cortical columns, then the implications for the role of the hippocampus in recognition are considerable. The proposal is, however, speculative, and in contrast to it, Halgren (1984) has suggested that cortico-hippocampal and cortico-amygdalar links may be randomly convergent and divergent, consistent with his idea that the limbic system integrates previously unconnected cortically processed information.

One implication of the possible specificity of cortico-hippocampal connections is that each hippocampal lamella should be concerned with recognition and recall of highly specific kinds of information that have been processed in their cortical projection areas. How the hippocampus performs this service is not, however, immediately apparent! Even so, it may become possible to develop model systems composed of a few hippocampal lamellae and the cortical regions that project to them, and to record changes in the activity of their neurons during the acquisition of recognition for appropriate material. Mishkin's (1982) hypothesis gives an equal role in recognition to the amygdalar circuit. Slightly less is currently known about the details of cortical projections to this structure. What can be said of both hippocampus and amygdala is that they receive projections from both posterior and frontal association cortices, and that there are reciprocal projections back to the cortex from both structures. It would seem, then, that both these 'memory structures' receive inputs about the kinds of information for which recognition and recall are disturbed in amnesics.

One topic that has been conspicuously absent in this section on animal models of amnesia is that of retrograde amnesia. The reason is that there has been hardly any experimental work on the problem. It is important that there should be such work not only to establish that the models completely reproduce the human syndrome, but also for two other reasons: to determine more precisely the conditions under which temporally graded retrograde amnesia is found, and to determine whether anterograde and retrograde amnesia can occur as separate syndromes and, if so, what lesions are responsible for the syndromes. The first aim could be better achieved with animals than with humans not only because lesions can be specified exactly, but also because the degree of rehearsal of the information to be remembered can probably be more easily controlled. Animals can be trained to exactly the same extent on each item to be remembered, and the items can be selected so that they are unlikely to be subsequently rehearsed. In other words, it should be possible to create memories that differ only with respect to how long before lesioning they were acquired. If the resultant retrograde amnesia was not graded, tasks could be selected so that rehearsal was greater in proportion to an item's age in memory.

Three relevant studies have been done using rats, and one has involved monkeys. In the first, Winocur (1985) found results suggestive of a temporally graded retrograde amnesia. Rats were exposed to a demonstrator rat that had just been fed a special diet. Exposure to olfactory cues emanating from such demonstrator rats gives the exposed rats a preference for the special diet eaten by the demonstrator. At various stages after their exposure, the rats were given hippocampal lesions. Whereas the control rats remembered the preference best immediately after exposure, next best after a delay of 19 days, and worst after a delay of 24 days, the hippocampally lesioned rats showed the opposite trend. Tested 14 days after surgery, they remembered least about preferences acquired immediately before surgery, and progressively more about preferences acquired 5 and 10 days before it. Even at the longest delay, however, their performance was not normal. The hippocampal lesions also caused anterograde amnesia for this task, although it is difficult to imagine what would be an equivalent task in humans! The second study involved training eight monkeys on five sets of 20 two-choice object discrimination problems (Salmon, Zola-Morgan, & Squire, 1987). Different sets were given 32, 16, 8, 4, and 2 weeks prior to bilateral hippocampal and amygdala removals that were performed on four of the animals. Six weeks before surgery, all the monkeys were also trained on the 'American Polo', or 'Lifesaver', motor skill task, in which they had to manoeuvre a Polo-like sweet along a bent metal rod. Training on the five sets of object discriminations had been shown to be about equal by testing retention 1 day after the acquisition of each set. Three weeks after the operation, remote memory was tested in all the animals by giving a single trial with each of the 100 object pairs. Although the control animals showed little evidence of forgetting even the earliest learnt discriminations, the lesioned animals were profoundly amnesic for the discriminations learnt in all the time periods, presumably evincing little sign of sparing of the oldest memories. In contrast, memory for the motor skill was relatively well retained in both groups. The failure of this study to find clear evidence of temporally graded retrograde amnesia contrasts with the results of Winocur. The second study was, however, performed on a species whose brain organization is more similar to that of humans, and it also seems likely that the different-age memories may have been equally learnt and *rehearsed* (although this may also have been true of Winocur's study). If this is so, then Salmon et al.'s study supports the view, expressed in chapter 6, that temporally graded amnesias are found only when older memories have been more rehearsed than newer ones. It would be interesting to see whether temporally graded retrograde amnesia would be found if the experiment was repeated so that the amount of rehearsal was in proportion to the age of a memory.

Both these experiments involved fairly extensive lesions (although Winocur lesioned only the hippocampus, which may possibly explain why he found graded amnesia, as inclusion of amygdalar damage might have abolished the temporal gradient). The other two studies were different because they involved smaller lesions to the hippocampus or its inputs and did not produce any detectable retrograde amnesia. In the more recent of these two studies, Staubli, Fraser, Kessler, and Lynch (1986) found that small entorhinal cortex lesions that disconnected olfactory inputs from their hippocampal targets caused an anterograde amnesia for an olfactory discrimination learning task in the experimental rats, but did not cause measurable retrograde amnesia for the same task, even when it had been learnt only 1 hour before the lesion had been made. In the earlier of the two studies, Jarrard (1980) reported that lesions confined to the CA1 field of the hippocampus impair only acquisition of complex tasks without affecting retention of pre-operatively acquired ones. The suggestion that this lesion may cause a selective anterograde amnesia clearly needs more rigorous examination. It does, however, relate interestingly to what was found with a human case, discussed in chapter 6, in whom damage was confined to the CA1 field (see Squire, 1986). This man showed moderately severe anterograde amnesia, but little, if any, retrograde amnesia. If appropriate toxins can be found to selectively impair the CA1 field of the hippocampus in animals, or if the temporary anoxia caused by carotid artery occlusion proves to generate a sufficiently confined CA1 lesion, it would be important to see whether lesioned animals show no signs of retrograde amnesia even with more sensitive tests. Both Jarrard's and Staubli et al.'s findings are tantalizing because they suggest that isolated anterograde amnesia may be caused by lesions confined to parts of the hippocampus or its inputs. But it will clearly be necessary to show that these effects occur in primates as well as in rodents and that they are found with kinds of memory likely to be affected in human amnesics.

One further use of the monkey model of organic amnesia is illustrated by the work of Mishkin and his colleagues. They have shown that monkeys fail to achieve adult performance levels on the delayed non-matching-to-sample task until they are nearly 2 years old, whereas at 3 months of age, they are as good as adults at learning certain kinds of discrimination problems (Mishkin, Malamut, & Bachevalier, 1984). This research suggests that the hippocampal and amygdalar circuits, hypothesized to mediate recognition, may take years to mature, whereas the brain systems that mediate habit memories mature much more quickly. If this suggestion is correct, then maturation of the human recognition system may be even slower, as human development is extended over a longer time than that of the rhesus monkey. Two implications of this idea remain to be properly tested in humans. First, very young children should behave in some ways like organic amnesics and will perhaps continue to do so to a lessening degree until they are perhaps 3 or 4 years of age. Second, the effects of lesions of the limbic–diencephalic structures early in life will not be apparent until several years later. As language can be very rapidly acquired within the first 2 or 3 years of life, it is possible that the *initial* acquisition of language is spared after lesions that cause organic amnesia in adults. Although early language acquisition may be little affected by limbic–diencephalic lesions, it seems likely that, in other ways, early lesions of these structures will cause far more severe impairments of semantic knowledge than are typically found in adult amnesics, and so may cause a far more drastic disruption of the cognitive functions that depend on this knowledge. Indeed, victims of early limbic–diencephalic lesions may well constitute a group of subnormal children. It has been suggested that autism may be caused by early lesions to the limbic structures of the medial temporal lobes, partly because memory deficits have been reported in some children with this disorder (see Mayes & Meudell, 1983), although this is a minority view. Animal models of organic amnesia may be used to test the view that early limbic–diencephalic lesions have delayed effects on recognition that may not become apparent for several years, but that the effects on behaviour may eventually be more devastating than if the same damage occurred later in life. This view should also be tested in humans, as should the idea that early language acquisition is immune to limbic–diencephalic lesions. A recent case report of a child with an anomia for animals may be interesting in this context (Temple, 1986). The child appeared to have learning problems, suggestive of a mild organic amnesia, so the anomia could have resulted from a failure to show normal learning of animal names. Why the learning problem should be relatively selective for animal names is, however, very puzzling and makes it likely that the child's early brain damage may have extended into PTO association neocortex.

The evidence reviewed in this section from monkey models of amnesia gives reasonable support for the proposal that damage to both hippocampal and amygdalar circuits is necessary to the occurrence of severe, permanent amnesia. There is some uncertainty about whether the amygdala and, possibly, other parts of the amygdalar circuit play as important a role in recognition and recall as the hippocampus and, possibly, other parts of the hippocampal circuit, which can be resolved only by painstaking lesion techniques. There is also no strong evidence that the system extends as far as the ventromedial frontal cortex. The circuits contain abundant feedback loops, so it is conceivable that limbic, diencephalic, and ventromedial frontal stages of the circuits make different contributions to recognition and recall. Precisely what these contributions may be will be considered further in the final section, which briefly examines lesion and physiological studies of the regions where lesions produce amnesia. The next section elaborates a little further on the possibility that lesions affecting neurons that release particular transmitters may sometimes be involved in amnesia.

Pharmacological models of amnesia

In chapter 6, some evidence was reviewed that suggests that dysfunctions of cholinergic and noradrenergic neurons may sometimes contribute to organic amnesia, although this disorder is most often caused by damage to limbic–diencephalic structures. The cholinergic neurons lie in the basal forebrain and project widely to neocortex, amygdala, and hippocampus, whereas the critical noradrenergic neurons lie in the locus coeruleus and project widely to neocortical and limbic system structures. It is widely believed that these projections do not transmit specific information to limbic and neocortical structures, but serve to modulate their activity. For example, there is evidence that individual noradrenergic neurons send projections to many forebrain neurons and that the effect of noradrenergic stimulation is to increase a neuron's signal-to-noise ratio, so that it can encode inputs more effectively. There is also some evidence that noradrenergic stimulation of the hippocampus facilitates the development of LTP, which might be expected if the signal-to-noise ratio of hippocampal neurons were improved (see Gold, 1984). It might therefore be postulated that cholinergic modulation of limbic and, possibly, neocortical structures by basal forebrain neurons and different kinds of modulation of these structures by noradrenergic neurons projecting from the locus coeruleus improve the efficiency of the structures that play a central role in recognition and recall. Damage to the basal forebrain or locus coeruleus might, then, be expected to exacerbate an existing amnesia or, possibly, produce a mild amnesia if no other damage was involved.

The human evidence for this hypothesis depends on two kinds of evidence. First, the examination of the brain damage in amnesics to determine whether basal forebrain or locus coeruleus damage might be contributing to the memory failure. Second, studies with drugs that facilitate or inhibit cholinergic or noradrenergic activity in the brain to determine how these drugs affect memory. The first source of evidence is not a particularly strong one. For example, although it is popularly supposed that atrophy of basal forebrain cholinergic neurons is the major cause of the relatively selective amnesia found in the early stages of Alzheimer's disease, brain damage is so widespread that it is very hard to identify what lesions cause the memory deficit in this disease. Many of these patients not only have losses of neurons that use other transmitters, including noradrenalin, but more seriously, compared with elderly matched controls, have massive damage to the perforant pathway (see Figure 6.1). The damage is so extensive that the hippocampus is effectively isolated from its cortical input of processed sensory information about the external world (see Hyman, Van Hoesen, Damasio, & Barnes 1984). The damage was found in end-stage patients (in whom most of the cholinergic deficits have also been identified), but may well be present in early-stage patients with relatively selective amnesias. If this was so, then drugs that boost cholinergic (and, indeed, noradrenergic) activity in the brain would have little effect on memory because they could not reverse the isolation of the hippocampus from its cortical input. It is possible, however, that in elderly Alzheimer patients, atrophy is more confined to the cholinergic basal forebrain. When young and old Alzheimer patients were matched on their dementia rating scores, it was found that the older patients showed much less brain pathology, and that the best correlate of degree of dementia in these older patients was the degree of reduction of choline acetyltransferase, the enzyme necessary for synthesizing acetylcholine, found in high concentrations in the basal forebrain. In these more elderly patients, basal forebrain lesions may, therefore, be somewhat more selective, but the evidence that they provide is still not good enough to conclude confidently that their amnesia is caused by a cholinergic dysfunction. The evidence favouring a role for a noradrenergic dysfunction in amnesia is perhaps a little better. As discussed in chapter 6, it has been shown that a correlation exists between a measure of memory in alcoholic amnesics and the levels of a noradrenergic metabolite in their cerebrospinal fluid, which may indicate that memory is worse in patients with more damage in the locus coeruleus. In my laboratory, it was also found that the more amnesic of two patients differed from the other patient mainly in having more damage to this nucleus and to no other brain region.

The second source of evidence derived from human studies involves pharmacological manipulations of patients and normal subjects. Some of these studies were referred to in chapter 6. Attempts to model amnesia by giving anticholinergic drugs have met with some success (see Drachman, 1977), but the literature abounds with empirical conflicts, which suggests that many important factors are currently being left uncontrolled in such studies. Although there is evidence that anticholinergic drugs disturb new learning and leave measures of short-term memory, such as the digit span, unaffected, until recently there was no evidence about whether the kind of retrograde amnesia seen in organic amnesics is also found. Broadly similar effects on memory in young volunteer subjects have been reported following injections of benzodiazepines, which is interesting because these drugs, like the anticholinergics, may influence activity in limbic system structures as well as other brain regions. Thus Brown, Lewis, Brown, Horn, and Bowes (1982) found that benzodiazepine injections caused anterograde amnesia, but not retrograde amnesia. This absence of retrograde amnesia in the presence of anterograde amnesia has now been reported with anticholinergic drugs, such as scopolamine, as well (Troster, Staton, Rorabaugh, & Beatty, 1987). Retrograde amnesia was assessed with objective questionnaires that tapped memory for remote events. These attempts to produce a drug model of amnesia also face a general problem – that the anticholinergic drugs affect cholinergic neurons other than those in the basal forebrain. It is hard to know the extent to which dysfunction in these other cholinergic neurons contributes to any memory disturbances observed. The matter will be important if it is shown that the memory problems of drugged patients are caused by failures of encoding not found in any organic amnesics. It is interesting to note that the first reports of amnesia caused by anticholinergics came from the maternity clinic, where such drugs were used to induce a 'twilight sleep' state, after recovery from which little was remembered. This may have been because little was encoded during the drug-induced state.

Cholinergic drugs have also been shown to improve memory in young and old normal people. Thus cholinergic agonists, such as arecoline and physostigmine, and cholinergic precursors, such as choline and lecithin, have been found to improve memory in healthy young people, and the agonists arecoline and physostigmine have been shown to improve memory in healthy old people, although the effective dose seems to vary markedly across subjects (see Bartus, Dean, Pontecorvo, & Flicker, 1985). Administration of such drugs to amnesic patients has been largely confined to those with Alzheimer's disease, although there are reports of a favourable effect of physostigmine with two post-encephalitic amnesics (see Catsman-Berrevoets, Van Harskamp, & Appelhof, 1986). This drug is actually known as an anticholinesterase, because it prevents available acetylcholine from being broken down in the synaptic gap by the enzyme acetylcholinesterase. When there are only moderate amounts of the transmitter in the synapse, the effect of an anticholinesterase is to facilitate transmission. The effects of physostigmine on the memory of patients with Alzheimer's disease have generally been disappointing. The acetylcholine precursors choline and lecithin have usually, although not always, been found to be ineffective, at least when given alone, whereas the effects with physostigmine and agents, such as arecoline, that directly stimulate the acetylcholine receptor sites on post-synaptic neurons have been a little more encouraging (see Kopelman, 1986). More recently, the anticholinesterase drug 1, 2, 3, 4, -tetrahydro-9-aminoacridine (THA), which remains active for longer than physostigmine when taken orally, has been reported to produce striking memory improvements in patients in the early stages of Alzheimer's disease (Summers, Majovski, Marsh, Tachiki, & Kling, 1986). If these results can be confirmed, they would provide strong support for the view that damage to cholinergic neurons in the basal forebrain contributes significantly to the memory deficits of Alzheimer patients, at least in the disease's early stages. Currently, however, the case for the view, provided by the effects on patients of cholinergic agonists, such as THA, must be regarded as not proved. When these drugs are ineffective, it may be that patients have damage to the 'memory structures' that are modulated by the cholinergic neurons. They also have low levels of the enzymes needed to manufacture acetylcholine, which may explain why the choline and lecithin precursor treatments have little effect. As these patients show atrophy in neurons that release several different transmitter systems, it has been suggested by more optimistic workers that a cocktail of drugs may have a more beneficial effect.

It is a pity that drugs that facilitate cholinergic activity have not been tried more with amnesic patients, who have less extensive damage than Alzheimer's disease patients and, unlike them, have a non-progressive disease so that assessment of drug effects is somewhat easier. It is nevertheless probable that cholinergic agonists will have somewhat different effects on stable amnesics and normal people because the patients will, in many cases, have sustained damage to the 'memory structures' that are modulated by cholinergic projections from the basal forebrain. Something similar is apparent with drugs that affect noradrenergic activity. In chapter 6, it was mentioned that a drug that affects noradrenergic activity improves certain measures of memory in alcoholic amnesics. This drug, clonidine, is used as an antihypertensive agent. There had been anecdotal reports for a number of years that it causes forgetfulness in the patients who take it to reduce their blood pressure. Frith, Dowdy, Ferrier, and Crow (1985) confirmed these reports by showing that injections of the drug in normal volunteers causes an impairment in learning paired associate words and reduced subjective estimates of arousal.

Why does the drug have opposite effects in normal people and alcoholic amnesics? The answer is not certain, but probably is related to the fact that clonidine is an agonist that stimulates a particular kind of receptor for noradrenalin, the alpha-2-receptor. There are alpha-2-receptors that are pre-synaptically located on neurons that release noradrenalin. When these are activated naturally or by cloni-dine, the release of noradrenalin is inhibited. This action of clonidine in normal people is believed not only to inhibit noradrenalin release, but also to produce sedation and the negative effects on learning. But there are also post-synaptic alpha-2-receptors on neurons that receive noradrenergic inputs. Clonidine also stimulates these receptors, which increases the effectiveness of the noradrenergic inputs, but this effect is overridden in normal people by the drug's action on the pre-synaptic sites. If in alcoholic amnesics, there is relatively selective degenera-tion of the pre-synaptic sites, which lie on the terminals of the locus coeruleus neurons, then the net effect of clonidine should be to increase noradrenergic activity and improve aspects of memory. Although this interesting example is a case where a drug affects amnesics beneficially, but normal subjects negatively, one would expect that cholinergic and noradrenergic agonists should often have less beneficial effects on amnesics than controls if the cholinergic and noradren-ergic dysfunction hypotheses are correct. This is because there should be fewer neurons in the 'memory structures' to benefit from the favourable modulations provided by the drugs.

In many ways, it is easier to study the effects of lesions that are relatively spe-cific to cholinergic and noradrenergic neurons in animals than it is in humans. There have also been many experiments in which cholinergic and noradrener-gic drugs have been used to examine the effects on memory in animals, and in future, it should be increasingly possible to apply these drugs directly to the target brain regions. In addition, animal studies provide a better opportunity to monitor directly biochemical measures of cholinergic and noradrenergic activity in the basal forebrain and locus coeruleus. For example, it has been shown that normally ageing monkeys and rodents develop adverse changes on measures of acetylcho-line synthesis; reduced numbers of acetylcholine receptors, as indicated by the lowered response to acetylcholine of neurons that are sensitive to the transmitter in normal brains; as well as losses of basal forebrain neurons and impairments on various learning tasks (see Bartus et al., 1985). The experiment of Mishkin and his colleagues (Aigner et al., 1984), in which the effects of basal forebrain le-sions on recognition in monkeys was examined, was described in the last section. Their conclusion that lesions confined to the nucleus basalis of Meynert do not in themselves cause a significant memory impairment is, however, still polemical. Bartus and his co-workers have reported that nucleus basalis lesions in rats can cause an impairment in spatial memory when a delay is introduced (see Bartus et al., 1985). The animals had, however, recovered from this deficit in retaining spatial information by 6 months after surgery, although there was no measurable change in acetylcholine function.

One of the most interesting developments in this area has been the use of im-plants of foetal brain tissue to reverse the impairments found in rats with reduced numbers of basal forebrain neurons that occur as a result of either old age or experimental lesions. It has proved possible to reverse some memory problems, of a kind likely to be found in amnesics, by implanting foetal basal forebrain neurons. For example, Gage, Bjorkland, Stenevi, Dunnett, and Kelly (1984) have shown that the learning impairments, but not the motor clumsiness, of aged rats can be reduced by placing grafts of foetal septum into the hippocampus of recipient rats. The grafts have been shown to establish connections with surrounding hippocampal neurons, probably raising the level of cholinergic stimulation that reaches them. The inputs to the grafted septal neurons do not appear to be normal (they are, after all, not in their natural brain location), so this stimulative effect is almost certainly not specific. The effects are, however, probably caused by the implantation of cholinergic neurons, as in a similar study of rats with spatial learning problems caused by lesions of the nucleus basalis of Meynert, learning was improved by cortically placed implants of basal forebrain neurons rich in acetylcholine, but not by similarly placed implants of foetal non-cholinergic hippocampal neurons.

Grafts of foetal cholinergic neurons improve memory in elderly rats, which are known to suffer atrophy of basal forebrain neurons rich in acetylcholine-releasing neurons. Similar grafts also improve memory in rats with experimental lesions of the basal forebrain. These findings provide a strong indication that these cholinergic basal forebrain neurons are important in the kinds of memory mediated by the limbic–diencephalic structures. The grafts are still impure, however, as they contain non-cholinergic neurons from the basal forebrain, so more refined techniques will need to establish more precisely the role of the cholinergic neurons. As implants work in rats, it has been suggested by some that they may work in humans. Indeed, implantation of dopaminergic adrenal medulla cells into the brain has already been tried as a treatment of advanced Parkinsonism. The gap between rat and human is, however, very large. The prospects for treating Alzheimer's disease in this way cannot be very good because even if the technical problems could be overcome, the disease affects many non-cholinergic neurons that mediate recognition and recall, and it is progressive. Treatment will ultimately depend on understanding the processes that cause so many neurons to die. Foetal-tissue grafting might stand more chance of working in patients with relatively selective and non-progressive lesions of the basal forebrain.

An involvement of basal forebrain cholinergic neurons in recognition and recall is, then, supported not only by human data, but also by evidence from animal lesioning and foetal-tissue-graft experiments. Cholinergic agonists and antagonists have also been found to have effects on monkeys and rodents similar to those seen in humans. The possible role of a dysfunction of noradrenergic locus coeruleus neurons has also been pursued in animal studies. Unfortunately, this research has not used learning tasks that tap forms of memory that are known to be impaired in human amnesics. Nevertheless, there is a strong indication that noradrenergic dysfunction does cause certain kinds of memory deficit. Not only do some noradrenergic antagonists impair learning in rodents, but, as Zornetzer and his co-workers have shown, removing the locus coeruleus in rats immediately after training extended the period during which electroconvulsive shock could disrupt memory – up to 168 hours from a normal maximum of about 1 hour (see Zornetzer, 1985). He also found that if middle-aged rats, over a 6-month period, either received electrical stimulation to the locus coeruleus or were regularly given a drug that increased activity in noradrenergic locus coeruleus neurons, their memory for a one-trial passive avoidance task was comparable with that of a group of young rats. According to Zornetzer, elderly rats normally forget faster on a variety of tasks than do younger animals, although they do not show severe learning problems. There is also considerable evidence that elderly animals show reduced activity of noradrenalin in their brains, which is associated with a marked loss of locus coeruleus neurons. Zornetzer and his co-workers have been able to show that the degree of loss of these neurons correlates significantly with how poorly elderly rats remember the passive avoidance task after 1 day. Aged monkeys have also been shown to suffer from memory problems and locus coeruleus atrophy. More interestingly, Arnsten and Goldman-Rakic (1985) have shown that although elderly monkeys' memory for a visual pattern discrimination was not improved by clonidine, the drug did improve their memory for a spatial task. Noradrenergic neurons may not therefore be involved in mediating all forms of memory. Furthermore, they may mediate those kinds of memory affected in amnesics. The possibility is supported by Squire and Zola-Morgan's (1985) finding, in their monkeys with conjoint hippocampal and amygdalar lesions, of an impairment in the same task on which Arnsten and Goldman-Rakic found improved performance in elderly monkeys treated with clonidine.

If cholinergic inputs from the basal forebrain and noradrenergic inputs from the locus coeruleus modulate the activity of the limbic system structures involved in recognition and recall memory, so that these structures perform their functions more efficiently, then it is of considerable interest what inputs control the modulating brain regions. Van Hoesen (1985) has pointed out that the nucleus basalis of Meynert receives input from virtually the entire limbic system, and certainly the hippocampus and amygdala, as well as from the hypothalamus. The nucleus, therefore, probably receives information about what the 'memory structures' are processing as well as information about internal bodily states from the hypothalamus.

The hypothalamic connection may be an important one, as this region manufactures the hormone and putative transmitter vasopressin. Studies in which animals have been given injections of vasopressin, sometimes directly into the brain, have suggested that this compound affects performance on several learning tasks and may influence the development of stable long-term memory. It has been argued that vasopressin has this effect because it changes noradrenergic activity in parts of the midbrain and forebrain (Kovacs, Bohus, & Versteeg, 1979). Kovacs and his colleagues have shown that administering vasopressin has no effect on the learning tasks normally sensitive to this compound if the locus coeruleus has been lesioned. Their hypothesis assumes that the noradrenergic influences that reach the limbic system and other forebrain regions stem from the locus coeruleus. Structures that are influenced by the noradrenergic projections from the locus coeruleus include the hippocampus and amygdala. If Kovacs and his colleagues are correct, then vasopressin released by neurons projecting to these structures, possibly from vasopressinergic neurons in the hypothalamus, increases the response of hippocampal and amygdalar neurons to noradrenalin released by the locus coeruleus. Such an action of vasopressin is known as neuromodulation. Its occurrence might increase the efficiency of the limbic system neurons that mediate recall and recognition. There is still controversy, of course, about what kinds of memory are influenced by noradrenergic agonists, but the view of Kovacs and his colleagues implies that vasopressin should affect similar kinds of memory. In humans, one would expect that patients who respond to noradrenergic agonists, such as clonidine, should also respond to vasopressin. What is the evidence?

The evidence is somewhat conflicting, but in one study with normal volunteer subjects, Weingartner et al. (1981) administered vasopressin by nasal inhalation and found improvements in recall and recognition. They also referred to preliminary results suggesting that vasopressin may improve memory in patients who had just received ECT and possibly even in early Alzheimer patients, although these latter observations clearly require replication. Timsit-Berthier, Mantanus, Jacques, and Legros (1980) studied the effects of nasally administered vasopressin given for 15 days to patients suffering from memory problems caused by closed head injury. Five of the patients showed improvement either fairly quickly or more slowly in the weeks after the end of treatment. Similar improvements have been noted in other studies of patients with memory problems arising from closed head injury, as well as the memory decline associated with normal ageing. Timsit-Berthier and her colleagues also noted that there were improvements in the patients' attentional capacity as well as in their general activity, motivation, and social adaptation. Four of the patients who showed memory improvement revealed a considerable increase in serum levels of neurophysin 1. This polypeptide is related to vasopressin and may be regarded as a marker for it.

Timsit-Berthier and her colleagues have investigated further the relationship among memory improvement, attentional improvement, neurophysin 1 levels, and vasopressin treatment in patients with memory failures caused by closed head injury. In addition to using behavioural measures of attention, they have adopted electrophysiological measures that are believed to correlate with attention in humans. For example, one of the measures is the contingent negative variation (CNV), a negatively shifting component that can be recorded from the scalp, the amplitude of which indicates the strength of attentional anticipation of a coming stimulus. It was found that administering vasopressin to patients prevented the spontaneous reduction in CNV amplitude that had previously been seen when anticipated stimuli were presented in a repetitive series. Other electrophysiological measures were also affected, which suggests that vasopressin acts to enhance the ability to maintain alert attention, so important for good memory. A clear correlation was found among CNV measures, serum neurophysin 1 levels, and memory improvement. Whether or not patients would show an improvement in memory was predicted by their initial levels of neurophysin 1. If these were low, then there was a good chance of improvement.

These results indicate that vasopressin is likely to improve memory only in people with low basal levels of this hormone/transmitter, which are associated with poor ability to generate and maintain an adequate amount of focused attention. Vasopressin treatment somehow raises basal levels in a way that may persist after treatment, and this increases attentional capacity. The result is that the ability to learn and remember also increases. Although this account is, in principle, consistent with the view that vasopressin influences memory via its action on the noradrenergic neurons of the locus coeruleus, there are some problems. For example, Arnsten and Goldman-Rakic (1985) found that their elderly monkeys showed improvements in spatial memory when given clonidine, despite the fact that the drug actually had a mild sedative effect on them. This seems to conflict with Timsit-Berthier's finding that vasopressin increases attentional arousal (Timsit-Berthier et al., 1980), if this increase is mediated via the noradrenergic neurons of the locus coeruleus. Whatever the resolution of this problem, it is clear that Timsit-Berthier would predict that vasopressin therapy will improve memory in organic amnesics only if they have low basal levels of vasopressin and probably show mild attentional problems. This picture is most likely to apply to alcoholic amnesics. Indeed, McEntee and Mair (1984) have shown that clonidine increased the size of the orienting responses and accelerated habituation in two of their alcoholic amnesics. (Their task was different from that used by Timsit-Berthier and her colleagues, which may explain why Timsit-Berthier seemed to find slowed habituation, whereas McEntee and Mair found faster habituation. Timsit-Berthier's subjects were instructed to attend to the target stimuli, but McEntee and Mair's were not.) It is known that these patients normally show smaller orienting responses and are slower to habituate than control subjects. These results therefore suggest that alcoholic amnesics may have an attentional problem (possibly additional to their major memory difficulty), which could be improved by treatment with a noradrenergic agonist. If correct, vasopressin and noradrenergic agonists may have similar effects, and the results of Arnsten and Goldman-Rakic may be for some reason anomalous in finding clonidine to produce an improvement in spatial memory associated with mild sedation.

If cholinergic basal forebrain neurons and noradrenergic locus coeruleus neurons do modulate limbic structures important for recognition and recall, it still needs to be determined how this modulation is performed and, even more importantly, how the limbic–diencephalic structures contribute to recall and recognition. This problem is further considered in the next section.

Functions of the limbic and diencephalic structures lesioned in amnesia: animal studies

What operations are performed on the processed information that reaches the hippocampus and amygdala from the association cortices that are so essential for subsequent recognition and recall of that information or a subtle transform of it?

In chapter 6, it was tentatively concluded that the systems damaged in amnesia process background and format contextual information and integrate it with target information that has been at the focus of attention. In other words, processed information from association cortices (regions like TE) is integrated with other information in the hippocampal and amygdalar circuits. The cortically derived information will be stored in the association cortex in regions like TE, and the contextual information will be stored most probably in the medial temporal lobe limbic system. A related possibility is that contextual information is stored in the limbic system, which unifies the otherwise isolated nuggets of cortically stored information. An extreme version of this view, apparently adopted by Teyler and DiScenna (1986), is that the limbic system (particularly the hippocampus) stores a record of all the neocortical modules activated when an event or a fact is represented in the neocortex, and that initially at least, there are no storage changes in these neocortical modules. A third possibility is that the limbic circuits modulate the cortical storage of the information they receive, so that their influence would be essential to guarantee stable storage; that is, they boost consolidation of the storage processes needed for recognition and recall. This possibility, which is the opposite of Teyler and DiScenna's view, in that it denies the occurrence of limbic system memory storage, has been favoured by Hirsh (see Gray, 1982).

Proper assessment of these views depends on having a good knowledge of the anatomical connections of the regions concerned, of their physiology, and of the effects of relatively small lesions within the critical structures. Much is now known about the connections of the hippocampus in non-human primates and in rodents. It has already been suggested that it can be divided into slices, or lamellae, which may receive information from highly specific cortical regions. The hippocampus seems to feed information back into the same cortical regions that project to it. How precise this loop between hippocampal lamellae and their cortically linked sites actually is needs to be determined more precisely. In addition to these input–output links with overlying cortex, the hippocampus has two-way connections with other subcortical sites. Inputs to the system come prominently from the septum, a good proportion of whose input to the hippocampus is cholinergic. The septum itself receives inputs from a variety of brain sites, and functional evidence has suggested that these inputs are concerned partly with arousal level and internal states. In addition, there are the noradrenergic inputs from the locus coeruleus, discussed in the last section, and serotonergic inputs from the raphe nuclei, also in the brain-stem. These monoaminergic neurons project not only to the hippocampus, but also to the neocortex, amygdala, and other forebrain areas. The overall pattern of hippocampal inputs suggests that it receives processed information mainly about the external world from the neocortex and information related to internal states and arousal from the subcortex.

Apart from its reciprocating outputs to overlying association cortex, the hippocampus sends fornical projections funnelled through the subiculum to subcortical sites. Notable among these sites are the mammillary bodies and anterior nucleus of the thalamus. Both of these nuclei send reciprocal projections back to the hippocampus (Amaral & Cowan, 1980). Interestingly, although it is the medial nucleus of the mammillary bodies that receives a hippocampal projection, it is from the cells that cap and surround this nucleus that a projection returns to the hippocampus (Amaral & Cowan, 1980). This reciprocating closed-loop pattern of connections is highly typical of both hippocampal and amygdalar circuitry, although the dorsomedial nucleus of the thalamus does not seem to send a projection back to the amygdala. Other midline thalamic nuclei do, however, have reciprocal connections with the amygdala. A pattern of reciprocating projections also seems to exist between the amygdala and the nucleus basalis of Meynert in the basal forebrain. The pattern is even apparent within the architecturally regular structure of the hippocampal system. For example, the subiculum receives information from the neocortex (see Figure 6.1), which is recirculated to the subiculum through both long and short loops. The amygdala also projects to the hippocampus via the entorhinal cortex, which overlies it, as well as receiving a direct projection from the subiculum, and the dorsomedial thalamus projects to the anterior thalamic nucleus. This suggests that the amygdalar and hippocampal systems may interact quite closely, a possibility that is further supported by evidence that the part of the amygdala that receives the subicular input itself projects to the dorsomedial thalamus, and that the amygdala projects to the cingulate cortex, which projects, in turn, not only to the subiculum, but also to the dorsomedial thalamus. Clearly, these anatomical connections should be considered in assessing Mishkin's (1982) hypothesis, which implicitly assumes independence of hippocampal and amygdalar circuits. Finally, if the circuit is followed round, there appear to be projections from the ventromedial frontal cortex onto the limbic structures of the medial temporal lobe. In the long run, any theory of amnesia will have to explain the significance of the various loops that characterize the hippocampal and amygdalar circuits. Some of these loops are illustrated in Figure 7.5.

Studies of the effects of lesions in animals have been used to identify more precisely the functions of structures that lie within the limbic–diencephalic regions where lesions cause amnesia. One topic that was left unresolved in chapter 6 was whether forgetting is faster in any amnesic patients than it is in normal people. The presence of such a deficit would have important implications for theories of the functional deficit(s) that underlie amnesia. The study most directly relevant to this issue was performed by Zola-Morgan and Squire (1982), who compared rate of forgetting on the delayed non-matching-to-sample task in monkeys with conjoint hippocampal and amygdalar lesions and monkeys with medial diencephalic lesions. Lesioned animals were shown test objects for longer than controls in an attempt to match initial performance. Whereas the animals with conjoint lesions forgot faster than controls, those with diencephalic lesions did not. The difference may, however, have been an artefact associated with the fact that memory was actually worst in the animals with limbic system lesions. This possibility is a serious one because a similar claim that hippocampally lesioned rats forgot more rapidly the last rewarded position in a positional reversal task was later shown to

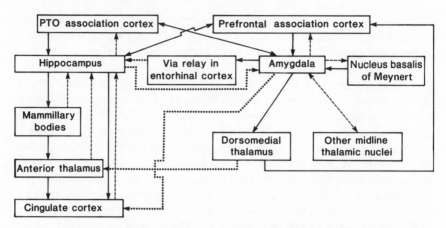

Figure 7.5 Three kinds of projections between limbic–diencephalic structures, association neocortex, and the nucleus basalis of Meynert. The solid arrows represent the major projections postulated by Mishkin. The dashed arrows represent some of the feedback projections that exist in Mishkin's two circuits. The dotted arrows represent the projections known to exist between the hippocampal and amygdalar circuits.

be an artefact caused by not completely matching learning in control and lesioned animals. When matching was appropriate the effect disappeared (see Mayes & Meudell, 1983).

Despite this uncertainty, Winocur (1985) has argued that faster forgetting occurs in hippocampally lesioned rats. He trained rats with hippocampal and dorsomedial thalamic lesions as well as controls on a simple passive avoidance task, where the animals learnt not to lick a water spout that was associated with electric shock. He claimed that the three groups learnt the task equally well and that at short delays, there were no recall differences. By 21 days, however, the hippocampal rats showed significantly more forgetting than the other groups. Although the animals with dorsomedial lesions were not impaired at recalling this task, Winocur believes on the basis of other evidence that they suffer from an encoding problem, which when it affects a task will manifest as a learning failure apparent with minimum delays. One puzzle with the hippocampal results was that no learning deficit was found. Indeed, even at 1 week, the lesioned animals showed no impairment in recall. This is not seen in human amnesics, who, of course, show a dramatic memory loss as soon as their attention is distracted. Apart from the possibility that there is a species difference, this discrepancy might arise either because the task used by Winocur was relatively preserved in amnesia, or because damage in all the lesioned animals was confined to either the hippocampal or the amygdala circuit. A recent study by Staubli et al. (1986) indicates that the effect of apparently normal initial learning followed by pathologically fast forgetting is not task-specific in rodents. In this study, it was found that a small entorhinal cortex lesion that disconnected olfactory inputs from their hippocampal targets did not seem to appreciably impair learning of an olfactory discrimination but did cause abnormally fast forgetting of what had been learnt. Whether both passive avoidance learning and olfactory discrimination learning would be unaffected in amnesia remains, however, a moot point.

An ingenious study by Dunnett (1985) suggests that the normal learning and faster forgetting found by both Winocur (1985) and Staubli et al. (1986) may, indeed, depend on lesions being confined to the hippocampal rather than the amygdalar circuit. He created an adaptation of the delayed matching task for rats and examined the effects on performance in this task of ibotenic acid lesions of the nucleus basalis of Meynert (which sends cholinergic projections to the amygdala) and transections of the fornix (which blocks cholinergic inputs to the hippocampus). Compared with the controls, the rats with nucleus basalis lesions showed an equal depression of recognition at all retention intervals, whereas those with fornix transections had no impairments at the shortest delays, but a progressively greater one as the interval was increased. When the anticholinergic drug scopolamine was given to intact animals shortly before a testing session, there was a recognition impairment apparent at the shortest delays, which became greater as the delay was increased. As scopolamine affects both cholinergic systems disrupted by the more specific lesions, one would expect it to have their combined effects.

A number of comments on this interesting study need to be made. First, the maximum delay used did not exceed 64 sec, so the retention intervals used are in no way comparable with those employed by Winocur. With such short delays, it could well be that one should not expect an impairment with a hippocampal dysfunction in the rats with the shorter delays of a few seconds because this may correspond to short-term memory in humans. The issue is blurred, however, because scopolamine does not affect human short-term memory, and yet in Dunnett's (1985) study, it impaired rats' recognition at even the shortest intervals. This may mean that the rats do not have a short-term memory system similar to that of humans, and the effects of fornix lesions in rats are different from anything that has been observed in humans – that is, normal recognition at first, followed by pathologically fast forgetting. Second, the nucleus basalis lesions disrupted not only inputs to the amygdala, but those to the neocortex as well, so it is impossible to know which disruption was responsible for the memory deficit at the shortest delay. It would be interesting to examine the effects of amygdalar lesions on Dunnett's task. Third, the finding does not agree with that of Aigner et al. (1984), which was described in the earlier section of this chapter, that discusses animal models of organic amnesia. These workers found a recognition deficit only when they lesioned both nucleus basalis and fornix in monkeys. The discrepancy may be due to a species difference but requires resolution. If it is caused by a species difference, then, unfortunately, the rat results suggesting that selective hippocampal dysfunction does not affect initial learning but does cause faster forgetting will not be relevant to humans.

Although the studies just discussed do not lead to any unequivocal conclusion, they do strongly indicate that the possibility of a fast-forgetting form of amnesia should be kept open. The evidence that selective hippocampal lesions do not affect learning and memory initially, but cause an increasingly severe retention deficit as the delay from learning lengthens, is, however, more contentious. It appears to conflict with some of the available data on non-human primates and with what is known about human amnesics who have lesions confined more or less to the hippocampus. Although it has been claimed that recall is worse affected than recognition in these patients and that recall may show pathologically fast forgetting, it is also believed that they show poor initial learning (see Squire, 1986; Volpe et al., 1986). Both human and animal data are, however, consistent with the idea that amnesia becomes worse if there is damage to the amygdala as well as to the hippocampal circuit. Does the animal-research literature give any indication of what contribution the two circuits make to recognition and recall memory?

There is, in fact, interesting evidence that the hippocampal and amygdalar circuits are involved in distinct aspects of contextual memory. To anticipate: Lesions of the hippocampus have particularly dramatic effects on spatial memory, and lesions of the amygdala affect temporal judgements, cross-modal judgements, and, possibly, the association of external events with reward. The idea that the hippocampus plays a central role in spatial memory is particularly associated with O'Keefe and Nadel (1978), and a considerable amount of data has been gathered showing that hippocampal lesions impair spatial memory in a variety of tasks.

A recent illustrative study is particularly relevant to the problems of amnesia. Parkinson and Mishkin (1982) tested spatial memory in monkeys with either hippocampal or amygdalar lesions. Animals were trained to remember the locations of particular objects on the basis of a single trial before the operations were performed. In the final stages of this training, two objects were placed on two randomly selected wells, and animals had to displace both objects in order to obtain a test trial 12 sec later in which a food reward could be obtained. On the test trial, one of the two previously seen objects was again presented on the well that it had been placed on 12 sec before. Another exact duplicate object was placed either on the other well or on a third well, which had not been covered by an object 12 sec before. Animals had to choose the original object in its original position in order to be rewarded. When the duplicate object was placed on the other well, successful performance depended on memory for both object and position, whereas when it was placed on the third well, successful performance depended on memory for position alone. Once trained, the monkeys were lesioned and allowed 10 days to recover before being retrained on this final stage of the task. The animals with amygdalar lesions fairly quickly reattained their pre-operative levels of performance. In contrast, the hippocampally lesioned animals continued to perform at a chance level until retraining was stopped. It made no difference whether successful performance depended on memory for position alone or on memory for position and object. Unlike Mishkin's (1982) results with object recognition, this study implies that the hippocampus and amygdala are not equally involved in spatial memory. Rather, the data imply that the hippocampus makes a selective contribution to the rapid learning of information about objects' positions. The effect is more dramatic than that of hippocampal lesions on object recognition, as the deficit is devastating even at a 12-sec delay. This suggests that these lesions cause a disproportionate spatial memory deficit of the kind discussed in chapter 6. It should be noted, however, that this view about the role of the hippocampus in spatial memory is still polemical, and contradictory positions have been espoused recently (see Gray, 1982; Jarrard, 1986).

Despite opposing views, the suggestion that a disproportionate spatial memory deficit follows lesions to the hippocampal circuit is reinforced by Aggleton and Mishkin's (1985) data on the effects of mammillary body lesions. Although the researchers did not find a significant decrement in object recognition, monkeys with these lesions were impaired at learning a spatial discrimination reversal, with the extent of the impairment correlating with the amount of mammillary body tissue destroyed. In a similar vein, Holmes, Jacobson, Stein, and Butters (1983) reported that mammillary body lesions in monkeys impaired spatial, but not object reversal, learning, and impaired spatial alternation when long delays were used. As similar results have recently been reported after fornix lesions, it will be interesting to determine whether anterior thalamic nucleus lesions also affect spatial memory in this disproportionate way. Evidence from rats with selective lesions of either the anterior thalamic or the dorsomedial thalamic nuclei does, however, strongly suggest that such thalamic lesions do not affect spatial memory, although both hippocampal and mammillary body lesions do in this species (Greene & Naranjo, 1986). If the anterior thalamus is not involved in spatial memory, one must assume that the circuit relevant to this form of memory feeds information directly from the mammillary bodies back to the hippocampus and from there, perhaps to the association neocortex. Such a feedback path exists in mammals (see Amaral & Cowan, 1980) so that information relevant to spatial memory might not be projected forward to thalamic structures. The severity of the deficits suggests that the hippocampal system may have some role in processing spatial information. It should not be assumed that the hippocampus is not concerned with processing other kinds of contextual information. In humans, who show more hemispheric specialization than other animals, only right hippocampal lesions impair spatial memory (see Milner, Petrides, & Smith, 1985). The left hippocampus may have some analogous role with processing whatever corresponds to space in the verbal domain, as was originally proposed by O'Keefe and Nadel (1978). Independent of this possibility, it is known that hippocampal lesions impair associations not only between a stimulus and its location, but also between stimuli and bodily responses that are associated with them (see Rolls, 1986). It seems plausible that such movements might act as contextual cues for target stimuli and that they may be processed with minimal attentional effort when target stimuli are being processed.

If Mishkin (1982) is correct, however, these contextual-processing problems are insufficient in themselves to cause a general recognition failure that is permanent and severe (and this assumes, of course, that remembering context is important for general recognition of target material). One recent finding that may jar with the idea that the amygdalar circuit is not involved with spatial memory is that of Isseroff, Rosvold, Galkin, and Goldman-Rakic (1982). They found that dorsomedial thalamic lesions disrupt spatial memory in monkeys. There is uncertainty about this result, however, because Aggleton and Mishkin found no deficit in similarly lesioned monkeys using the same task (Aggleton, personal communication), and this lesion does not appear to disrupt spatial memory in rats (Greene & Naranjo, 1986). If thalamic nuclei lesions do not cause spatial memory deficits, this might provide some basis for distinguishing between medial temporal and diencephalic amnesia, although the effect of mammillary body lesions on spatial memory would present a problem for this possibility.

Amygdalar lesions also disturb selective kinds of information processing. Murray and Mishkin (1985a) compared the ability of monkeys with amygdalar or hippocampal lesions at making cross-modal associations. The same monkeys were trained on both visual and tactual versions of the delayed non-matching-to-sample task before being operated on. As usual, the monkeys that were given amygdalar lesions and those that were given hippocampal lesions were found to perform equally well on both versions of the task. When, however, an object was touched but not seen during its initial presentation, and seen but not touched during the test trial itself, the amygdalar animals were impaired relative to the hippocampal ones. The amygdala receives modality-specific information directly in the case of olfaction, and indirectly from the cortex in the cases of vision, touch, audition, and gustation, and it projects back onto these modality-specific cortical areas. The experimenters therefore speculated that modality-specific information is stored in the cortex and that cortico-amygdalar-cortical pathways create connections between representations that are stored in this modality-specific fashion. If this interpretation is correct, the amygdala could be regarded as both processing and, perhaps, storing cross-modal associations. When it is damaged, cross-modal sensory cues would no longer be available to aid retrieval of target material. Such cues may well fall in the attentional background during the encoding of stimuli and so can be reasonably regarded as contextual in nature. It needs to be determined whether dorsomedial thalamic lesions have a similar effect or whether this deficit is specific to amygdalar lesions. In this regard, it is interesting to note that human amnesics with diencephalic lesions may have a disproportionate problem in remembering cross-modal associations.

Study of tactual recognition in monkeys with hippocampal or amygdalar lesions has yielded one other serendipitous finding. Murray and Mishkin (1985b) tested both visual and tactual recognition and, unlike in other studies, found that the amygdalar animals were more impaired. Retrospective analysis revealed that the size of this atypical effect was correlated with the size of the object sets used in the tests. In this study, objects were not trial unique; that is, they were shown more than once, and frequency of presentation was inversely related to set size. The effect therefore seemed to indicate that the amygdalar lesion caused a greater effect when animals were required to remember which of two stimuli they had seen more recently, rather than which object was completely novel. This suggestion that amygdalar lesions selectively affect memory for how recently an event occurred is compatible with evidence that human patients with dorsomedial thalamic lesions are disproportionately bad at judging the temporal order of events. As there are reports that lesions of the hippocampal circuit also affect memory for the temporal order of events [for example, some of Hirst & Volpe's (1982) patients had suffered an anoxic episode, so probably had fairly selective lesions to the CA1 field of the hippocampus], it needs to be determined whether amygdalar circuit lesions have a more drastic effect on this form of memory. Whatever the result of this line of investigation, Murray and Mishkin's finding does hint that the deficit in memory for the temporal order of events seen in alcoholic amnesics may not be secondary to incidental frontal lobe damage.

The amygdala may also play a role in the formation of associations between objects and rewards and punishments (see Rolls, 1986). It is known that the amygdala receives cortical inputs of sensory information that has already received a considerable amount of processing, and it has connections with the hypothalamus, which mediates many aspects of reward, punishment, and emotion. Neurons in the amygdala are activated by rewarding brain stimulation of the hypothalamus, and its direct stimulation can produce rewarding and punishing effects in rats and monkeys. Lesions of parts of the amygdala prevent the acquisition of learnt taste aversions and may also impair the ability to associate sensory signals with reward and punishment. It could well be that the amygdala's links with the hypothalamus enable it to process and store stimulus–reinforcement associations, just as its links with sensory association cortex enable it to process and store cross-modal information. Whether other parts of the amygdala circuit have the same or related functions needs resolution. There is, however, similar, but much less extensive evidence that the orbitofrontal cortex in the monkey may be important in the extinction of associations between stimuli and reinforcement. Whether the inability to establish appropriate links between target events and reinforcement will remove an important source of cues to aid recognition and recall is an open question. But it is not unreasonable to suggest that the emotional or other reinforcement significance of target material constitutes its background context and may normally be processed with minimal attentional effort.

The amygdala comprises several nuclei with somewhat different input–output connections, so that future work may well show that lesions to it may disturb further kinds of contextual information processing. The same point has already been made about lesions of the hippocampal circuit. The two circuits may process and store different (but perhaps partly overlapping) kinds of information that may be regarded as contextual because they are normally encoded with minimal attentional effort. The absence of one circuit's contribution removes cues that are useful in accessing target material from memory, but the cues provided by the other circuit are largely able to compensate for this. When both circuits' contribution to the availability of contextual cues is abolished, however, there is a serious disturbance of recognition and recall. The animal studies discussed provide some support for this view, but it needs much more buttressing. The most important aspect of the hypothesis that needs better support is the assumption that spatial memory, cross-modal memory, and so on are critical for recognition and recall. Evidence on this point may be particularly hard to gather because the relationship between individual kinds of contextual memory and target recognition may well be weak. A strong relationship might hold only between some composite measure of contextual memory and recognition.

The hypothesis just outlined is consistent with the idea that amnesia comprises several subdisorders. The animal literature also gives some support for the view that medial temporal lobe amnesia, but not diencephalic amnesia, is associated with pathologically fast forgetting. This unconfirmed possibility is not necessarily in conflict with Mishkin's (1982) view. Hippocampal and amygdalar processing and feedback to overlying association cortex would be prevented by direct medial temporal lobe lesions, and these activities might be essential if forgetting is to occur at a normal rate. Diencephalic lesions would not necessarily destroy this activity, but would prevent diencephalic influences from reaching the cortex either by feedback loops through the limbic system or by the ventromedial frontal cortex. The lost influences might differ from those lost following limbic system lesions because the diencephalic structures receive somewhat different inputs.

The context-memory-deficit hypothesis as applied to hippocampal functions states that the hippocampus is concerned with processing information of specific kinds. It is not concerned with processing information not of those kinds. There is considerable evidence from both lesion studies and anatomical knowledge of the pattern of cortical inputs to the structure that one of its major processing roles may involve integrating representations of objects with certain aspects of their contextual background. These certainly include spatial location and probably include responses made in association with objects. This suggestion that the hippocampus integrates representations of objects with certain kinds of contextual background is also supported by electrophysiological studies (Rolls, 1986). Rolls recorded the activity of 1,510 hippocampal neurons in monkeys that were performing learning and memory tasks known to be impaired following damage to the hippocampal circuit. In a task in which animals had to remember both objects and their positions, he found that nearly 6% of recorded neurons responded differentially, depending where on a screen objects were shown, and 1% of the neurons responded more the first time that an object appeared in a specific position. The response latencies of these neurons was considerably quicker than the animals' learnt behavioural responses. In another task, in which monkeys had to learn to associate visual stimuli and bodily responses, Rolls found that over 10% of the neurons he recorded from responded to specific combinations of stimuli and responses. Nearly the same number of neurons responded when a stimulus occurred with a particular response, but not when it occurred with another response in a different task or when another stimulus was paired with that response. Rolls was also able to show that the responses of some hippocampal neurons were modified in the course of learning new associations between stimuli and responses, which suggests that information about such associations is actually stored in the structure. Rolls hypothesized that inputs from different cortical regions encoding object representations and representations of contextual information may be integrated in the hippocampus, where the new association is stored. For example, information about visual objects from area TE and spatial information originating in the parietal cortex may be combined in the hippocampus.

The view that emerges from Rolls's work is that the hippocampus may play a critical role in integrating certain kinds of contextual information with object representations rather than in the actual encoding of certain types of contextual information *per se*. It is reasonable to assume that these integrations are very important if the object information is later to be recognized. This hypothesis makes clear that the hippocampus is concerned with processing only certain classes of information. Recently, however, Rawlins (1985) has argued that the hippocampus is necessary for processing all classes of information when these stimuli need to be associated with other stimuli that are temporally separated from them. To be able to make such associations, it is vital to hold a representation of the first stimulus in memory until the second stimulus appears. Rawlins argued that when the temporal gap between the stimuli is short and few items need to be remembered, a non-hippocampal short-term memory system can retain the stimuli. In his view, hippocampal damage disrupts a much larger capacity intermediate memory store, so that lesioned animals can form associations only between stimuli that are closely adjacent in time. Once associations are formed, however, they are immune from hippocampal damage and are presumably stored in the cortex or in other brain regions.

To support his hypothesis that the hippocampus is an intermediate memory store for sensory information of all kinds, Rawlins reanalysed old lesion data and cited some of his own to show that tasks normally insensitive to lesions may become sensitive when the temporal interval between stimuli that need to be associated is increased. In contrast, tasks that are normally sensitive to lesions become insensitive when the temporal interval between stimuli that need to be associated is reduced. For example, reference memory tasks are contrasted with working memory tasks because in the former (but not the latter), task requirements do not change across trials, and some theorists have argued that such tasks are insensitive to the effects of hippocampal lesions. Rawlins showed, however, that when the temporal gap between events that need to be associated is increased, lesioned animals reveal a memory deficit. Similarly, working memory tasks that are normally sensitive to lesions become insensitive if the temporal gap is minimized.

Although Rawlins (1985) has shown that changing the temporal parameters is a major factor in determining whether a task is sensitive to hippocampal lesions and that existing distinctions between sensitive and insensitive tasks ignore this factor at their peril, the evidence does not compel the adoption of an intermediate memory hypothesis with the properties suggested by Rawlins. An alternative possibility, which Rawlins himself considers, is that the hippocampus is a rehearsal or consolidation system for memories that are stored elsewhere, possibly in the cortex. This hypothesis seems to account for the data as well as the intermediate memory notion (for a development of this position, see Gray & Rawlins, 1986).

Rawlins's intermediate memory hypothesis, like that which can be derived from Rolls's (1986) data, and unlike the rehearsal and consolidation view developed by Gray and Rawlins, proposes that the hippocampus itself stores information, albeit for a relatively short period of time (which is not too clearly specified). His proposal has the advantage that there is evidence of plastic changes taking place in the hippocampus, as was discussed in chapter 1. Thus the plastic changes associated with LTP (see chapter 1) are known to occur at synaptic sites where cortical input arrives in the hippocampus. The LTP data are also consistent with the view that the hippocampus stores only certain kinds of information, such as associations between spatial features and objects. It is known that the increase in neuronal sensitivity to stimulation found in some hippocampal cells (LTP) decays over a period of days or weeks, and there is evidence that this rate of decay correlates with that of a spatial memory problem learnt by rats (McNaughton & Barnes, 1985). Both decay faster in old rats. It has also been observed that exposure of rats to complex environments produces an enhancement of responses in many hippocampal neurons that closely resembles LTP induced by electrical stimulation. The change reaches asymptote after 3 days' exposure to the complex environment and decays when the animals have been back in their home cages for 2 weeks (McNaughton & Barnes, 1985). This suggests that the massive sensory input to which animals are exposed in the complex environment may cause the storage of memories, some of whose physiological bases are the LTP responses.

The evidence that memory storage takes place in the hippocampus is therefore quite strong. There appear to be other processes of plastic change apart from LTP that last between 100 msec and several minutes (see commentaries on Rawlins, 1985). A considerable body of biochemical evidence also supports the idea that memory changes occur in the hippocampus and that the neurons where these changes occur are influenced by the cholinergic input from the medial septum (see Routtenberg, 1984). This influence may lead to a strengthening of the synaptic changes essential for memory formation. Routtenberg also suggests that acetylcholine release onto the critical hippocampal cells is itself controlled by opioid transmitters (naturally occurring substances with effects like those of morphine and heroin) that act on the cholinergic neurons. These conclusions are consistent with evidence that anticholinergic drugs or opioid stimulation can cause amnesia in animals. The hippocampus, then, may store information for periods of time ranging from less than 1 sec to weeks, months, or even longer. This ability is compatible with its being an intermediate store, as postulated by Rawlins, but it is equally compatible with its storing certain kinds of contextual information, or perhaps the integration of such information with target information. Both versions of the contextual memory hypothesis require that hippocampal storage continue only until the storage of the target information is reorganized so that it can be retrieved without the mediation of the limbic–diencephalic structures damaged in amnesia. Neither Rawlins's nor the context memory accounts specify very precisely what duration of retention they require, although it seems probable that the second hypothesis will involve longer durations. Unfortunately, very little is known about the course of forgetting for unrehearsed long-lasting memories. It could be that, unless heavily rehearsed, several weeks is their natural lifetime, whether stored in the hippocampus or the cortex. If they are to last for months – or years, in the case of humans – this may only be because they have received periodic boosts from a rehearsal process. An LTP-like change maintained in this way might endure for years. In other words, the hippocampus may have the ability to store information for the period of time required by Rawlins's hypothesis, but it can probably also store information for any period of time, ranging from less than 1 sec to years.

A more crucial distinction between the intermediate store and the context memory hypotheses is perhaps related to the kinds of information that the hippocampus stores. Whereas Rawlins (1985) argues that the hippocampus is a large-capacity intermediate store for any kind of information, which enables items spaced widely apart in time to be associated, the context memory view postulates that only certain kinds of contextual information or their integration with target information are stored. There is unquestionably much data linking the hippocampus with spatial memory. As indicated above, these data are derived not only from lesion studies, but also from studies that recorded the activity of hippocampal neurons in behaving animals. Since O'Keefe and Nadel (1978) formulated their spatial hypothesis, it has been argued that the hippocampus contains a type of neuron (probably the rather large pyramidal neurons) that fires maximally when animals are in certain spatial locations, defined by cues distant to the apparatus in which the animals are being tested; that is, these cues constitute the background context.

The firing of the cells has been shown, however, to depend not only on these distant cues, but also on other, more proximate ones. Thus in one experiment (Kubie & Ranck, 1983), rats were tested in an operant chamber, a radial maze, and a large home pen, with the same distant cues in all three apparatuses. There were, however, very few consistencies in the same 'place' with the different apparatuses. The response of the hippocampal neurons therefore seems often to depend on cues unique to each apparatus as well as the background cues. These and other results imply that the hippocampal pyramidal neurons are sensitive to both distant spatial cues and other, less clearly defined kinds of background context. Kubie and Ranck have in fact argued from these and related data that the hippocampus plays an important role in processing spatial and other kinds of contextual information that normally falls on the periphery of attention. One striking feature of such stimuli is that they tend to be tonic – that is, continuously present during any given series of episodes. Olfactory cues are tonic in this way, and the olfactory bulbs have substantial projections to the hippocampus. There is also considerable anecdotal evidence that smells act as important memory cues, so the sensitivity of the hippocampus to different olfactory backgrounds would be well worth investigating.

It may be that the hippocampus is particularly well suited for processing and storing spatial and other contextual cues that are continuously present across a number of episodes, but it cannot, of course, be assumed that this is all it can process and store. For example, Rolls (1984) has reported that some hippocampal neurons respond selectively to the conjoint occurrence of specific stimuli and particular bodily movements. It is difficult to see how the ability of hippocampal neurons to encode such conjunctions can be construed as the processing of tonic contextual information, although it can be argued that such processing abilities may help create spatial maps (see Rolls, 1986). The issue needs more research, but particular stress has to be placed on whether there are any kinds of processing with which the hippocampus is not concerned. If the hippocampus is centrally involved with processing continuously present contextual information so that it helps to create a framework in which target information can be set and without which that information will float relatively inaccessible to retrieval, lost in limbo, it may still act as a kind of intermediate store of the kind postulated by Rawlins (1985). An intermediate store of this kind may enable contextual features to be associated with one another and with target information, although spaced widely apart in time. In other words, an ability to store briefly a wider range of stimuli may increase the hippocampus's capacity to process and store tonic contextual information that is probably integrated with target information. If this possibility applies, one would expect that hippocampal lesions should cause retrograde as well as anterograde amnesia. Rawlins's hypothesis does not predict retrograde amnesia following lesions; so if they occurred, this would be evidence that the hippocampus was involved in storing contextual information that played a role in retrieval for some time after information acquisition. Surprisingly, no studies have examined whether total hippocampal lesions in monkeys cause retrograde amnesia, and only one has examined this in rats (see Winocur, 1985), which found a temporally graded memory deficit.

Several commentators on Rawlins (1985) pointed out that temporal discontiguity between events that need to be associated in order to solve a task is not a necessary condition for making that task sensitive to hippocampal lesions. This is consistent with the proposal that the hippocampus may be not only an intermediate store, but also a store for particular kinds of contextual memory. There are other effects of hippocampal lesions that are not clearly predicted by either the intermediate store or the context memory hypotheses. For example, the effects of hippocampal lesions are in many respects similar to those produced by anxiolytic drugs, such as the benzodiazepines. These and related effects have been explained by Gray (1982) by the proposal that the hippocampus is a comparator that compares events in the outside world with predicted events transmitted round the septohippocampal system and Papez circuit. The activation of a mismatch leads to behavioural inhibition, increased arousal, and increased attention. Although these processes may well improve memory for novel or unpleasant events, it is hard to see how they can affect memory for more commonplace events. At most, therefore, damage to the system should selectively disturb memory for certain particularly striking events. but in amnesia, there is a severe global disturbance of memory for all events, trivial as well as striking. It seems, then, most parsimonious to assume that, if Gray is correct in his proposal that the hippocampus is part of this kind of comparator system and that hippocampal lesions also cause amnesia of at least moderate severity, the two things must be partially or completely independent (see Gray & Rawlins, 1986). If so, the hippocampus may be a system that acts as an intermediate store for a wide range of stimuli, part of a system that stores certain kinds of contextual information, and part of a system that acts as a comparator between actual and expected events in the world.

Assuming that the hippocampus does subserve these three kinds of function, it is likely that they will interact. The intermediate store will not only enhance the ability to process and store contextual information, but also increase the ability of the comparator to match predicted and actual events to each other. These possibilities remain to be explored. One implication of the comparator hypothesis is of particular interest from the point of view of the role of the hippocampus in memory. In primates, and particularly in humans, there is evidence of an increase in frontal connections to the hippocampal system (including inputs from the ventromedial frontal cortex). It has been suggested by Gray (1982) that these inputs could activate the mismatch system whenever the planning system rated an event as one to which attention should be paid. Subsequent memory for the event would be improved. If the system was damaged, there would be a mild memory loss additional to the one caused by disruption of the context-processing system.

If there is such a functional impairment, however, it could not be modelled in rats, which lack some of the frontolimbic projections to subserve it. Nevertheless, even rodents show a memory effect that has been related to the hippocampus. They display a temporary improvement in the retrieval of previously acquired information when presented with novel events. Perception of these novel events is believed to activate the hippocampal mismatch system, which may, via its fornical links to the hypothalamus, activate the release of Beta-endorphin. Beta-endorphin is a chemical messenger (perhaps a neurotransmitter), produced mainly in the hypothalamus, that has some actions like those of the opiate drugs morphine and heroin, probably because it binds to the same receptor sites in the brain as do these drugs. It is believed that when Beta-endorphin is released via activation of the hippocampal mismatch signal, it improves retrieval of already established memories, although the mechanism of this action is still not well understood (see Izquierdo & Netto, 1985). Similar effects have been reported by Izquierdo in humans where the perception of novel stimuli temporarily improves recall of previously established memories. One would expect that damage to the hippocampal system would compromise the processing that underlies this effect and thus cause mild retrieval deficits in certain situations.

The hippocampus is, of course, only one of the structures, albeit a pivotal one, lesions of which cause amnesia, and if Mishkin (1982) is correct, then the resulting amnesia is worse if the damage extends into the amygdala circuit as well. The physiology of these other structures in relation to memory has been somewhat less explored than has been that of the hippocampus. Rolls and his collaborators have, however, done relevant work (see Rolls, 1986). In his work recording the responses of neurons to stimulation, Rolls makes use of anatomical knowledge and traces the responses of a series of neurons between input and output. In some work on stimulus–reinforcement learning, he followed the course of visual information from the inferotemporal cortex through the amygdala to the lateral hypothalamus. As he recorded neurons along this pathway, he found increasing evidence of units that responded selectively to associations between previously neutral visual stimuli and food reward. In further studies, Rolls and his collaborators have attempted to identify neurons that relate to recognition memory in monkeys. The animals were shown visually presented objects twice a day. The first time, the object was novel; on the second occasion, it was familiar. The interval between presentations contained from zero to 17 intervening items and was up to 15 min long. The monkeys licked to obtain fruit juice if they recognized that they had seen an object before. A population of neurons was found at the anterior border of the thalamus that responded to the objects only if they were familiar. It was also shown, at least for some of these neurons, that they responded equally to familiar stimuli that were associated with reward and familiar stimuli that were associated with punishment. Unlike neurons in the lateral hypothalamus, these neurons therefore seemed to respond on the basis of familiarity rather than of stimulus–reinforcement associations.

As well as establishing this double dissociation, Rolls showed that these neuronal responses to familiarity decayed over time and that the rate of decay varied across the neurons sampled, with the decline, like forgetting, following an approximately exponential function. The electrophysiological 'familiarity' response was apparent 100 to 200 msec after stimulus presentation, and both this response and behavioural recognition could be made after stimuli had been exposed for 100 msec. It was also found that repeated exposure of items could extend neuronal 'memory' for more than 100 intervening trials. The neurons in their far anterior thalamic location probably receive connections from other thalamic regions, such as the dorsomedial nucleus, where damage is believed to cause amnesia in humans and monkeys. The evidence therefore suggests that the anterior thalamus plays a role in recognition memory, although the precise nature of this role will require further work for its elucidation. It also needs to be determined whether similar response patterns are found in other limbic–diencephalic structures, damage to which causes amnesia. One would expect not only such similar response patterns, but also evidence that each region has its own distinctive functions. There is evidence for this, as Rolls and his collaborators have found that the nucleus basalis of Meynert contains some neurons that seem to respond to novel stimuli (indicating that they are sensitive to stimulus familiarity and are therefore recognition units, like those found in the anterior thalamus), others that are activated by visual stimuli associated with reward, and yet others that become active when a cue is presented that enables animals to pay attention. Rolls (1986) argues that these results show that the nucleus basalis sends signals to the neocortex and amygdala when a new stimulus is shown, when a stimulus associated with reward is shown, or when a stimulus indicating that the monkey should attend is shown. The effect of these signals may be to enhance information consolidation in the cortex and amygdala.

Rolls has found further evidence of distinctive processing in the amygdala and in the orbitofrontal cortex (which forms part of the ventromedial frontal cortex). The responses of some neurons in the amygdala show that they receive processed information from more than one sensory modality, which is compatible with lesion evidence implicating this structure in cross-modal judgements. Orbitofrontal neurons also respond to combinations of visual and somatosensory stimuli, but in addition, neurons in this area respond in a way that is compatible with this structure playing a role in determining whether a stimulus previously associated with reward is still so associated. The role of the orbitofrontal cortex in recognition and recall is, of course, still controversial, so it also has to be shown that these processing abilities are related to recognition. The rationale of this kind of research is, nevertheless, clear. The flow of information from neocortex through limbic–diencephalic structures needs to be traced, so that the processing and mnemonic abilities of neurons in different parts of the system can be described and related to lesion effects. Confident conclusions can be drawn only after both single-unit-recording and lesion studies have indicated that specific structures play a role in memory. Only in this way will it be possible to identify what the system's components do and how they interact. In addition, the recording methodology may be used to clarify some of the unresolved issues of amnesia research. For example, if amnesia does not affect recall of older pre-traumatically acquired semantic and episodic memories, then neurons in the hippocampus and related structures should not become active when such memories are recalled, although they should when more recent memories are.

The different components of the limbic–diencephalic structures, lesions to which cause amnesia, presumably perform functions that are not identical. But according to the extension of Mishkin's (1982) hypothesis, considered in this chapter, the hippocampus, mammillary bodies, anterior thalamus, and, possibly, cingulate cortex may be concerned with processing and storing certain kinds of contextual information, whereas the amygdala, medial thalamic structures, and, possibly, orbitofrontal cortex may be concerned with processing and storing other kinds of contextual information. The structures in each of these circuits presumably process related kinds of information, which they feed to other structures in the circuit.

All the structures in the limbic–diencephalic region are, however, very highly interconnected, so it is perhaps not surprising that a different account of the organization of the areas involved in recognition has recently been advanced (see Markowitsch, 1985). Unlike Mishkin, Markowitsch has argued for two distinct and differently organized circuits that mediate recognition. The first involves a projection from association neocortex to the hippocampus, and from there to the mammillary bodies and anterior thalamus, whereas the second involves a projection from association neocortex to the amygdala, and from there to the cingulate cortex and the dorsomedial nucleus of the thalamus. In other words, one of the structures from Mishkin's hippocampal circuit (the cingulate cortex, which some research has certainly linked with spatial processing) has been included in Markowitsch's amygdalar circuit. As has already been pointed out, the structures in Mishkin's hippocampal and amygdalar circuits are strongly interconnected, and the cingulate cortex is no exception, as it is linked to both amygdala and dorsomedial thalamus in addition to structures in the hippocampal circuit. One needs to examine the results of lesions and physiological recording studies, however, in order to determine which links indicate the most important functional connections.

Markowitsch not only postulates somewhat different circuits from Mishkin, but also suggests that the hippocampal circuit normally dominates the amygdalar one. According to Markowitsch, the strength of this dominance and, indeed, whether it is reversed varies from person to person, and is controlled by unspecified genetic and experiential factors. When it operates, the dominant system inhibits the activity of the subordinate one. In support of this view, Markowitsch cites lesion research on cats, performed with his colleagues, in which damage to any two of the three main structures in the hippocampal circuit severely disrupted performance on several learning tasks, whereas lesions that included the whole circuit did not impair learning or had a lesser effect. He interpreted this result to mean that the partially destroyed hippocampal circuit not only functioned ineffectively, but also still inhibited the amygdalar circuit from working properly, whereas a total lesion removed the inhibition and enabled the amygdalar circuit to perform its unspecified mnemonic functions. It should be noted, however, that this dramatic effect may well be found only in cats, as Markowitsch himself indicates that in humans, lesions of all three main hippocampal circuit structures causes a severe amnesia. Second, he claims that similar lesions in different patients may result either in severe amnesia or in little or no impairment. The evidence for this interesting claim is nevertheless very weak, partly because it is still hard to be sure that lesions in different patients are truly comparable.

Although Markowitsch's (1985) hypothesis will probably turn out to be incorrect, it does serve to illustrate how difficult it is to analyse the functions of highly interconnected brain structures. To stand any chance of understanding these functions, lesion studies must be combined with anatomical analysis and studies that record physiological and biochemical activity in relevant structures. Hypotheses about the brain regions involved in amnesia may yet undergo a revolution, but at the moment, it can be concluded that storage takes place in at least some of these structures. The best supported account of what is stored is probably provided by Mishkin's (1982) hypothesis, according to which the hippocampal circuit processes and stores spatial and other less well-specified forms of contextual information, whereas the amygdalar circuit processes and stores temporal, crossmodal, emotional, and probably other kinds of contextual information. These kinds of contextual information are very likely integrated with target information, which is stored primarily in the association neocortex. Indeed, it may even be the case that the coherence of the neocortically stored target information is initially maintained by the contextual markers that are stored in the limbic system. Until the integrity of the target information can be maintained without these contextual markers, as a result of repeated rehearsals, the retrieval of the target information will not be effective unless the contextual features linked to it are also retrieved. The ability to process and store contextual information may be enhanced by nor-adrenergic inputs to the cortex from the locus coeruleus and cholinergic inputs to the hippocampus and amygdala from the basal forebrain structures. Cholinergic inputs from the nucleus basalis of Meynert and adrenergic inputs from the locus coeruleus may also enhance the ability of the cortex to store target information.

8   Less well-characterized memory disorders

Research on short-term memory disorders, disorders of well-established memory, frontal memory disorders, and organic amnesia is still in a very open stage of development. Hypotheses about the functional deficits underlying these deficits as well as the lesions that cause them may well undergo a sea change in the face of new discoveries over the next few years. All the interpretations advanced in previous chapters are tentative suggestions that seem plausible in the light of available evidence. Currently, it is unwise to become strongly attached to hypotheses about the bases of organic memory disorders, but quite a bit has been learnt about their main features. The same cannot be said about disorders of the kinds of implicit memory that are probably preserved in organic amnesics. Nor can it be said about the memory disorders that form an often variable part of certain complex psychiatric and neurological disturbances, such as schizophrenia and Parkinson's disease. This chapter considers first the small amount of research that has been directed at exploring whether brain damage can cause selective impairments of priming, skill acquisition and retention, and conditioning (all kinds of implicit memory in which the evidence of remembering is indirect rather than direct). The evidence concerning the memory deficits associated with the complex psychiatric and neurological syndromes is then briefly reviewed in order to ascertain whether the memory deficits reported in these conditions can be interpreted as compounds of the elementary memory disorders, discussed earlier in the book.

Are there specific disorders of memory for
skills, conditioning, and priming?

Skill learning, some forms of conditioning, and some forms of priming (all forms of implicit memory) seem to be unaffected in organic amnesics. This implies that lesions of certain limbic–diencephalic structures do not affect these kinds of learning and memory. It could be that lesions in other brain areas disrupt priming, skill learning, and conditioning, but if they do, it needs to be determined whether they are selective or also disrupt other functions and, in particular, whether they disrupt other kinds of memory, such as recognition and recall (explicit memory). This question is most relevant to possible deficits in priming for two reasons. First, the kinds of priming that are most clearly preserved in amnesics probably depend on the activation of already well-established semantic memories. Most likely, such priming could be disturbed by lesions that damage the storage of such well-established semantic memories, in which case explicit memory for some semantic memories would inevitably be impaired. Second, priming involves a change in the way recently presented items are processed and may be a vital stage in normal recognition and recall. If so, any lesion that disrupts priming should also disrupt recognition and recall – that is, cause the symptoms of organic amnesia. It has recently been reported that patients with Alzheimer's disease who are still only mildly demented show reduced word-completion priming, whereas alcoholic amnesics with equally bad recognition of recently shown words show normal word-completion priming (see Shimamura, Salmon, Squire, & Butters, 1987). This is interesting because these Alzheimer patients suffer both from loss of well-established memories and from the symptoms of organic amnesia. Of course, it needs to be shown more convincingly that priming deficits occur only in conjunction with these other two kinds of memory loss. Consistent with this possibility, in my laboratory, we have recently found that normal subjects whose ability to process words semantically is artificially reduced by requiring them to perform an arithmetic task simultaneously, show both reduced word-completion priming and reduced recall and recognition of the semantically processed words. The relevance of this finding to Shimamura and his colleagues' observations with Alzheimer patients remains to be explored.

This issue can be resolved only by studying patients with more selective lesions than those found in Alzheimer patients. There is, however, some evidence that disorders of well-established memory can occur without obvious deficits in priming, as might be expected if the processes underlying priming are necessary, but not sufficient, for the achievement of recognition. It has been shown that patients with Wernicke's aphasia, whose verbal comprehension is extremely poor as a result of damage confined largely to the left association neocortex, perform better on a test of lexical decision making that depends on semantic processing than on an explicit test of knowledge about word meanings (Blumstein, Milberg, & Shrier, 1982). Thus if shown a triad of words, two of which are meaningfully related, these patients are unable to indicate which are the related words (for example, of *doctor, nurse,* and *mouse,* the first two are related). But if given a list of words and non-words and asked to decide as quickly as possible which are words, their lexical decision is facilitated when a word is preceded by a semantically related term, as when *nurse* is preceded by *doctor*. No correlation was found between the abilities to do this priming task and the one involving verbal comprehension, respectively. It may be remembered from chapter 4 that Shallice (1986) has proposed that preserved priming in the face of poor recognition of previously well-established information may indicate that the deficit is one of retrieval rather than of storage. Although Shallice himself is sceptical about the data presented above, if they are correct and the validity of Shallice's criterion is accepted, then Wernicke's aphasia could be caused by a failure to retrieve semantic information rather than a disruption in storage. On the same grounds, it might be argued that Alzheimer patients show impaired priming because their storage of semantic information has been disrupted. Interpreting Wernicke's aphasia as a retrieval failure for explicit forms of memory, such as recognition, makes sense if one accepts that the retrieval processes necessary for accessing semantic information for purposes of recognition may be more complex than those underlying priming. If priming is disrupted only by failures of semantic storage and such information is stored largely in PTO association neocortex, then it should be affected only by lesions of this cortical region (and, possibly, frontal association cortex). Milberg (personal communication) has, however, recently found preliminary evidence that Broca's aphasics, who have fairly good comprehension but very poor verbal output abilities, may show very little semantic priming, in contrast to their good comprehension. If confirmed, this might be very interesting because the lesion that causes Broca's aphasia includes the basal ganglia as well as the left frontal association cortex (Kolb & Whishaw, 1985). It is therefore conceivable that basal ganglia lesions may impair some kinds of priming preserved in amnesics. If so, one would expect to see priming deficits in patients with Huntington's chorea and Parkinson's disease, who suffer from atrophy of basal ganglia neurons. Although patients with Parkinson's disease have not been tested, Shimamura et al. (1987) found that patients with Huntington's chorea show normal word-completion priming. On current evidence, therefore, it seems likely that those forms of priming that depend on the activation of already established memories may be disrupted only by lesions of PTO and, possibly, frontal association neocortex. It is unknown whether this disruption is always associated with poor recognition and recall, and whether deficits in priming are always storage rather than retrieval failures. Failures of retrieval are perhaps more likely to be found in those forms of priming, reportedly sometimes preserved even in severely amnesic patients, that depend on the acquisition of new information (see chapter 6). Although uninvestigated, these forms of priming may be disrupted by different lesions from those that affect activational priming. It is, however, unproved that the two forms of priming are mediated differently, and both may depend on processes that are essential to explicit memory.

Although the evidence is still scanty, it seems more likely that skill learning and conditioning may be disrupted by lesions that do not affect other kinds of memory. Preliminary evidence has been provided by Martone, Butters, Payne, Becker, and Sax (1984), who contrasted the performance of alcoholic amnesics and Huntington's choreics on the mirror-reading skill-acquisition task used by Cohen and Squire (1980). Whereas the amnesics learned the skill of reading novel mirror-reversed words at a normal rate, but failed to recognize those words with which they had practised in developing the skill, the patients with Huntington's chorea achieved a significantly lower level of skill development, but recognized the practice words as well as their controls. This double dissociation appears to support the view that recognition memory can function normally even when skill learning is impaired. The interpretation faces several problems, however. First, the choreics would almost certainly have shown impaired recall of the practice words (see Butters, 1985). Second, they suffer from frontal lobe atrophy as well as basal ganglia degeneration, and there is reason to suppose that large frontal lesions will disrupt the planning that may be important in the early stages of acquiring a skill. Third, Huntington's choreics make involuntary movements, including involuntary eye movements, and if Martone et al.'s patients were doing so to an appreciable extent, their ability to decipher mirror-reversed words would probably have been affected. The patients' eye movements were not monitored, and it was not shown that they could perform normally on other tasks equally dependent on the ability to control such eye movements, but not involving skill acquisition, so it remains possible that the skill-learning deficit was a secondary result of a motor control problem. This interpretation is perhaps less feasible for another study of motor skill learning in patients with Huntington's disease (Heindel, Butters, & Salmon, 1987). Subjects were trained on a pursuit rotor task in which they had to keep a stylus in contact with a small rotating disc. Patients with Huntington's chorea were impaired at learning this task when compared with normal controls and Alzheimer patients, despite the fact that before training, performance levels were matched to those of their comparison subjects.

Two other studies have looked at the effects of basal ganglia lesions on skill acquisition in humans. In the first, Frith, Bloxham, and Carpenter (1986) examined the ability of Parkinson patients to learn two novel motor skill tasks that involved tracking a moving target with a joystick. In the first task, subjects had to learn to anticipate a slightly unpredictable target, and in the second, they had to track a target whose movements were mirror-reversed relative to those of the joystick. For both tasks, there were two practice sessions, separated by 10 min. The Parkinson patients performed worse overall than their controls, but this could have resulted from their general motor dysfunction. Unlike the controls, however, they did not show a dramatic improvement in the first 0.5 min of the practice sessions. As the benefit of this improvement was only temporary, it was interpreted by the experimenters as an indication that the patients could not form motor sets in which they learnt to apply existing motor programs in a new way on the basis of information that they had acquired about the task. In contrast, the patients did show normal improvement between the practice sessions, which the experimenters interpreted as evidence that they could automatize the motor skills normally. As the failure to develop a temporary motor set might have been caused by a frontal lobe dysfunction that may occur in Parkinson patients, this study does not provide strong support for the view that basal ganglia lesions selectively disrupt skill acquisition. The view needs to be further examined in studies that focus on the different components of skill acquisition and attempt to control for the motor disorders found in patients with basal ganglia lesions. In the second study of skill acquisition in patients with basal ganglia lesions, Saint-Cyr, Taylor, and Lang (1987) found a double dissociation in the performance of a group of Parkinson patients and some organic amnesics on standard verbal memory tests (on which the amnesics were worse) and learning of variants of the Tower of Hanoi (tasks that depend on the acquisition of a cognitive skill and on which the amnesics showed normal learning, but the Parkinson patients were impaired). The results were interpreted as favouring a role of the basal ganglia in skill acqui-

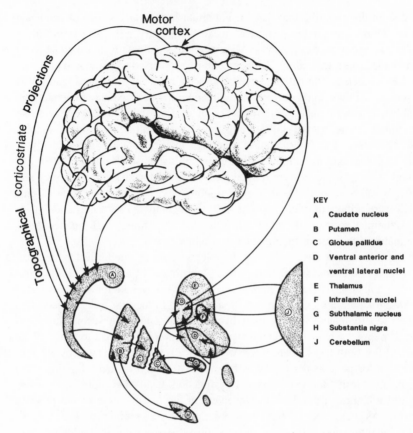

Figure 8.1 The complex pattern of connections among the neocortex, basal ganglia, and cerebellum. It can be seen that there are massive neocortical projections to the caudate nucleus that have some degree of topographical organization. The figure does not show some of the connections between the cerebellum and the neocortex.

sition, but other possibilities (for example, the deficit could have resulted from a frontal lobe dysfunction) were not excluded.

Although the evidence for a role of basal ganglia structures in skill learning and retention is still weak, Mishkin and his co-workers (see Mishkin, Malamut, & Bachevalier, 1984) have argued that habits may be stored in these structures. If so, one would expect that the appropriate basal ganglia lesion would have a devastating effect on habit memory. The argument is based on a knowledge of anatomical connections, some physiological considerations, and some lesion evidence drawn from animal studies. The concept of a habit is derived from behaviourist learning theory and involves the formation of a link between stimulus elements and a particular response as a result of that response's being followed by reinforcement. It is postulated that the link is forged slowly over many trials rather than rapidly, as with recognition memory. The basal ganglia could well be the site of storage for such links because there is a heavy and, to some extent, topographically organized projection from many neocortical regions to one important basal ganglia structure, the caudate, which projects to the putamen. The putamen projects, in turn, to other extrapyramidal regions that ultimately control movement (Figure 8.1). Clearly, the pathway from cortex to basal ganglia provides a means of creating links between processed sensory inputs and motor outputs. The suggestion is further supported by evidence that visual stimuli increase metabolic activity not only in visual cortex regions, but also in many parts of the basal ganglia. Evidence from lesions is rather sparse, but there is some evidence from animal studies that performance on a slowly acquired pattern discrimination is unaffected by lesions that cause amnesia, but disrupted by damage to parts of the caudate nucleus and putamen (see Mishkin et al., 1984). Rolls (1986) has also found suggestive evidence from recordings of the activity of single neurons in the head of the caudate nucleus of monkeys. These neurons do not seem to respond to the association between visual stimuli and reinforcement (unlike some neurons in the hypothalamus), nor do they necessarily respond to movements. Rather, they respond when specific responses are made to specific stimuli, as occurs with habits in which stimuli rapidly and inflexibly trigger specific responses.

The view that habits depend on a cortico-basal ganglia system whereas recognition memory depends on cortico-limbic-diencephalic structures has some interesting implications. First, the distinction can be matched to the old dispute between cognitivist and behaviourist learning theory. If so, it implies that animals and humans can acquire both habits (behaviourist) and expectations (cognitivist) during conditioning and perhaps through other learning experiences. The point is of particular significance when applied to conditioning experiments, because there is evidence that the likelihood of forming habits or expectations (in which the nature of the reinforcement would be represented, so that if the reinforcement were to be changed in any way, behaviour would also be likely to change in a way not seen when learning had produced only a habit) depends on the conditions of training. It should therefore be possible to manipulate these conditions during conditioning experiments in order to increase or decrease the likelihood that habits are formed. If the view of Mishkin and his co-workers is correct, then basal ganglia lesions should be more disruptive when behaviour depends mainly on habits, whereas limbic–diencephalic lesions should be more disruptive when behaviour is guided mainly by expectations. A second implication, related to the first, is that both kinds of information may be stored simultaneously, as they are derived from similar, although not identical experiences. Phobic patients may, for example, have a maladaptive habit, stored in a cortico-basal ganglia system, and a rational expectation, stored in a cortico-limbic-diencephalic system.

A third implication of the distinction between habit and recognition memory is that they might have different evolutionary and developmental histories. There is evidence that monkeys do not achieve adult levels of performance on the delayed non-matching-to-sample task until they are nearly 2 years old, whereas even at 3 months of age, they are as proficient as adults at learning long lists of discrimina tion problems (Mishkin et al., 1984). The former task taps recognition memory, but the latter involves learning to associate objects with reward or non-reward and is acquired very gradually. These findings therefore strongly suggest that the system mediating recognition memory does not mature until a long time after birth, whereas that mediating habit formation matures much earlier. The fourth implication of the habit–recognition distinction concerns the relationship among habits, skills, and conditioning. Depending on the circumstances of learning, conditioning may involve the formation of either habits, expectations, or both to varying degrees. Like habits, skills seem to depend on the formation of 'automatic' sensorimotor links, but the degree of similarity between the two forms of memory remains poorly understood. Whether the automatization that occurs in habits and skills is similar needs to be explored, as does the way in which stimulus–response links become concatenated in skill development.

Whether the view of Mishkin and his co-workers is broadly correct may be known in a few years' time. Basal ganglia lesions in animals have been reported to impair learning on several kinds of task, but the results are difficult to interpret because the lesions may affect basic motor control. For example, although neurotoxic lesions of specific parts of the basal ganglia disrupt the ability of rats to make skilled movements with their forepaws, it is unknown whether this occurs because the animals' memory for the skill has been impaired or because their general motor control has been reduced (Sabol, Neill, Wages, Church, & Justice, 1985). It will be very difficult to deal with this kind of methodological problem, which all studies using lesions face. The use of physiological and biochemical measures made whilst animals are learning and performing skills may be essential if the lesion studies are to be interpretable. For example, extension of the work of Rolls (1986) might confirm that at least some caudate neurons encode relationships between stimuli and responses, and are not activated whenever similar responses are elicited by different stimuli. Damage to such neurons might be expected to impair the execution of habits and skills without causing a general deficit in movement control.

Although it is argued above that the basal ganglia store kinds of information relevant to the expression of certain habits and perhaps skills, there is an older tradition that relates the cerebellum to the storage of information that underlies these kinds of performance ability (see, e.g., Leiner, Leiner, & Dow, 1986). Recent evidence, discussed in chapter 1, suggests that cerebellar lesions in animals impair the acquisition and retention of certain kinds of classical conditioning in a selective way.

Despite the fact that there are no published studies that examined the effects of cerebellar lesions on habit memory in humans, one study currently in progress is investigating the effects of cerebellar lesions on the classical conditioning of the eyelid-closure response in people. This conditioning task involves the presentation of a tone (the conditioned stimulus) immediately before a puff of air is blown in one of the subject's eyes (the unconditioned stimulus that reflexly causes an eyelid closure). After a number of such pairing trials, normal subjects begin to show closure of the eyelid to the tone alone; that is, they show a conditioned response. The procedure allows one to present the unconditioned stimulus to one eyelid at a time. This is an advantage because the anatomical connections of the cerebellum mean that the sensory input from each eyelid projects mainly to the cerebellar hemisphere on the same side of the body. Indeed, the main sensory *and* motor projections between each eyelid and the cerebellum are ipsilateral. If a conditioned response capacity for that eyelid was stored in the cerebellum, then it would probably be stored in the cerebellar hemisphere ipsilateral to the conditioned eyelid. One of the patients studied suffered a vascular accident that, together with the subsequent surgery, led to selective destruction of the right cerebellar hemisphere, sparing only 1.5 cm of tissue adjacent to the midline, although the extent of damage to the deep cerebellar nuclei is currently uncertain. Interestingly, in this patient with a large unilateral cerebellar lesion, unconditioned eyelid responses were produced by both eyes, but a conditioned response did not develop in the eye controlled mainly from the lesioned half of the cerebellum, despite exposure to a large number of training trials. When training was transferred to the other eye, however, conditioned responses appeared within a few trials (O'Boyle, personal communication). Although confirmation is needed that these results are not secondary to subtle sensory or motor deficits, this study suggests that the human cerebellum plays a role in classical conditioning similar to that found in other mammals, such as the rabbit. Several theorists have also proposed ways in which memory changes in the cerebellum might form the basis for skill acquisition. There is a massive projection, containing an estimated 20 million fibres, that runs from the human neocortex via the pons to the cerebellum. The cerebellum also projects back to many regions of neocortex via certain nuclei in the thalamus. This structure therefore receives much sensory information processed by the neocortex, and outputs to both spinal and motor cortex regions that control movement. It therefore seems reasonable to hypothesize that both basal ganglia and cerebellar structures are involved in habits and skills, and that lesions of each of them may have selective, but possibly different effects on skill and habit formation and retention.

It has been claimed that the human cerebellum has shown a three- or fourfold increase in size during the last million years. The newly evolved regions have developed strong connections with association cortex, particularly frontal association cortex. Leiner et al. (1986) have speculated that these connections enable the newly evolved cerebellar regions to play a role in the formation and expression of mental as well as motor skills. They cite evidence that some patients with cerebellar lesions have difficulty with anticipatory planning behaviours and sometimes fail to show motor symptoms, and that one was unable to maintain mental images when performing actions. Thus it may be that parts of the cerebellum interact with the frontal association cortex in mediating planned behaviours. These parts may store action programmes that the frontal cortex can draw on in a variety of situations. It is possible that some apraxias, in which a learned and usually skilfully performed action can no longer be properly carried out, are caused by frontal cortex lesions that prevent access to a cerebellar stored action programme. A similar effect may be produced by basal ganglia lesions, as there is a strong frontal cortex projection to the caudate nucleus, and Rolls (1986) has found that neurons in the head of the caudate nucleus and the dorsolateral frontal cortex are activated under similar circumstances.

Memory disorders associated with complex psychiatric and neurological syndromes

Several neurological and psychiatric conditions are associated with poor memory. Unfortunately, no systematic attempts have been made to see whether the memory deficits correspond to the elementary memory disorders and to identify the kinds of brain damage with which they are related. Such analyses are also important because memory impairments may be a variable feature of some conditions. For example, some, but not all, patients with the demyelinating disease of multiple sclerosis (M.S.) have poor learning and memory abilities. A plausible hypothesis would be that such deficits can be linked to the extent and location of the demyelinating process in patients. There is now some direct evidence supportive of this hypothesis. Sheremata (1984) used a PET scan to measure regional cerebral glucose metabolism in five M.S. patients and five matched controls whilst they were performing a series of verbal learning tasks. The one patient who performed within the normal range on these tasks also showed normal metabolic activity in her temporal and frontal lobes, whereas the other patients showed reduced metabolic activity in these regions. Metabolism was measured in temporal and frontal regions because it was recognized that lesions in these sites may cause serious memory problems. Sheremata was able to show, by using MRI, that reduced metabolic activity in the temporal and frontal lobes was associated with demyelinating, subcortical white matter lesions beneath these lobes. He also found that verbal learning was accompanied by an increase in the level of metabolic activity of these two lobes. This finding strongly supports the view, defended in this book, that lesions of these lobes impair memory because the lobes perform functions vital for normal memory.

This evidence makes it seem likely that memory deficits in M.S. are caused by dysfunction in brain regions that have specific mnemonic functions. The disease is, however, variably associated with a range of other cognitive, emotional, and personality abnormalities, which might contribute to observed memory problems. For example, mild depression is quite common in M.S. patients, so they may not be motivated to try very hard on learning tasks. This is a common finding with clinically depressed patients, who often perform poorly on tasks that require the expenditure of a considerable amount of mental effort; that is, they depend on processing that would be seriously disrupted by the simultaneous performance of another demanding task. Indeed, Roy-Byrne, Weingartner, Bierer, Thompson, and Post (1986) have reported that depressed patients are most impaired at memory tasks that need the expenditure of effort, but perform normally at memory tasks that depend on automatic processing, such as the making of frequency judgements about recently experienced events. Poor memory in M.S. patients, then, may be partly caused by specific information-processing and storage failures, resulting from lesions of the medial temporal and prefrontal association cortex, and partly caused by depression, which leads to less effort being applied to memory tasks. Separation of these factors is likely to prove hard. It depends on the identification of brain lesions in M.S. patients. It also depends on whether depression and the specific lesions can be shown to produce distinct patterns of memory breakdown.

During depression, there may well be a brain dysfunction, perhaps caused by reduced activity in the neural systems that use noradrenalin and serotonin as neurotransmitters. Whatever precise functional deficits these transmitter abnormalities cause, the end result seems to be a reduction in the patient's expenditure of attentional effort. In severe depression, any memory deficits will merely be part of a picture of widespread cognitive impairments. Indeed, it is sometimes difficult to distinguish between ageing depressives and dementing patients. The poor performance of depressed people on memory tasks should perhaps be viewed as an attentional disorder, secondary to a motivational disturbance, which disrupts many memory and cognitive functions. Even so, a distinct depressive pattern of memory failure can be discerned. The deficits fall into two groups. First, there are the deficits that can be seen as arising from reduced expenditure of effort, and, second, there are deficits characterized by poor memory for pleasant experiences, which have a different explanation. Much more research needs to be done on the first group of deficits, but they clearly include impairments not only in learning new information, but also in retrieving information from the distant past (Frith et al., 1983). Short-term memory does not, however, seem to be affected. It is generally believed that recall tasks usually require a greater expenditure of effort than recognition tasks, so one would expect depressives to be more impaired at recall. Although Frith et al. (1983) found that both recall and recognition were impaired in depressed patients, there is evidence that recall is more severely affected than recognition (see Roy-Byrne et al., 1986).

Several studies have reported that depressed people are relatively worse at recalling pleasant than unpleasant information, whether depression occurs as a clinical state or is induced by experimental manipulations (see Bower, 1981). As the depression becomes more severe, the greater is the proportion of unhappy to happy memories that can be recalled. This second group of depressive memory problems is probably an example of state-dependent forgetting. This form of forgetting is believed to affect recall but not recognition, and occurs when there is a change in a subject's physiological state between the time of initially experiencing an event and the time of recall. The effect of this change is to make certain cues that were encoded during learning less available at retrieval. These cues relate not only to a subject's mood and physiological state, but also to the background context present during learning, as context-dependent forgetting is also found.

When a patient's mood improves, he becomes more able to retrieve mood-related cues that were encoded at an earlier, happier date.

There is some evidence that depressives' facility with recalling unpleasant memories may arise because the patients' depressed mood matches these negative memories and so aids retrieval. This kind of state-dependent account of why depressives are better at recalling unpleasant memories than pleasant ones cannot, however, explain why recall of unpleasant memories should be normal in depressives. But precisely this has been reported. Indeed, it has been found that patients' memory for emotionally unpleasant material may actually be as good as or even better than that of controls (see, e.g., Dunbar & Lishman, 1984). This suggests that, at least in some depressives, when material corresponds to their mood, they effectively engage in effortful, elaborative encoding as well as retrieval because their interest is aroused. This interest may also be sufficient to overcome the lapses of attention that have been noted in tasks with little memory load (see Frith et al., 1983). Although more research is needed, the impaired memory seen in depressives can be regarded as a function of state-dependency and reduced employment of attentional effort. The identification of the precise cause of the reduced employment of effort remains uncertain, although it appears to be reversible if patients' interest is aroused by exposure to unpleasant material that also matches their mood.

The other major psychotic disorder, schizophrenia, has been associated with memory impairments similar to those shown by depressives. These memory impairments are exacerbated by the anticholinergic drugs that schizophrenics are sometimes given to counteract the side effects of their antipsychotic medication, but cannot be due solely to such drugs. This claim is based on two kinds of evidence. First, patients on antipsychotic medication alone also show memory deficits, as, indeed, do people with schizophrenic symptoms who are not even receiving neuroleptic medication. This evidence indicates that memory problems, even in mild schizophrenics, cannot possibly be solely caused by anticholinergic medication, let alone neuroleptic medication or a combination of the two. Second, the severity of the memory problems of chronic schizophrenics, who tend to have more severe cognitive deficits than other schizophrenics, is too great to be explained by the level of anticholinergic medication they are receiving. The memory deficits observed are surprisingly similar to those seen in depressives. Thus schizophrenics have been reported to show normal short-term memory, poor recall, normal or near normal recognition, particular difficulties with active organizational processes in encoding and retrieval, and more severe deficits of memory when material with a high semantic content is learnt (Gjerde, 1983). There is some evidence that chronic schizophrenics show poor memory for information that should have been acquired in the distant past (Liddle & Crow, 1984; Stuss et al., 1982). The chronic schizophrenics who were impaired at remembering remote events were also shown, in one study, grossly to underestimate their own ages (Liddle & Crow, 1984). This problem may be caused partly by a temporal discrimination deficit similar to that which has been reported in patients with frontal association neocortex lesions. The deficit in remembering remote events, which may also occur in depression (see Frith et al., 1983), could be caused by a failure to exert effort during retrieval. It has been suggested that chronic schizophrenics may not acquire information normally even before their psychiatric symptoms become evident because they are suffering from a lifelong pathological process affecting their brains. Schizophrenics have also been reported to perform very badly on the Brown-Peterson task (Stuss et al., 1982). As discussed in previous chapters, this task requires subjects to retain information for short periods of time, during which they engage in an interfering activity. Good performance on this task probably requires the ability to alternate rapidly between rehearsing the items and doing the distracting task. This rapid alternation is likely to demand considerable amounts of attentional effort, which schizophrenics are unable to employ. Depressed patients should also perform poorly on the Brown-Peterson task, although this remains to be properly demonstrated.

There is even some evidence that schizophrenics resemble depressives in showing a greater memory impairment for emotionally pleasant or neutral material than for unpleasant material. Thus Koh (1978) reported that young patients showed normal recall of recently presented words with unpleasant connotations, but were impaired at recalling words with neutral or pleasant connotations. This result needs replication, however, particularly with respect to the reportedly normal recall of unpleasant words. Consistent with the view that poor schizophrenic memory results from reduced employment of attentional effort, Koh also found evidence that patients' recall deficit is reduced or even abolished when they are encouraged to engage in elaborative processing through the use of orienting tasks that appropriately direct their attention. Calev, Venables, and Monk (1983), however, have reported results that suggest that although the memory deficits of mild schizophrenics with an average of 2 years' hospitalization may be caused solely by a failure to engage normally in effortful processing, those of chronic schizophrenics also involve other factors. Thus encouraging normal elaborative semantic encoding did not completely restore recall of the chronic patients, who also forgot abnormally fast over 24 hours when recall was tested.

Calev et al.'s results raise two questions about the schizophrenic memory deficit. The first is whether different subgroups show distinct memory problems. The subgroups between which differences are most likely to exist are process and reactive schizophrenics. Reactive schizophrenics usually develop the disease rapidly, respond well to drugs, have a good prognosis, show unclear evidence of heredity, and display mainly positive symptoms, such as hallucinations, paranoid delusions, and thought disorder; process schizophrenics have an insidious onset of symptoms, respond poorly to drugs, have a poor prognosis, evidence hereditary disposition, and display mainly negative symptoms, such as poverty of speech and flattening of affect (Crow, 1980). Process schizophrenics also show more signs of brain damage. Although there has been little research comparing the memory deficits of these two groups, it is interesting that recognition in process schizophrenics has been found to be particularly poor, and Calev et al. found that they forgot abnormally fast over a period of 2 days. This finding weakly supports the claim that process schizophrenics have pathology of the limbic system structures of the medial temporal lobe, because lesions of this region have also been reported to cause abnormally fast forgetting (see Parkin & Leng, 1987; chapter 6).

The second question raised by Calev et al.'s (1983) result concerns the causes of the schizophrenic memory deficit. The disease is generally believed to be caused by a brain dysfunction that in reactive schizophrenics, at least, may involve some kind of abnormality of those neurons in the limbic system of the temporal lobe that are sensitive to the neurotransmitter dopamine, which is released by other neurons that have their cell bodies in the ventral tegmentum of the midbrain. In support of this view, it is notable that there is an association between temporal lobe epilepsy, in which the lesion focus is in the left hemisphere, and the tendency to develop schizophrenic-like symptoms (Flor-Henry, 1976). This evidence does not link reactive schizophrenia specifically to a dopaminergic abnormality in the limbic system, but there is further evidence consistent with the existence of such an abnormality (for a review, see Carlson, 1985). The abnormality of the limbic system structures in the medial temporal lobe may be caused by an initial lesion or by developmental abnormality in parts of the prefrontal lobe. This view is supported by several strands of evidence. First, schizophrenics perform poorly on tests that are sensitive to frontal lobe lesions (Kolb & Whishaw, 1983). Second, techniques including EEG, CAT, MRI, and PET are broadly consistent with the claim that prefrontal cortex in schizophrenics may be abnormally small, show some atrophy, and show reduced levels of activity, particularly when the individual performs a task sensitive to frontal lesions (see Weinberger, Berman, & Zek, 1986). Third, animal studies suggest that certain frontal lesions cause a secondary overactivity in dopaminergic neurons in the limbic system (see Weinberger et al., 1986). It is interesting to note that the negative symptoms characteristic of process schizophrenia are very similar to the deficits found in some frontal lobe syndromes, whereas the positive symptoms characteristic of reactive schizophrenia also sometimes occur in temporal lobe epilepsy and may be caused by limbic system anomalies. It could be, therefore, that process and reactive schizophrenia are caused by different frontal lobe pathologies, the first of which causes negative symptoms, typical of frontal lobe lesion, and the second of which causes dopaminergic overactivity in the limbic system. Much more work needs to be done before it will be known whether these speculations are well founded.

There are two main hypotheses about the causes of schizophrenic memory impairments. The first is that they are caused by specific information-processing and storage failures, resulting from dysfunctions of the limbic system structures in the medial temporal lobes and the frontal lobes. According to this hypothesis, patients should suffer from a combination of the frontal lobe memory problems and organic amnesia. The second hypothesis is typified by the view of Gjerde (1983), who argues that schizophrenics are hyperaroused, which causes inefficient employment of attentional effort, which, in turn, causes the pattern of memory deficit seen. The hyperarousal might be caused by overstimulation from the psychiatric symptoms, such as hallucinations, and so might be said to be secondary to these symptoms, which would have a still unexplained organic cause. Differentiation between these two broad positions will depend on the use of techniques like the PET, and on the kinds of memory assessment discussed in chapter 2. Even so, both views may be applicable to patients, but to different degrees, in a way that relates to their schizophrenic subgroup. Furthermore, the two views may be very hard to distinguish because (as was discussed in chapter 5) frontal lobe lesions appear to disturb the control of effort and attention, and so may produce effects similar to those of hyperarousal.

The memory deficits found in patients with M.S., depression, and schizophrenia are all associated, to varying degrees, with the reduced application of effort during encoding and retrieval. This reduced effort may have different origins in the three conditions, but in each case makes it harder to measure the contribution to the deficit of specific processing and storage failures. It remains plausible to argue that one possible cause of the reduced application of effort during encoding and retrieval seen in these patients is a dysfunction of the prefrontal association neocortex. Damage to this large region of the brain not only affects those kinds of memory, such as recall, that are most obviously dependent on the exertion of effort during learning and retrieval, but also specifically disrupts the ability to remember the temporal order of events (as was discussed in chapter 5). It might be argued, therefore, that if dysfunction of the frontal lobes causes the memory problems seen in M.S., depression, and schizophrenia, the patients with these disorders should be disproportionately bad at temporal discrimination tasks. The issue needs to be systematically tested, but in a preliminary study of schizophrenia, Shoqeirat (1986) found that reactive schizophrenics were not disproportionately poor at a temporal discrimination task on which performance would be expected to be impaired following certain frontal lobe lesions. This finding needs replication, but suggests that memory deficits of reactive schizophrenics are not caused by frontal lobe deficits, whereas those of process schizophrenics could well be. It is, however, also possible that the dysfunction affects a part of the frontal cortex in reactive schizophrenics that is not involved in the mediation of temporal discrimination judgements.

Parkinson patients, like those with M.S., depression, and schizophrenia, also show memory deficits that might be attributed to the reduced employment of effort at encoding and retrieval. Patients with this disease have been reported to show normal recognition of recently presented material, but poor recall (see Flowers, Pearce, & Pearce, 1984). This performance pattern is probably not caused by the anticholinergic medication on which these patients are sometimes placed. It is also apparent in patients without obvious signs of dementia (which is more common in Parkinson's disease patients than in non-Parkinson subjects of the same age). This deficit pattern may be caused by a disturbance within the frontal association neocortex because, as was discussed in chapter 5, the motor disorder of Parkinsonism results from a progressive atrophy of dopaminergic neurons in the substantia nigra (a structure in the midbrain that projects to the caudate nucleus in the basal ganglia). Not only does the caudate nucleus project to the frontal association neocortex, but there is evidence that patients with Parkinson's disease show atrophy of other dopaminergic neurons near the substantia nigra in the midbrain, and that these neurons project directly to frontal association neocortex. A frontal neocortex dysfunction could therefore be responsible for the Parkinsonian memory deficit. Preliminary support for this possibility comes from a study by Sagar et al. (1985), which found that although Parkinson patients could recognize past news events normally, they were very poor at dating them. Other tests indicated that their ability to order events temporally was impaired, even when memory load was minimal. Parkinson patients, therefore, have a temporal discrimination deficit similar to that seen in patients with frontal lobe lesions. Systematic cognitive and memory assessments will, however, be required to determine whether the deficits underlying the memory failures caused by Parkinsonian and frontal lobe lesions are really the same.

Whereas the primary symptom of Parkinsonism is slowness in initiating or stopping voluntary movements and the disease may be caused by industrial toxins that destroy the dopaminergic neurons of the substantia nigra (for a discussion of this hypothesis, see Ferry, 1987), Huntington's chorea is a disease in which the victim suffers from progressively more severe involuntary movements, which are accompanied by a worsening dementia, and is determined by a dominant gene. In chorea, the motor symptoms are caused by atrophy of the caudate nucleus in the basal ganglia, and the dementia may be caused partly by the atrophy of the prefrontal cortex that is also found in the disease. Choreics also have a memory disorder, which has been well studied (see Brandt & Butters, 1986). Patients' verbal recall seems to be more severely affected than their verbal recognition, and deficits in elaborative encoding have been described. Patients show poor retrieval of public events acquired before brain atrophy began, and the deficit is equivalent whatever the age of the memories. These deficits could be caused by the frontal lobe atrophy and/or reflect a reduced employment of effort: but the patients also appear to be poor at learning new skills, although their word-completion priming is preserved as was discussed earlier in this chapter. This deficit in learning new skills may be caused by atrophy of the caudate nucleus. Analysis of the functional deficits shown by these patients is hard because they suffer from many cognitive deficits.

Parkinson's disease and Huntington's chorea are progressive atrophic disorders, but 'healthy ageing' is associated with atrophy of brain structures, including association neocortex and limbic system. Mean scores on some memory tests decline by about 20%, although variability of memory among the elderly is far greater than among the young. It is generally supposed that the elderly experience a general reduction in their cognitive resources, which impairs all their cognitive functions, including memory. On this view, the performance of the elderly on memory tasks should be precisely predictable from their scores on intelligence tests, as these most closely depend on available cognitive resources. It would also be expected that old people's memory should be more impaired when it depends on elaborative encoding and retrieval processes, whereas memory dependent on automatic processes should be more nearly normal. There is some evidence for these predictions (for example, recall may be more impaired than recognition), but it is open to methodological criticisms (see Meudell, 1983). More importantly, this monolithic account of the origin of the memory failures in healthy ageing is also open to theoretical criticisms. First, the decline in intelligence that occurs with ageing probably impairs not only the general resource component of cognition (which involves planning and monitoring), but also specific processing abilities, such as arithmetic skills. The former impairment might affect effortful processing, whereas the latter might affect mainly automatic processes. Memory for temporal sequence and frequency of occurrence, forms of memory usually said to depend on automatic processing, have indeed been reported to decline with age (Kausler, 1987). Second, the memory deficits of ageing probably have more than one cause, and the relative importance of the different causes probably varies across individuals. The elderly suffer from atrophy of the frontal cortex and the hippocampus and amygdala within the medial temporal lobes, so one should expect them to show some of the features of organic amnesia and the frontal lobe memory syndrome. Indeed, there seems to be greater neuronal loss with age from prefrontal cortex and hippocampus than from most brain regions. Thus 15 to 20% of prefrontal cortex neurons are lost between young adulthood and old age, and there may be a greater rate of loss from the CA1 field of the hippocampus (for a review, see Squire, 1987). These atrophic changes have recently been associated with expected memory deficits. Between their 60s and their 70s, healthy elderly subjects have been found to get disproportionately worse at recall relative to recognition, cease to show normal release from proactive interference in the Brown-Peterson task, and get particularly bad at recency judgements, as would be expected with frontal lobe atrophy (Winthorpe, personal communication). In addition, the elderly are more likely to experience depression, which may impair their memory on tasks requiring the expenditure of effort. These possibilities remain to be properly tested, but if correct, must indicate that ageing causes several kinds of elementary memory deficit, the severity of each of which varies from person to person.

It is arguable that there is no such thing as healthy ageing. Just because age-related brain atrophy is normal does not mean that it is not caused by disease. 'Healthy ageing' is merely a cloak for our ignorance of the disease processes involved. It has even been suggested that the brain atrophy of 'healthy ageing' is merely the benign end of a continuum, at the other end of which lies Alzheimer's dementia, the most common cause of abnormal cognitive deterioration associated with ageing. A distinction is, however, usually made between the early (onset before age 65) and late (onset after age 65) forms of Alzheimer's disease, and there appear to be some qualitative differences between normal ageing and the early-onset form of Alzheimer's disease (see Roth & Iversen, 1986). The causes of early- and late-onset forms of the disease are unknown, although recent work suggests that there may be one or more genetic predisposing factors. At the microscopic level, plaques and neurofibrillary tangles are found in greatest density within frontal and temporal association cortex and in limbic system structures, such as the hippocampus, cingulate cortex, and amygdala, although other brain regions are affected as well. Plaques are abnormally shaped axon terminal buttons that contain at their core a protein–starch complex known as amyloid and high levels of aluminium silicate. They seem to represent a distortion of the synaptic connections of affected neurons. Neurofibrillary tangles are twisted lengths of those parts of the affected neurons' cytoskeleton that transport substances between the neurons' cell bodies and axonal endings. Tangles are therefore almost certainly associated with disruption of this transport system. Plaques and tangles are found at very much lower levels in the brains of healthy elderly individuals. They probably kill the cells they disrupt, as their presence is associated with neuronal death, which follows the appearance of plaques and tangles. Neuronal loss is concentrated in the regions most affected by plaques and tangles. Clearly, the disease does not cause a non-specific destruction of all neocortical and subcortical neurons. It is particularly associated with the loss of neurons that release the neurotransmitters acetylcholine, noradrenalin, and somatostatin, and it has long been known that biochemical markers of cholinergic activity are reduced in patients with Alzheimer's disease. Also, there is evidence that the levels of these markers may correlate with measures of memory and dementia (see Iversen & Rossor, 1984).

Although any suggestion about the mechanism underlying the degenerative changes seen in Alzheimer's disease must currently be speculative, one recent proposal is particularly interesting (Maragos, Greenamyre, Penney, & Young 1987). Glutamate, which is a major excitatory neurotransmitter in the brain, is found to be present in reduced concentrations in the late stages of Alzheimer's disease. Maragos and his colleagues have argued, however, that in the disease's early stages, there is overactivity of this neurotransmitter; the effect of this is that those neurons excited by glutamate are poisoned, develop plaques and tangles, and then die. There is independent evidence that glutamate neurotoxicity occurs and that it can cause changes like neurofibrillary tangles as well as neuronal death. Also, the neurons excited by glutamate are believed to be those most at risk in Alzheimer's disease, including large pyramidal cells in the association neocortex and neurons that themselves release glutamate, which may explain why levels of the neurotransmitter are reduced in the late stages of the disease. It could be that some or all Alzheimer patients inherit an abnormal biochemical control system for glutamate metabolism, which may not become manifest until late in life.

Alzheimer's disease is a dementia, so that patients suffering its later stages show drastic spatial disorientation, aphasia, loss of skills, inability to interpret sensory events, and even eventually incontinence, epilepsy, and paralysis. However, when the disease first becomes apparent, the most prominent symptom is memory failure. In broad terms, this memory failure resembles organic amnesia because it involves both a dramatic loss of the ability to learn and retain new information and a loss of the ability to remember information that was acquired pre-morbidly. But there is evidence that in addition to these symptoms, the patients progressively lose the ability to remember previously very well-established semantic information – a deficit that is not found in most organic amnesics (Weingartner, Grafman, Boutelle, & Martin 1983). Further, it has been shown that even in the early stages of Alzheimer's disease, patients show reductions in word-completion priming (Shimamura et al., 1987). As the brain damage in Alzheimer's patients is progressive and includes the limbic structures of the medial temporal lobes, the prefrontal association cortex, and, particularly, the temporal lobe region of PTO association cortex, it is likely that the memory deficit involves several independent kinds of memory disturbance. Other kinds of brain dysfunction may also be involved in the memory losses seen. Thus many believe that biochemical disorders of the cholinergic neurons and, perhaps, noradrenergic neurons play a role in the memory disruption. Acetylcholine-releasing neurons project widely to the neocortex and hippocampus from three areas of the basal forebrain: the nucleus basalis of Meynert, the diagonal band of Broca, and the medial septum (see Figure 6.2). Noradrenalin-releasing neurons also project widely to these sites from the locus coeruleus, a small nucleus in the brain-stem. As was discussed in chapter 7, there is some evidence that lesions of these nuclei may disrupt memory and that pharmacological blockade of acetylcholine (and possibly noradrenalin) have similar effects. It remains to be determined, however, whether or not the memory deficits produced are the same as or different from those seen after lesions of the hippocampus and amygdala or the association cortex. It also needs to be shown that Alzheimer's disease does not involve kinds of memory breakdown not observed in the elementary memory disorders so far identified.

One kind of organic memory disorder that has not been included in the list of elementary memory deficits has been reported following section of the corpus callosum for the treatment of intractable epilepsy. It is still polemical whether there is any memory deficit after callosotomy, partly because if there is one, it is mild in nature so that comparisons of patients' memory before and after surgery are vital. Research into this putative memory deficit has been minimal because whereas millions of people suffer from Alzheimer's disease (including about 10% of the population over 80) and other dementias, the number of people who have undergone callosotomy can be no more than a few tens. Very few comparisons of patients' memory have been made both before and after surgery, and they have not used a wide enough battery of tests to determine whether the memory loss resembles that seen in the better established elementary memory deficits (see Huppert, 1981). If there is a memory deficit, it may reflect the need for effective encoding and retrieval to access and interrelate information that is stored in both left and right neocortices. A recent study, which examined memory both before and after total callosotomy in nine patients, highlights the difficulty of determining whether callosotomy itself causes a genuine memory deficit (Sass, Novelly, & Spencer, 1987). Although there was no overall significant effect of the operation on memory, there were clinically significant declines in memory

Table 8.1. *Taxonomy of memory disorders associated with psychiatric and neurological breakdown*

Name of disorder	Probable cause	Characteristics of memory failure	Nature of brain damage	Elementary or complex disorder
1. Depression	Possibly stress reaction associated with inherited disposition	Poor learning and memory where effort is involved	Possibly underactivity of brain noradrenergic systems	Reduced motivation; perhaps patients less able to apply effortful attention
2. Schizophrenia	Evidence of inheritance and may relate to early viral exposure	Poor learning and memory where effort is involved (e.g., recall worse than recognition)	Possibly fronto-temporal dysfunction	Both frontal and medial temporal lobe dysfunctions could be important, but there may be an independent deficit in applying effort
3. Multiple sclerosis	Possibly autoimmune reaction to certain viruses	Variable, but similar to above	Variable demyelination may affect fronto-temporal systems	Possibly combination of frontal lobe dysfunction and mild organic amnesia
4. Parkinson's disease	Possibly toxic damage and effects of normal ageing	Recall affected, not recognition; evidence of poor memory for event order	Atrophy of dopaminergic neurons of substantia nigra	Possibly frontal lobe dysfunction

5. Huntington's chorea	Inherited, neuronal degenerative disorder	Poor skill learning; recall worse than recognition; retrograde amnesia with old memories as poor as younger ones	Loss of caudate and frontal lobe neurons	Probably frontal lobe lesion deficit, but skill problem may arise from a caudate lesion
6. Normal ageing	Unknown degenerative disorder	Mild anterograde and retrograde amnesia; evidence of reduced processing ability	Widespread cortical and subcortical atrophy	Poor memory may be mainly caused by loss of processing ability, but organic amnesia and frontal deficits may sometimes be salient
7. Alzheimer's dementia	Unknown degenerative disorder	Severe anterograde and retrograde amnesia; some well-established memories lost; processing can be grossly impaired	Atrophy severely affects association cortex and limbic system	Probably organic amnesia, loss of well-established memory, and frontal problems
8. Callosal agenesis	Usually, surgical	Problems with new learning, but their existence is polemical	Corpus callosum and hemispheres	Elementary
9. Functional amnesia	Emotional traumas giving motive to forget the past	Retrograde amnesia that may be general or quite specific	Usually none	Non-organic

observed in isolated cases. It remains to be seen whether these cases suffered extra brain damage or whether the corpus callosum plays a role in memory for some people, but not for others.

The list of organic memory disorders described in this chapter is not intended to be complete, but is summarized in Table 8.1. Other organic disorders also appear to be associated with memory deficits. For example, the aphasias (language disorders caused by brain damage) are commonly reported to have memory failures associated with them. These include failures of short-term verbal memory, difficulties in retrieving previously well-established verbal information, and other learning problems that are probably caused by an inability to use language properly to help with the distinctive encoding of new information (see Kolb & Whishaw, 1985). Other organic disorders arise from unclearly specified brain damage and involve several cognitive deficits apart from memory failures. For example, acute intoxication or prolonged exposure to organic solvents can cause impairments that are most marked on tests of visuospatial intelligence, short-term memory, and long-term memory for visual information (Eskelinen, Luisto, Tenkanen, & Mattei, 1986). Much more research will have to be done before the precise nature and causes of the memory breakdown in such cases is understood. Overall, however, it can be argued that the memory deficits associated with psychiatric and neurological syndromes are compounds of the elementary memory disorders, reviewed in this book. It is possible that the callosotomy memory syndrome, if it exists, may prove to be a distinct elementary memory deficit and that the memory decline associated with reductions in general intelligence, as in normal ageing, may not be due entirely to a frontal cortex dysfunction compounded with difficulties in remembering information previously well-established in memory. But both these possibilities require far stronger support.

9   Overview

In this book, five possible groups of elementary organic memory disorders have been discussed. It is still controversial whether the disorders considered are truly elementary or whether at least some of them are composed of two or more independent disorders that could be separately compromised by more selective lesions. For example, the organic amnesia caused by medial temporal lobe lesions may differ from that caused by diencephalic lesions, and lesions of the hippocampal and amygdalar circuits may disrupt recognition for somewhat different reasons. This kind of issue is hard to resolve, partly because lesions in humans are adventitious and tend not to honour boundaries between functionally distinct brain regions, so that it is often difficult to distinguish between cognitive deficits that are essential to a memory deficit and those that are incidental to it.

Despite the problems, five groups of organic memory deficits can be identified. The first group of memory deficits is caused by lesions to PTO association neocortex. This neocortical region includes parts of the parietal, temporal, and occipital lobes and is not specialized for obvious motor or sensory functions. Instead, as its neurons lie several relays away from the sensory input, it is probably concerned with the later stages of analysis and interpretation of sensory information. Lesions to it can cause breakdowns that comprise several kinds of fairly selective short-term memory deficits specific to certain types of information. These disorders, which are discussed in chapter 3, probably arise for a number of reasons, although it still needs to be shown convincingly that they are ever caused by isolated disruption of short-term storage, rather than of specific encoding and retrieval processes.

Second, PTO association cortex lesions also cause deficits in memory for previously well-established information. These are considered in chapter 4. One of the most interesting features of these disorders is that they may be confined to highly specific kinds of information, such as that concerned with animate things or even with fruits and vegetables. These patterns of breakdown must reveal something about the organization of complex semantic and episodic memory in the neocortex.

Third, frontal cortex lesions seem to disrupt memory because they affect the ability to plan and organize encoding and retrieval. For example, they disrupt recall, but have little or no effect on recognition, which depends less on planning than does recall. It is polemical, however, whether all their effects on memory can be explained in this way, because at least some frontal neocortex lesions disrupt memory for the temporal order and frequency of occurrence of events, kinds of memory usually believed to depend on automatic encoding and retrieval processes rather than on effortful and planned processing. These impairments are discussed in chapter 5.

Fourth, lesions of certain limbic and diencephalic structures impair one or a number of memory-related functions so that there is impaired recognition and recall of pre-traumatically acquired (retrograde amnesia) and of recently presented information (anterograde amnesia). Recall and recognition are collectively known as explicit memory, in contrast to implicit memory, because the presence of memory is indicated directly by verbal or non-verbal means, such as drawing or pointing, whereas implicit memory can be indicated only indirectly through behaviour. These organic amnesic deficits are discussed in chapter 6, and in chapter 7, animal and pharmacological models of the organic amnesias are considered. It remains unsure whether retrograde and anterograde amnesia can occur in isolation, although several cases of isolated retrograde amnesia have been reported. Similarly, the evidence that hippocampal and amygdalar lesions in the medial temporal lobe cause faster forgetting than diencephalic lesions needs to be convincingly confirmed. Nevertheless, lesions of the hippocampal and amygdalar circuits almost certainly compromise recognition for different reasons, and it is tentatively concluded that both types of lesion somehow impair distinct aspects of contextual memory.

Fifth, there is growing evidence that lesions of the basal ganglia, cerebellum, and other non-limbic–diencephalic subcortical sites may affect learning and memory for skills and certain kinds of conditioning in fairly selective ways. Review of the available evidence about these disorders in chapter 8 indicates that although forms of implicit memory, such as skill memory and conditioning, are affected by basal ganglia and cerebellar lesions, there is no evidence that a third form of implicit memory, priming, is affected by these lesions. It is known, however, that at least some kinds of priming are affected by PTO and, possibly, frontal association neocortex lesions that also disrupt storage of previously well-established semantic memories. Other less well-specified memory disorders, which probably comprise compounds of several of the elementary memory disorders, perhaps intermixed with further cognitive disorders, are also discussed in chapter 8. Alzheimer's dementia fits this description well, as it seems to involve components with the features of organic amnesia, difficulty with previously well-established memories, and possibly short-term memory difficulties, together with other cognitive failures. Interpretation of memory problems in the major psychiatric syndromes is less certain, although there is a view that the symptoms of schizophrenia are caused by dysfunction of the limbic system structures within the medial temporal lobes and of the frontal association neocortex. If correct, schizophrenics should show both a mild organic amnesia and frontal lobe memory problems. The pattern of deficit seems to depend, however, on the schizophrenic subgroup to which the patient belongs.

One view that can explain the five main groups of elementary memory disorders is that the brain can be pictured as a large set of modular systems, each of which processes particular kinds of information in particular ways and sends the results to other modular systems. Some or all of these systems store and retrieve the kinds of information that they process. Furthermore, the kind of information that particular modules process, as well as the way they process such information, develops as a result of experience. For example, some lesion evidence suggests that certain left neocortical regions are specifically devoted to reading processes in adults. They clearly cannot subserve this precise function in pre-reading-age children or in non-literate adults, although the functions that they do subserve in such groups must make these regions suitable for processing the kinds of information essential to reading. A modular interpretation of the five groups of elementary memory disorders would run as follows. Sensory information is fed into the posterior neocortex, where it is processed through a large number of modular channels, working both in series and in parallel. Even within one sensory modality, such as vision, modules will extract information about colour, orientation, movement, and the like in parallel. The results of these separate analyses are later integrated within PTO association cortex, so that more complex information may be represented and, eventually, meaningful analysis can be achieved. It is possible that there are auxiliary modules that serve to keep the 'mainstream' modules active for a short period of time so that the information they have just processed is maintained. If these auxiliary modules were lesioned, then immediate memory for particular kinds of information would be impaired because of a selective disruption of short-term storage. Alternatively, immediate memory might be impaired because a 'mainstream' module was damaged and thus less efficient in processing information. Rehearsal impairments are best interpreted as partial disconnections between sensory-processing modules and motor output ones.

The meaningful interpretation of sensory inputs involves accessing well-established semantic and episodic memories, stored in a variety of modules in PTO association neocortex. As lesions can sometimes produce very selective deficits in semantic memory, it has been argued that different kinds of semantic memory are housed in distinct regions of PTO association cortex. For example, it has been suggested that concepts defined predominantly in terms of their functions are stored in regions that only partially overlap with the regions in which other concepts, defined predominantly in terms of their sensory features, are stored. Whether or not this functional–sensory dichotomy can be related to the different location of lesions that disrupt memory for distinct kinds of concept, it seems appropriate to argue, more generally, that the storage of concepts depends on the storage of a range of sensory and other attributes and that, for different classes of concept, the relative importance of the various attributes will not be the same. If this is so, and different kinds of attribute are stored in distinct parts of the association neocortex, then lesions in particular PTO association neocortex regions will disrupt memory for some conceptual categories more than others. This kind of view implies that particular categories of semantic memory are stored in small and discrete regions of PTO cortex. The lesions that cause these highly specific deficits tend, however, to be typically rather extensive. It could be, therefore, that storage of discrete categories of information, such as 'fruit and vegetables' or 'inanimate things', is not in a compact region, but is widespread in a net-like fashion over PTO cortex and perhaps unified by specific kinds of biochemical activation that project from subcortical regions. The neocortex certainly contains receptors for many putative peptide transmitters or neuromodulators of subcortical origin.

This speculation may relate to another interesting hypothesis about the way in which semantic memory breaks down following PTO association neocortex lesions. It is well known that when in a particular motivational state, one tends to retrieve motivationally relevant information more efficiently and more frequently. Different memories come to mind when an individual is hungry, thirsty, or sexually aroused. It seems possible that the limbic–diencephalic structures aroused in such states selectively activate particular PTO sites through pathways that release specific peptide or other transmitters. These pathways would have been activated early in development when the individual was in an appropriate motivational or emotional state. If their activation lowered the thresholds of receiving neurons, then these neurons would very probably encode and store information associated with those specific states. This kind of viewpoint may also help explain why lesions can differentially compromise memory for concepts concerned with animate and inanimate things. Even in people, animate objects are more likely than inanimate objects to be associated with hunger, whether they are food objects themselves or merely similar to other objects that are food objects. Furthermore, hunger is not a unitary state; there are specific hungers, and satiety may be specific to certain kinds of food. One might therefore predict that memories for subcategories of animate objects may be grouped together. Not only may there be anomias specific to 'fruits and vegetables', there may also be other memory impairments that affect further subcategories of animate objects, corresponding to the specific hungers. Although this view – that acquisition of certain categories of semantic knowledge may be primed and unified by particular motivational states – can help account for some of the highly selective disorders of semantic memory that have been reported, the occurrence of these disorders very probably also depends on other, as yet unknown, processes. Furthermore, the motivational hypothesis is surely irrelevant to some of the deficits in remembering previously well-established memories that have been reported. For example, it is difficult to relate specific motivational states to knowledge of such categories as colour and number.

These proposals partly explain how different categories of knowledge come to be separately stored in the course of development, but how this knowledge is represented remains a contentious issue. In chapter 4, Allport's (1985) suggestion was considered. According to it, concepts do not have some kind of separate representation, but are stored as an associated network of sensory attributes. It remains to be shown whether such a network can incorporate all the properties of semantic memory. If correct, Allport's view somewhat blurs the distinction between failures of retrieval and failures of storage because, according to his view, retrieval is the reactivation of the pattern that represents a particular piece of semantic knowledge through the encoding of cues that form part of that pattern.

If this is so, then the main way in which a retrieval failure can occur is when the links among the individual components of a semantic network are broken. Such a lesion seems unlikely to occur in isolation, but if it did occur, it could clearly be seen as a disruption of storage as well as retrieval.

On Allport's view, retrieval deficits for previously well-established memories are more likely to be caused by frontal lobe lesions that disrupt the ability to plan more complex retrieval processes. Elaborating the meaning of any sensory input probably involves an interaction between modules in PTO association cortex and modules in the frontal cortex. If this interaction is disrupted, then the encoding of new kinds of semantic and episodic information will be impeded. The way in which frontal cortex mediates these and other kinds of planned activities is still very poorly understood. Clearly, it is not very useful to state that the frontal cortex plays a central role in planning. We need to know in detail how it achieves this. Any explanation will have to ascribe many subfunctions to different frontal regions. Whether lesions of these different regions will impair distinct aspects of memory remains an open question. If all the memory deficits are caused by failures in planning ability, and all frontal lobe lesions disrupt planning, albeit for different reasons, then all frontal lobe lesions might affect memory in the same way. There is some evidence against this possibility, however, as dorsolateral prefrontal cortex and orbitofrontal cortex lesions may affect memory differently, and it is also possible that some frontal lobe lesions affect memory for kinds of activity, such as temporal judgements, that some people believe do not involve planned encoding and retrieval. Indeed, Schacter (1987a) has argued that lesions of frontal association neocortex disrupt memory for automatically processed contextual features, but do not affect those kinds of memory, such as recall of target information, that depend on effortful and planned processing. The case for this view still needs to be convincingly made, however, and the opposing view – that a major effect of frontal lobe lesions is to disrupt those kinds of memory most dependent on effortful processing – is more strongly supported. A further possibility that has yet to be tested is that frontal lobe lesions affect planning because they disrupt memory for well-established information about which actions are appropriate in a variety of situations. If so, it would need to be determined whether the information was stored in the frontal cortex or in more recently evolved regions of the cerebellum.

Subsequent recall and recognition of the kinds of semantic and episodic information that must be stored largely in PTO and, possibly, frontal association cortices is massively impaired unless processed information from these cortices is sent to one or more modules in the limbic–diencephalic structures that are lesioned in amnesics. These structures may relate target features of the sensory input to their background and format contexts or, perhaps, integrate the different components of the input by linking them with their common contextual markers. Another closely related view, adopted by Teyler and DiScenna (1986), is that the hippocampus stores an index of the presumably thousands of neocortical modules that are activated by particular events and that, initially at least, no storage changes occur in these neocortical modules. The memory changes are confined to the hippocampus, where LTP-like modifications enable a record of the activated neocortical modules to be stored. LTP, or long-term potentiation, is itself an increase in neural excitability, originally noted in the hippocampus and most prominent there, that is triggered by high-frequency electrical stimulation of the perforant pathway leading into the hippocampus from the entorhinal cortex. Interestingly, the increased excitability can persist for weeks, and other evidence relates it to the plastic changes underlying memory. Like one form of the context-memory-deficit hypothesis, Teyler and DiScenna's view proposes that the hippocampus plays a role in integrating the complex information represented in the neocortex. Unlike the context-memory-deficit hypothesis, however, Teyler and DiScenna's view focuses on the hippocampus and does not allow the other limbic and diencephalic structures a role in storing contextual information and integrating the complex information represented in the neocortex. Also unlike the context-memory-deficit hypothesis, which postulates that contextual information, stored in limbic–diencephalic structures, integrates neocortically stored target information, their view denies that there is initially any neocortical storage. The context-memory-deficit hypothesis about the role of the structures damaged in amnesia is preferred because its proposal that all the limbic–diencephalic structures damaged in amnesia (rather than just the hippocampus) store contextual information is better supported by the evidence. More important perhaps, its other postulate – that target information is stored neocortically, even at initial learning – seems very likely to be true. Although it would be easy to generalize Teyler and DiScenna's hypothesis to allow a role for limbic and diencephalic structures other than the hippocampus, if neocortical storage does occur at initial learning, then their view is wrong in a critical respect. There does, however, seem to be evidence that as memories are rehearsed following initial learning, they are gradually reorganized so that they can eventually be recalled without the mediation of the limbic–diencephalic structures damaged in amnesics. Such memories are presumably stored entirely in the neocortex and may also be recalled and recognized solely through the offices of the neocortex.

There is, then, an important distinction to be drawn between very well-learnt and repeatedly rehearsed explicit memories, such as those that constitute much of our mental dictionaries and encyclopaedias, and less well-rehearsed explicit memories, which particularly include those that have been recently acquired. There is no sharp division between these two forms of explicit memory. Rather, the latter kind is gradually transformed into the former through a process of rehearsal, which leads to their being stored entirely in the neocortex so that they can be recalled and recognized without the involvement of limbic–diencephalic structures. The limbic–diencephalic structures damaged in amnesia seem to be unnecessary not only for well-rehearsed explicit memory, including both semantic and episodic information (as shown by normal recall and recognition of such information in amnesics), but also for implicit memory of even little rehearsed and novel information (that is, priming of novel information). This second claim is supported by evidence that amnesics show normal priming of information that is already stored in established semantic memory and growing evidence that they can show normal priming of novel information, which could not have been in their memory. Thus it seems likely that much semantic and episodic information may be stored neocortically, even without extensive rehearsal, and that this information is stored in a form appropriate for implicit memory (indicated only indirectly), but not for explicit memory (indicated directly by recall and recognition). The offices of the limbic–diencephalic system are vital for recall and recognition of this information. In this book, it is argued that the reason for this dichotomy between implicit and explicit memory is that the system stores contextual information, which integrates semantic and episodic information stored in the neocortex. Explicit memory initially depends on the retrieval of this contextual information stored in the limbic–diencephalic system, although through rehearsal, it can eventually be manifested without the participation of this system.

As there is evidence that amnesics show normal implicit memory for both novel target and contextual information, which is probably stored in the neocortex, another hypothesis remains tenable. This hypothesis postulates that the limbic–diencephalic system is necessary for the making of familiarity judgements, which are made on the basis of whether or not information is processed more rapidly than it would have been if novel. The hypothesis is based on a modification of Jacoby's (in press) view that recognition sometimes involves a familiarity judgement predicated on the speed with which an item is processed. The modification suggests that recognition always involves such a judgement, but that the speeded processing sometimes also depends on retrieving contextual information. It is proposed, then, that recognition is a function of increased item-processing speed, which is dependent on a priming-like process that is preserved in amnesics and on a judgement process that is impaired in amnesics. The priming process is neocortically based, whereas the judgement process must depend, in part, on limbic–diencephalic structures. This view is, however, much less well supported than the one that argues that explicit memory depends on retrieving contextual information stored in the limbic–diencephalic system, partly because confirmation is still needed that priming of novel information is completely normal in amnesics. If amnesics have a general problem in making familiarity judgements, it is also hard to explain why their explicit memory for old, rehearsed information can be normal or nearly normal. It does, however, seem likely that priming depends largely on neocortical mechanisms, as neocortical lesions are known to disrupt it.

Finally, sensory information processed in the neocortex is sent to the basal ganglia and other subcortical structures, such as the cerebellum. These subcortical structures are involved in initiating motor outputs, so that modified neocortical connections to them form the basis of new habits and skills (both forms of implicit memory). These and other subcortical motor systems also receive sensory inputs that have been processed in subcortical sensory regions, and new connections with these subcortical sensory regions will form the bases of simpler kinds of habits and skills. In contrast, more complex habits and skills will probably involve the establishment of new connections between the neocortical sensory regions and the basal ganglia and cerebellar regions that initiate motor outputs. Mishkin and his colleagues (see Mishkin, 1982) have argued that whereas the sensory inputs involved in recognition memories are integrated in order to contribute to the creation of semantic memories that are stored neocortically, the sensory inputs involved in habits are represented as a set of specific components, such as size, shape, and colour, each of which forms an association with a particular motor output. If this is correct, then one should expect to find marked differences between the microstructures of the neural inputs from cortical sensory regions into the limbic system and into the basal ganglia.

In chapter 1, the currently popular view that information is stored where it is processed and represented was discussed. If correct, it should be impossible to find brain lesions that impair only storage. Although some have argued that certain short-term memory deficits may be of this kind, this position is disputable, and all the other kinds of impairment can readily be construed as disturbances of processing as well as storage. This is of interest because it indicates that memory for complex information can be devastated when the processing and storage of only specific aspects of that information are directly disrupted. Thus amnesics have poor recognition and recall of all kinds of semantic and episodic information because they have a problem with the processing and storage of certain sorts of contextual features, and patients with frontal lobe lesions have difficulty recalling similar types of information because they do not process and store the sorts of semantic information whose encoding requires effort and planning.

The existence of five main groups of memory disorders indicates that different kinds of information are represented and stored in different brain systems. It is an open question whether the kinds of logical operation that these systems perform on their inputs are radically distinct from or basically similar to one another. If they are radically distinct, then the different regions may encode and retrieve the information they store in very different ways, and the ways they represent that information in storage may also be very different. If the logical operations they perform are similar, then one must assume that the various memory systems, identified through the analysis of lesion effects on remembering, are distributed in order to avoid overloading the storage capacity of individual brain regions. The pattern of their distribution in the brain would be determined simply by the distinct parts of the brain to which different kinds of information are projected. One way of broaching this extremely difficult problem might be to compare the micro-anatomical structure of regions, such as association neocortex, hippocampus, basal ganglia, and cerebellum, to determine whether the patterns of connections observed suggest similar or different kinds of information processing. An easier and different question that can probably be answered sooner is whether the microscopic biochemical and physiological changes that underlie memory in different brain regions are the same or different. Work on LTP, discussed in chapters 1 and 7, illustrates one way in which this issue may be examined. It might be found, for example, that LTP-like changes occurred only with information storage in the neocortex and limbic system, with storage in other regions depending on different processes. Indeed, Lynch and Baudry (1984) have advanced an argument of this kind.

If this book were to be rewritten in 20 years' time, many of its main conclusions would be different. Obviously, it is not possible to predict where the changes will be, but undoubtedly some of the future developments will be based on a better understanding of anatomical connections between brain regions and the kinds of information processing that activate these regions. In other words, it will be based on knowledge of the flow of information processing through the brain. This knowledge will be derived not only from animal research, but also from the application of increasingly refined neurotechnology to the human brain whilst subjects are engaged in cognitive and memory tasks.

Glossary

Alzheimer's disease. The most common form of dementia, in which cognitive functions are progressively lost. In the early stages of Alzheimer's disease, there is often a relatively selective amnesia, probably accompanied by some loss of previously well-established memory and perhaps poor short-term memory. It is caused by degenerative processes that particularly occur in the parietotempero-occipital (PTO) association neocortex (q.v.), the cholinergic basal forebrain (q.v.), and limbic system (q.v.) structures, such as the hippocampus and amygdala. Neurons in the degenerating regions show plaques and neurofibrillary tangles. The cause of the degeneration is unknown, but appears to have a genetic component.

Amnesia. Also known as organic amnesia and sometimes as global amnesia, amnesia is a memory disorder in which intelligence and short-term memory may be preserved in the face of very poor recall and recognition (explicit memory [q.v.]) of recently presented information (anterograde amnesia) and very poor recall and recognition of information that was acquired before brain damage occurred (retrograde amnesia). It results from several aetiologies and is caused by lesions to a number of related brain regions, including the hippocampus and, possibly, the amygdala in the limbic system (q.v.) of the medial temporal lobe and midlying structures in the diencephalon.

Aneurysm. A vascular dilation in an artery or a vein that fills with blood and is caused by a local defect in the elasticity of the vessel's wall.

Anterior communicating artery aneurysm amnesia. A form of amnesia that results from the bursting of an aneurysm on the anterior communicating artery and/or the repair operation associated with such aneurysms. The location of the critical lesion is polemical, but it has been argued that both frontal association neocortex and cholinergic basal forebrain (q.v.) may be affected. The symptoms are also variable in terms of both the extent of 'frontal' symptomatology and the degree of amnesia.

Automatic processing. It is commonly argued that processing activities, such as encoding and retrieval, draw on attentional capacities to differing extents. Although the theoretical interpretation of this claim is unclear, it can be defined operationally because automatic processes are minimally disrupted by the simultaneous performance of other demanding tasks, regardless of the precise nature of these tasks. Similarly, automatic processing minimally disrupts the performance of these other tasks. In contrast, effortful processing (q.v.) activities are disrupted by and disrupt other demanding tasks that are simultaneously performed.

271

Background context.   When a subject attends to episodic or semantic target information, that information falls within a spatiotemporal framework known as its background context or background spatiotemporal context. Background context, together with format context (q.v.), constitute extrinsic context (q.v.), which is contrasted with intrinsic context (q.v.). It has been argued that background context is processed automatically, and, certainly, it usually falls on the periphery of attention. It includes not only the precise spatial and temporal parameters of events and facts, but also other features of the background in which they occur – for example, its colour or the objects present in it.

Basal ganglia.   A group of large nuclei that lie deep in the forebrain and include the caudate nucleus, putamen, and globus pallidus. The basal ganglia play an important role in movement control and may help mediate the development of skills and habits. The caudate receives a massive topographical projection from overlying neocortex and projects indirectly not only to downstream motor systems, but also back via the thalamus to frontal motor cortex regions.

Broca's aphasia.   A disorder in which both written and spoken verbal output is non-fluent, effortful, and telegraphic despite reasonably good comprehension of substantive words, such as nouns. Broca's aphasia is caused by a lesion that includes a region of the left frontal cortex, although to produce a permanent disorder, the damage probably has to be more extensive, perhaps including parts of the basal ganglia (q.v.).

Brown-Peterson task.   An often used test of recall over delays of a few seconds in which items are presented to subjects, usually in triads, after which they engage in some interfering activity, such as counting backwards by threes, until the end of the retention interval, when they are asked to recall the items just presented. Although recall typically declines steeply over a 30-sec delay, it is unlikely that the interfering tasks completely prevent rehearsal. They are more likely merely to make rehearsal more difficult. Alzheimer patients and some amnesics perform badly at the Brown-Peterson task. Their problems could be caused, at least in part, by frontal cortex lesions because patients with such lesions also perform poorly on the Brown-Peterson task. Performance tends to decline over trials, particularly when similar items are used on the trials. This effect has been exploited in the Wickens release from proactive interference paradigm, in which triads of items drawn from one category (for example, names of living things) are presented for four trials with testing at a fixed delay. On the fifth trial, a triad of items drawn from a different category (for example, they may all be names of kitchen implements) is presented and tested after the same delay. Normal subjects show improved recall under these conditions, whereas patients with frontal cortex lesions and some patients with amnesia (q.v.) do not.

Cholinergic basal forebrain.   Several nuclei in the deep-lying regions of the forebrain that contain mainly neurons that release the neurotransmitter acetylcholine. The cholinergic basal forebrain includes the medial septum, which projects to the hippocampus; the diagonal band of Broca, which projects to the hippocampus and amygdala; and the nucleus basalis of Meynert, which projects to the neocortex and amygdala. Damage to these structures is believed to contribute to organic amnesia (q.v.).

Declarative memory. Declarative memory is contrasted with procedural memory (q.v.). This distinction should be compared with that between episodic and semantic memory (q.v.), and between explicit and implicit memory (q.v.). Squire (1986), who has advocated the declarative–procedural distinction, defines declarative memory as explicit and accessible to conscious awareness, and consisting of facts, episodes, lists, and routes of everyday life. It therefore comprises both episodic and semantic memory. As such, memories can be declared by verbal statements or indicated non-verbally by an image (or presumably by pointing or drawing). The concept of declarative memory is very similar to that of explicit memory (q.v.).

Depression. There are probably several disorders in which extreme levels of despair are central. In some of these disorders, the depression is regarded as a psychosis because the connection between mood and reality seems to be broken. Severe depression is accompanied by physical symptoms, such as sleep disturbances and loss of appetite for food and sex, and is associated with a memory deficit that is in some ways similar to that shown by some patients with schizophrenia (q.v.) and by patients with frontal lobe lesions.

Effortful processing. Effortful processing is contrasted with automatic processing (q.v.). Thus effortful encoding and retrieval use considerable attentional capacity and hence disrupt and are disrupted by the simultaneous performance of another attention-demanding task. Effortful processing probably always requires planning and is therefore likely to be compromised by frontal cortex lesions that disrupt the ability to plan.

Episodic memory. Episodic memory is contrasted with semantic memory (q.v.) and refers to memory for individual episodes in personal life that have specific spatial and temporal contexts. It is therefore believed by some to depend on the retrieval of such contexts in a way not shared by semantic memory.

Explicit memory. Explicit memory is contrasted with implicit memory (q.v.), and the distinction between them is very similar to that between declarative and procedural memory (q.v.). Like declarative memory, explicit memory can be indicated directly either through a verbal statement or through non-verbal means, such as pointing. In other words, explicit memory is indicated by recall and recognition.

Extrinsic context. Synonymous with independent context, extrinsic context comprises both background and format context (q.v.). Its defining feature is that it is not supposed to affect the meaningful interpretation of corresponding target information. In this, it is contrasted with intrinsic context (q.v.), which is synonymous with interactive context. The distinction is probably one of degree, rather than being absolute. There is some evidence that extrinsic context is automatically processed, although this is polemical.

Format context.   Together with background context (q.v.), format context constitutes extrinsic context (q.v.). It comprises those forms of contextual features linked to the form of presentation of target items, such as the sensory modality in which they were presented and the way in which they were presented within that modality.

Huntington's chorea.   An inherited disorder that causes abnormal involuntary movements (chorea) and cognitive deficits, including poor memory. Huntington's chorea is progressive and results from an increasing atrophy of the caudate nucleus in the basal ganglia (q.v.) and, to a lesser extent, of the frontal association neocortex. The origins of the atrophy are unknown, but it resembles that seen after the brain is exposed to such neurotoxins as quinolinic acid.

Implicit memory.   Implicit memory is contrasted with explicit memory (q.v.), and the distinction between them is very similar to that between procedural and declarative memory (q.v.). Implicit memory can be indicated only indirectly in the way performances are executed. It includes skill memory, conditioning, and priming (q.v.).

Intrinsic context.   Intrinsic context is contrasted with extrinsic context (q.v.) and is defined as that kind of context that affects the interpretation of target information. For example, seeing the word *jam* in the intrinsic context of the word *traffic* will affect the semantic interpretation of the first word. It is probable that intrinsic context is processed effortfully and that its encoding and retrieval depend on the mediation of the planning functions of the frontal association neocortex.

Korsakoff's syndrome.   A form of organic amnesia (q.v.) caused by chronic alcoholism. It is controversial whether alcohol intake, thiamin deficiency, or both are the critical factors. Brain damage is often widespread, but invariably includes structures in the midline diencephalon, such as the mammillary bodies. It probably also includes the frontal association neocortex in most patients. This latter damage may be related to the much noted fact that Korsakoff patients often show additional cognitive and mnemonic deficits not found in other amnesics. In many cases, the disease is heralded by an initial Wernicke-Korsakoff episode, a confusional stage associated with a variety of motor symptoms as well as delirium. It is controversial to what extent the memory deficits have an acute onset concomitant with the Wernicke symptoms.

Leucotomy.   Shorthand for frontal leucotomy, an operative procedure, conceived by Moniz in 1936, in which nerve tracts connecting the frontal association cortex with deeper lying structures are severed. The procedure typically disconnects the frontal regions from midline diencephalic nuclei, such as the dorsomedial nucleus of thalamus, but much additional damage was undoubtably done because of the crude procedures that were often used (as with Freeman's ice-axe method!).

Limbic system. A term used to describe the structures that line the inside wall of the neocortex and that act as an interface between the neocortex and other structures in the brain-stem and diencephalon. The limbic system is sometimes considered to include these diencephalic structures because Papez proposed a hypothetical circuit that ran from the limbic system structures in the medial temporal lobe (most notably the hippocampus, although the amygdala also lies in this region) to diencephalic structures, such as the mammillary bodies and anterior thalamus, to the cingulate cortex, before the circuit was completed by a projection back to the hippocampus. Since Papez, this circuit has been associated with the control of emotional behaviour and with memory.

Long-term potentiation. An increase in the excitability of neurons that was originally noted in hippocampal neurons activated as a result of stimulating the perforant pathway leading from the entorhinal cortex into the hippocampus proper. There is evidence that long-term potentiation may also occur in other forebrain regions, and the plastic changes underlying it are related to memory storage.

Multiple sclerosis. Probably an autoimmune disease, in which the immune system attacks the myelin sheathing of neurons and disrupts neural functions. Multiple sclerosis is progressive, although its course is highly variable, being often subject to remission. Some, but not all, victims suffer memory deficits that seem to result from dysfunction in the frontal and temporal lobes.

Parkinson's disease. A progressive motor disorder characterized by tremors, rigidity, and slowness as well as difficulty in initiating voluntary movements. Parkinson's disease is caused by atrophy of dopaminergic neurons in the substantia nigra of the midbrain and of other neighbouring dopaminergic neurons. There is evidence that the motor deficits may be accompanied by cognitive problems, including poor memory, and that these deficits arise from dysfunction of the frontal association neocortex.

Post-encephalitic amnesia. A form of amnesia (q.v.) that results from a viral infection, particularly of the temporal lobes of the brain. Although the term covers infections by several different viruses, the herpes simplex virus is most commonly implicated, perhaps because it has a particular affinity for the temporal lobes and their underlying limbic system (q.v.) structures. The amnesia in patients with this disorder is probably caused by destruction of the hippocampus and amygdala, whereas the poor memory for previously well-established memories that they have been reported to show may result from destruction of the temporal association neocortex.

Priming. A form of procedural or implicit memory (q.v.) that is present whenever items are processed faster or differently as a result of having been recently perceived. Priming can occur with items that already exist in well-established memories and with items that were novel before their presentation. There is some evidence that both these forms of priming are preserved in organic amnesia (q.v.).

Procedural memory.   Procedural memory is contrasted with declarative memory (q.v.) by Squire (1986), and the distinction between them is very similar to that between explicit and implicit memory (q.v.). Procedural memory is accessible only through performance in an indirect or implicit fashion and comprises skill memory, conditioning, and priming (q.v.). These forms of memory are mediated by different brain regions and probably differ in other ways as well. They share the properties of being preserved in organic amnesia (q.v.) and of being accessible solely through performance.

PTO association neocortex.   Another name for posterior association cortex, used because it includes neocortex in the parietal, temporal, and occipital lobes. Association cortex is cortex that is not clearly specialized for motor or sensory functions and, as the name suggests, was originally supposed to be the region where inputs from different senses met and were associated with one another. Although this idea is unfashionable, PTO association neocortex lies several relays away from the cortical regions where sensory information is initially received, and so may reasonably be thought to be involved with the late stages of analysis of information, particularly with its meaningful interpretation.

Schizophrenia.   The most common form of psychosis, affecting 1% of the population. The patient suffers a break from reality that involves delusions, illogical thinking, incoherence and hallucinations. Symptoms are, however, variable, and subtypes of schizophrenia have been claimed to exist. Recently, it has been suggested that reactive and process schizophrenia differ. Reactive schizophrenia is characterized by rapid onset, good response to drugs, positive symptoms like hallucinations, few signs of heredity, and no indication of brain damage; process schizophrenia is characterized by insidious onset, poor response to drugs (and so tends to become a chronic condition), evidence of heredity, and negative symptoms like poverty of speech, cognitive deficits, and signs of brain damage. Memory disorders have been reported in schizophrenics, but it is still unclear to what extent they depend on subtype and to what extent they reflect the effects of the patients' poor ability to attend to external events.

Semantic memory.   Semantic memory is contrasted with episodic memory (q.v.), although both can be regarded as forms of explicit or declarative memory (q.v.). Semantic memory is of facts, the kind of information that can be kept in our mental dictionaries and encyclopaedias. Such information contains no explicit reference to the background context in which it was initially acquired or later rehearsed. It is polemical whether this fact indicates that contextual retrieval is never important in semantic memory. One problem in resolving this issue is that semantic memories are usually more rehearsed than episodic ones, although this is an incidental feature.

Wechsler Adult Intelligence Scale. A commonly used test for assessing the cognitive abilities of brain-damaged patients. The WAIS comprises two sets of subtests in a verbal scale and a performance (or visuospatial) scale, and taps several distinct cognitive functions. For example, the verbal scale contains tests that tap common knowledge, vocabulary, comprehension of common situations, mental arithmetic, short-term memory, and the ability to judge in what way items are similar to one another (a test of abstract-thinking ability). The performance scale contains more timed tests, and high scores on these tests probably depend less on using previously established knowledge and problem-solving strategies.

Wechsler Memory Scale. A battery of six subtests that are used to test memory in brain-damaged patients. The tests tap current general knowledge, personal orientation, mental control, digit span as a measure of short-term memory, copying drawings from memory, story recall, and paired associate learning. As a test of organic amnesia, the WMS has been criticized because it contains subtests, performance on which is unlikely to be disrupted in amnesics, and because it examines only recall, leaving recognition unassessed. As on the Wechsler Adult Intelligence Scale (q.v.), scoring on the test is standardized so that the mean is 100, with a standard deviation of 15 in the normal population. Amnesia (q.v.) is indicated when the intelligence score appreciably exceeds the memory score.

Wernicke's aphasia. A verbal disorder caused by lesions of the parieto-tempero-occipital (PTO) association neocortex (q.v.) of the left hemisphere, in which patients show impaired comprehension of spoken and written language and fail to produce meaningful verbal output. Wernicke's aphasia is clearly associated with difficulty in accessing the meaning of substantive words, such as nouns.

Bibliography

Aggleton, J. P., & Mishkin, M. (1983a). Visual recognition impairment following medial thalamic lesions in monkeys. *Neuropsychologia, 21*, 189–197.

Aggleton, J. P., & Mishkin, M. (1983 b). Memory impairments following restricted thalamic lesions in monkeys. *Experimental Brain Research, 52*, 199–209.

Aggleton, J. P., & Mishkin, M. (1985). Mamillary-body lesions and visual recognition in monkeys. *Experimental Brain Research, 58*, 190–197.

Aigner, T., Mitchell, S., Aggleton, J., De Long, M., Struble, R., Wenk, G., Price, D., & Mishkin, M. (1984). Recognition deficit in monkeys following neurotoxic lesions of the basal forebrain. *Society for Neuroscience Abstracts, 10*, 386.

Albert, M. S., Butters, N., & Brandt, J. (1981). Patterns of remote memory in amnesic and demented patients. *Archives of Neurology, 38*, 495–500.

Allport, D. A. (1984). Auditory verbal short-term memory and conduction aphasia. In H. Bouma & D. G. Bouwhuis (Eds.), *Attention and performance, X*. London: Erlbaum.

Allport, D. A. (1985). Distributed memory modular subsystems and dyphasia. In S. Newman & R. Epstein (Eds.), *Current perspectives in dysphasia*. Edinburgh: Churchill Livingstone.

Amaral, D. G., & Cowan, W. M. (1980). Subcortical afferents to the hippocampal formation in the monkey. *Journal of Comparative Neurology, 189*, 573–591.

Andrews, E., Poser, C., & Kessler, M. (1982). Retrograde amnesia for forty years. *Cortex, 18*, 441–458.

Arendt, T., Bigl, V., & Teanstedt, A. (1983). Loss of neurons in the nucleus basalis of Meynert in Alzheimer's disease, paralysis agitans and Korsakoff's disease. *Acta Neuropathologica, 61*, 101–108.

Arnsten, A. F. T., & Goldman-Rakic, P. S. (1985). Catecholamines and cognitive decline in aged nonhuman primates. *Annals of the New York Academy of Sciences, 444*, 218–234.

Assal, G., Buttet-Sovilla, J., Favre, C., Jacot-Descombes, C., & Lanares, J. (1985). Non-reconnaissance d'animaux familiers chez un paysan. Zoo-agnosie ou prosopagnosie pour les animaux. *Revue Neurologique* (Paris), *140*, 580–584.

Atkinson, R. C., & Shiffrin, R. M. (1971). The control of short-term memory. *Scientific American, 225*, 82–90.

Bachevalier, J., Parkinson, J., & Mishkin, M. (1985). Visual recognition in monkeys: Effects of separate vs. combined transection of fornix and amygdalofugal pathways. *Experimental Brain Research, 57*, 554–561.

Baddeley, A. D. (1982). Domains of recollection. *Psychological Review, 89*, 708–729.

Baddeley, A. D., & Hitch, G. (1974). Working memory. In G. H. Bower (Ed.), *The psychology of learning and motivation* (Vol. 8). New York: Academic Press.

Bahrick, H. P. (1984). Semantic memory content in permastore: fifty years of memory for Spanish learned in school. *Journal of Experimental Psychology: General, 113*, 1–47.

Bartus, T. R., Dean, R. L., Pontecorvo, M. J., & Flicker, C. (1985). The cholinergic hypothesis: An historical overview current perspective, and future directions. *Annals of the New York Academy of Sciences, 444*, 332–358.

Basso, A., Spinnlerm, H., Vallar, G., & Zanobis, M. E. (1982). Left hemisphere damage and selective impairment of auditory verbal short-term memory: A case study. *Neuropsychologia, 20*, 263–274.

279

Bauer, R. M. (1984). Autonomic recognition of names and faces in prosopagnosia: A neuropsychological application of the guilty knowledge test. *Neuropsychologia, 22*, 457–469.

Benson, D. F., Miller, B. L., & Signer, S. F. (1986). Dual personality associated with epilepsy. *Archives of Neurology, 43*, 471–474.

Blumstein, S. E., Milberg, W., & Shrier, R. (1982). Semantic processing in aphasia: Evidence from an auditory lexical decision task. *Brain and Language, 17*, 301–315.

Bower, G. H. (1981). Mood and memory. *American Psychologist, 36*, 129–148.

Brandt, J., & Butters, N. (1986). The neuropsychology of Huntington's disease. *Trends in Neuroscience, 9*, 118–120.

Bransford, J. (1979). *Human cognition: Learning, understanding and remembering*. Belmont, Calif.: Wadsworth.

Broadbent, D. E. (1984). The Maltese cross: A new simplistic model of memory. *Behavioral and Brain Sciences, 7*, 55–94.

Brown, J., Lewis, V., Brown, M., Horn, G., & Bowes, J. B. (1982). A comparison between transient amnesias induced by two drugs (diazepam and lorazepam) and amnesia of organic origin. *Neuropsychologia, 20*, 55–70.

Butters, N. (1984). Alcoholic Korsakoff's syndrome: An update. *Seminars in Neurology, 4*, 226–244.

Butters, N. (1985). Alcoholic Korsakoff's syndrome: Some unresolved issues concerning etiology neuropathology and cognitive deficits. *Journal of Clinical and Experimental Neuropsychology, 7*, 181–210.

Butters, N., & Albert, M. S. (1982). Processes underlying failures to recall remote events. In L. S. Cermak (Ed.), *Human memory and amnesia*. Hillsdale, N.J.: Erlbaum.

Butters, N., & Cermak, L. S. (1975). Some analyses of amnesic syndromes in brain damaged patients. In R. L. Isaacson & K. H. Pribram (Eds.), *The hippocampus* (Vol. 2). New York: Plenum Press.

Butters, N., Miliotis, P., Albert, M. S., & Sax, D. S. (1984). Memory assessment: Evidence of the heterogeneity of amnesic symptoms. In G. Goldstein (Ed.), *Advances in clinical neuropsychology* (Vol. 1). New York: Plenum Press.

Butterworth, B., Campbell, R., & Howard, D. (1986). The uses of short-term memory: A case study. *Quarterly Journal of Experimental Psychology, 38A*, 705–738.

Calev, A., Venables, P. H., & Monk, A. F. (1983). Evidence for distinct verbal memory pathologies in severely and mildly disturbed schizophrenics. *Schizophrenia Bulletin, 9*, 247–264.

Carlson, N. R. (1985). *Physiology of behavior*. Boston: Allyn & Bacon.

Catsman-Berrevoets, C. E., Van Harskamp, F., & Appelhof, A (1986). Beneficial effect of physostigmine on clinical amnesic behaviour and neuropsychological test results in a patient with a post-encephalic syndrome. *Journal of Neurology, Neurosurgery and Psychiatry, 49*, 1088–1090.

Cermak, L. S. (1982). *Human memory and amnesia*. Hillsdale, N. J.: Erlbaum.

Cermak, L. S., Blackford, S. P., O'Connor, M., & Bleich, R. P. (in press). The implicit memory of a patient with amnesia due to encephalitis. *Brain and Cognition*.

Cermak, L. S., & O'Connor, M. (1983). The anterograde and retrograde retrieval ability of a patient with amnesia due to encephalitis. *Neuropsychologia, 21*, 213–234.

Cohen, N. J. (1984). Preserved learning capacity in amnesia: Evidence for multiple memory systems. In L. R. Squire & N. Butters (Eds.), *Neuropsychology of memory*. New York: Guilford Press.

Cohen, N. J., & Squire, L. R. (1980). Preserved learning and retention of pattern analyzing skills in amnesia: Dissociation of knowing how and knowing that. *Science, 210*, 207–210.

Corkin, S. (1984). Lasting consequences of medial temporal lobectomy: clinical course and experimental findings in H. M. *Seminars in Neurology, 4*, 249–259.

Craik, F. I. M., & Lockhart, R. S. (1972). Levels of processing: A framework of memory research. *Journal of Verbal Learning and Verbal Behavior, 11*, 671–684.

Crow, T. J. (1980). Molecular pathology of schizophrenia: More than one disease process? *British Medical Journal, 280*, 66–68.

Damasio, A. R., Graff-Radford, N. R., Eslinger, P. J., Damasio, H., & Kassell, N. (1985). Amnesia following basal forebrain lesions. *Archives of Neurology, 42*, 263–271.

Davidoff, J. B., & Ostergaard, A. L. (1984). Colour anomia resulting from weakened short-term colour memory. *Brain, 107*, 415–430.

Davidoff, J., & Wilson, B. (1985). A case of visual agnosia showing a disorder of presemantic visual classification. *Cortex, 21*, 121–134.

Davis, H. P., & Squire, L. R. (1984). Protein synthesis and memory: A review. *Psychological Bulletin, 96*, 518–559.

De Renzi, E., & Nichelli, P. (1975). Transient global amnesia: Neuropsychological dysfunction during attack and recovery of two 'pure' cases. *Journal of Neurology, Neurosurgery and Psychiatry, 47*, 668–672.

DeWitt, E. D., & Goldman-Rakic, P. S. (1983). Intermittent thiamin deficiency in the rhesus monkey: 1. Progression of neurological signs and neuroanatomical lesions. *Annals of Neurology, 13*, 376–395.

Donchin, M. (1984). *Evidence that the process manifested by the P300 is associated with modifications in working memory.* Paper presented at the ICON III Conference, Bristol, England.

Drachman, D. (1977). Memory and cognitive function in man: Does the cholinergic system have a specific role? *Neurology, 27*, 783–790.

Dunbar, G. C., & Lishman, W. A. (1984). Depression, recognition-memory and hedonic tone: A signal detection analysis. *British Journal of Psychiatry, 144*, 376–382.

Dunnett, S. B. (1985, July). *Comparative effects of cholinergic drugs and lesions of the nucleus basalis or the fimbria-fornix on delayed matching in rats.* Paper presented at the meeting of the Experimental Psychology Society, Cambridge, England.

Eskelinen, L., Luisto, M., Tenkanen, K., & Mattei, O. (1986). Neuropsychological methods in the differentiation of organic solvent intoxication from certain neurological conditions. *Journal of Clinical and Experimental Neuropsychology, 8*, 239–256.

Eysenck, M. W. (1977). *Human memory: Theory research and individual differences.* Oxford: Pergamon.

Fedio, P., & Van Buren, J. M. (1974). Memory deficits during electrical stimulation of the speech cortex in conscious man. *Brain and Language, 1*, 29–42.

Ferry, G. (1987). New light on Parkinson's disease. *New Scientist, 113*, 56–60.

Fisher, R. P. (1979). Retrieval operations in cued recall and recognition. *Memory and Cognition, 7*, 224–231.

Flor-Henry, P. (1976). Lateralized temporal-limbic dysfunction and psychopathology. *Annals of the New York Academy of Sciences, 280*, 777–795.

Flowers, K. A., Pearce, L., & Pearce, J. M. (1984). Recognition memory in Parkinson's disease. *Journal of Neurology, Neurosurgery and Psychiatry, 47*, 1174–1181.

Fodor, J. A. (1983). *The modularity of mind.* Cambridge, Mass.: MIT Press.

Freed, D. M., Corkin, S., & Cohen, N. J. (1984). Rate of forgetting in H. M.: A reanalysis. *Society for Neuroscience Abstracts, 10*, 383.

Freedman, M., & Cermak, L. S. (1986). Semantic encoding deficits in frontal lobe disease and amnesia. *Brain and Cognition, 5*, 108–114.

Friedrich, F. J., Glenn, C. G., & Marin, O. S. M. (1984). Interruption of phonological coding in conduction aphasia. *Brain and Language, 22*, 266–291.

Frith, C. D., Bloxham, C. A., & Carpenter, K. N. (1986). Impairments in the learning and performance of a new manual skill on patients with Parkinson's disease. *Journal of Neurology, Neurosurgery and Psychiatry, 46*, 661–668.

Frith, C. D., Dowdy, J., Ferrier, I. N., & Crow, T. J. (1985). Selective impairment of paired associate learning after administration of a centrally-acting adrenergic agonist (clonidine). *Psychopharmacology, 87*, 490–493.

Frith, C. D., Stevens, M., Johnstone, E. C., Deakin, J. F., Lawler, P., & Crow, T. J. (1983). Effects of ECT and depression on various aspects of memory. *British Journal of Psychiatry, 142*, 610–617.

Gabrieli, J. D. E., Cohen, N. J., Huff, F. J., Hodgeson, J., & Corkin, S. (1984). Consequences of recent experience with forgotten words in amnesia. *Society for Neuroscience Abstracts, 10*, 383.

Gabrieli, J. D. E., Haimowitz, I., & Corkin, S. (1985). Constraints upon the acquisition of cognitive skills in amnesics: Studies with patient H. M. and patients with Alzheimer's disease. *Society for Neuroscience Abstracts, 11*, 458.

Gaffan, D. (1974). Recognition impaired and association intact in the memory of monkeys after transection of the fornix. *Journal of Comparative and Physiological Psychology, 86*, 1100–1109.

Gaffan, D., Saunders, R. C., Gaffan, E. A., Harrison, S., Shields, C., & Owen, M. J. (1984). Effects of fornix transection upon associative memory in monkeys: Role of the hippocampus in learned action. *Quarterly Journal of Experimental Psychology, 36B*, 173–222.

Gaffan, E. A., Gaffan, D., & Harrison, H. (1985, July). *Inferotemporal cortex: Visual identification and memory*. Paper presented at the meeting of the Experimental Psychology Society, Cambridge, England.

Gage, F. H., Bjorkland, A., Stenevi, U., Dunnett, S. B., & Kelly, P. A. T. (1984). Intrahippocampal septal grafts ameliorate learning impairments in aged rats. *Science, 225*, 533–536.

Gazzaniga, M. S. (1984). Advances in cognitive neurosciences: The problem of information storage in the human brain. In G. Lynch, J. L. McGaugh, & N. M. Weinberger (Eds.), *Neurobiology of learning and memory*. New York: Guilford Press.

Gjerde, P. F. (1983). Attentional capacity dysfunction and arousal in schizophrenia. *Psychological Bulletin, 93*, 57–72.

Glisky, E. L., Schacter, D. L., & Tulving, E. (1986). Computer learning by memory-impaired patients: Acquisition and retention of complex knowledge. *Neuropsychologia, 24*, 313–328.

Gold, P. E. (1984). Memory modulation: Roles of peripheral catecholamines. In L. R. Squire & N. Butters (Eds.), *Neuropsychology of memory*. New York: Guilford Press.

Goldberg, E., Hughes, J. E. I., Mattis, S., & Antin, S. (1982). Isolated retrograde amnesia: Different etiologies, same mechanisms? *Cortex, 18*, 459–462.

Goldman-Rakic, P. S. (1984). Modular organization of prefrontal cortex. *Trends in Neuroscience, 7*, 419–424.

Goodglass, H., Wingfield, A., Hydge, M. R., & Theurhauf, J. C. (1986). Category specific dissociations in naming and recognition by aphasic patients. *Cortex, 22*, 87–102.

Graf, P., & Schacter, D. L. (1985). Implicit and explicit memory for new associations in normal and amnesic subjects. *Journal of Experimental Psychology: Learning, Memory, and Cognition, 2*, 501–518.

Grafman, J., Vance, S. C., Weingartner, H., Salazar, A. M., & Amin, D. (submitted for publication). The effects of lateralized frontal lesions upon mood regulation.

Gray, J. A. (1982). *The neuropsychology of anxiety*. Oxford: Oxford University Press.

Gray, J. A., & Rawlins, J. N. P. (1986). Comparator and buffer memory: An attempt to integrate two models of hippocampal function. In R. L. Isaacson & K. H. Pribram (Eds.), *The hippocampus* (Vol. 4). New York: Plenum Press.

Greene, E., & Naranjo, J. N. (1986). Thalamic role in spatial memory. *Behavioral Brain Research, 19*, 123–131.

Halgren, E. (1984). Human hippocampal and amygdala recording and stimulation: Evidence for a neural model of recent memory. In L. R. Squire & N. Butters (Eds.), *Neuropsychology of memory*. New York: Guilford Press.

Halgren, E., Wilson, C. L., & Stapleton, J. M. (1985). Human medial temporal-lobe stimulation disrupts both formation and retrieval of recent memories. *Brain and Cognition, 4*, 287–295.

Hart, J., Berndt, R. S., & Caramazza, A. (1985). Category-specific naming deficit following cerebral infarction. *Nature, 316*, 439–440.

Hasher, L., & Zacks, R. T. (1979). Automatic and effortful processes in memory. *Journal of Experimental Psychology: General, 108*, 356–388.

Hawkins, R. D., & Kandel, E. R. (1984). Is there a cell biological alphabet for simple forms of learning? *Psychological Review, 91*, 375–391.

Hebb, D. O. (1949). *The organization of behavior*. New York: Wiley.

Heck, E. T., & Bryer, J. B. (1986). Superior sorting and categorizing ability in a case of bilateral frontal atrophy: An exception to the rule. *Journal of Clinical Psychology, 8*, 313–316.

Heindel, W. C., Butters, N., & Salmon, D. (1987). Impaired motor skill learning associated with neostriatal function. *Journal of Clinical and Experimental Neuropsychology, 9*, 18.

Hirst, W., (1985). Use of mnemonic in patients with frontal lobe damage. *Journal of Clinical and Experimental Neuropsychology, 7*, 175.

Hirst, W., Johnson, M. K., Kim, J. K., Phelps, E. A., Risse, G., & Volpe, B. T. (1986). Recognition and recall in amnesics. *Journal of Experimental Psychology: Learning, Memory, and Cognition, 12*, 445–451.

Hirst, W., & Volpe, B. T. (1982). Temporal order judgements with amnesia. *Brain and Cognition, 1*, 294–306.

Hirst, W., & Volpe, B. T. (1984). Automatic and effortful encoding in amnesia. In M. S. Gazzaniga (Ed.), *Handbook of cognitive neuroscience*. New York: Plenum Press.

Holmes, E. J., Jacobson, S., Stein, B. M., & Butters, N. (1983). Ablations of the mammillary nuclei in monkeys: Effects on postoperative memory. *Experimental Neurology, 81*, 97–113.

Horel, J. A. (1978). The neuroanatomy of amnesia: A critique of the hippocampal memory hypothesis. *Brain, 101*, 403–445.

Horel, J. A., Voytko, M. L., & Salsbury, K. G. (1984). Visual learning suppressed by cooling the temporal pole. *Behavioral Neuroscience, 98*, 310–324.

Horn, G. (1985). *Memory, imprinting and the brain*. Oxford: Oxford University Press.

Horton, D. L., & Mills, C. B. (1984). Human learning and memory. *Annual Review of Psychology, 35*, 361–394.

Huppert, F. A. (1981). Memory in split-brain patients: A comparison with organic amnesic syndromes. *Cortex, 17*, 303–312.

Huppert, F. A., & Piercy, M. (1978a). Dissociation between learning and remembering in organic amnesia. *Nature, 275*, 317–318.

Huppert, F. A., & Piercy, M. (1978b). The role of trace strength in recency and frequency judgements by amnesics and control subjects. *Quarterly Journal of Experimental Psychology, 30*, 346–354.

Huppert, F. A., & Piercy, M. (1979). Normal and abnormal forgetting in amnesia: Effect of locus of lesion. *Cortex, 15*, 385–390.

Hyman, B. T., Van Hoesen, G. W., Damasio, A. R., & Barnes, C. L. (1984). Alzheimer's disease: Cell specific pathology isolates the hippocampal formation. *Science, 225*, 1168–1170.

Isseroff, A., Rosvold, H. E., Galkin, T. W., & Goldman-Rakic, P. S. (1982). Spatial memory impairments following damage to the mediodorsal nucleus of the thalamus in rhesus monkeys. *Brain Research, 232*, 97–113.

Iversen, L. L., & Rosser, M. N. (1984). Human learning and memory dysfunction: Neurochemical changes in senile dementia. In G. Lynch, J. L. McGaugh, & N. M. Weinberger (Eds.), *Neurobiology of learning and memory*. New York: Guildford Press.

Izquierdo, I., & Netto, C. A. (1985). The brain beta-endorphin system and behavior: The modulation of consecutively and simultaneously processed memories. *Behavioral and Neural Biology, 44*, 249–265.

Jackson, J. L., Michon, J. A., Boonstra, H., DeJonge, D., & Harsenhorst, J. D. (1986). The effect of depth of processing on temporal judgement tasks. *Acta Psychologica, 62*, 199–210.

Jacoby, L. L. (in press). Memory observed and memory unobserved. In V. Neisser & E. Winograd (Eds.), *Real events remembered: Ecological approaches to the study of memory*. Cambridge: Cambridge University Press.

Jacoby, L. L., & Witherspoon, D. (1982). Remembering without awareness. *Canadian Journal of Psychology, 36*, 300–324.

Jarrard, L. E. (1980). Selective hippocampal lesions and behavior. *Physiological Psychology, 8*, 198–206.

Jarrard, L. E. (1986). Selective hippocampal lesions and behavior: Implications for current research and theorizing. In R. L. Isaacson & K. H. Pribram (Eds.), *The hippocampus* (Vol. 4). New York: Plenum Press.

Jetter, W., Poser, U., Freeman, R. B., Jr., & Markowitsch, H. T. (1986). A verbal long-term memory deficit in frontal lobe damaged patients. *Cortex, 22*, 229–242.

Johnson, M. K., Kim, J. K., & Risse, G. (1985). Do alcoholic Korsakoff's syndrome patients acquire affective reactions? *Journal of Experimental Psychology: Learning, Memory, and Cognition, 11*, 22–36.

Jones, G. V. (1979). Analyzing memory by cueing: Intrinsic and extrinsic knowledge. In N. S. Sutherland (Ed.), *Tutorial essays in psychology: A guide to recent advances* (Vol. 2). Hillsdale, N. J.: Erlbaum.

Jurko, M. F. (1978). Center median 'alerting' and verbal learning dysfunction. *Brain and Language, 5*, 98–102.

Kapur, N. (1985). Double dissociation between perseveration in memory and problem solving tasks. *Cortex, 21*, 461–465.

Kapur, N., Heath, P., Meudell, P., & Kennedy, P. (1986). Amnesia can facilitate memory performance: Evidence from a patient with dissociated retrograde amnesia. *Neuropsychologia, 24*, 215–221.

Kausler, D. H. (1987). Aging and automaticity of memory. *Journal of Clinical and Experimental Neuropsychology, 9*, 19.

Kay, J., & Ellis, A. (1987). A cognitive neuropsychological case study of anomia: Implications for psychological models of word retrieval. *Brain, 110*, 613–629.

Kellogg, R. T. (1980). Is conscious attention necessary for long-term storage? *Journal of Experimental Psychology: Human Learning and Memory, 6*, 379–390.

Kinsbourne, M. (1972). Behavioral analysis of the repetition deficit in conduction aphasia. *Neurology, 22*, 1126–1132.

Kinsbourne, M., & Warrington, E. K. (1962). A disorder of simultaneous form perception. *Brain, 85*, 461–486.

Koh, S. D. (1978). Remembering of verbal materials by schizophrenic young adults. In S. Schwartz (Ed.), *Language and cognition in schizophrenia*. Hillsdale, N. J.: Erlbaum.

Kohl, D. A. (1984). *An automatic encoding deficit in the amnesia of Korsakoff's syndrome*. Unpublished doctoral dissertation, Johns Hopkins University.

Kolb, B., & Whishaw, I. Q. (1983). Performance of schizophrenic patients on tests sensitive to left or right frontal, temporal, or parietal function in neurological patients. *Journal of Nervous and Mental Diseases, 171*.

Kolb, B., & Whishaw, I. Q. (1985). *Fundamentals of human neuropsychology* (2nd ed.). New York: Freeman.

Kopelman, M. D. (1985). Rates of forgetting in Alzheimer-type dementia and Korsakoff's syndrome. *Neuropsychologia, 23*, 623–638.

Kopelman, M. D. (1986). The cholinergic neurotransmitter system in human memory and dementia: A review. *Quarterly Journal of Experimental Psychology, 38A*, 535–574.

Kovacs, G. L., Bohus, B., & Versteeg, D. H. G. (1979). The effects of vasopressin on memory processes: The role of noradrenergic neurotransmission. *Neuroscience, 4*, 1529–1537.

Kowalska, D. M., Bachevalier, J., & Mishkin, M. (1984). Inferior prefrontal cortex and recognition memory. *Society for Neuroscience Abstracts, 10*, 385.

Kubie, J. L., & Ranck, J. B., Jr. (1983). Sensory-behavioral correlates in individual hippocampal neurons in three situations: Space and context. In W. Seifert (Ed.), *Neurobiology of the hippocampus*. New York: Academic Press.

Kunst-Wilson, W. R., & Zajonc, R. B. (1979). Affective discrimination of stimuli that cannot be recognized. *Science, 207*, 557–558.

Leiner, H., Leiner, A. L., & Dow, R. S. (1986). Does the cerebellum contribute to mental skills? *Behavioral Neuroscience, 100*, 443–454.

Levin, H. S., High, W. M., & Eisenberg, H. (1987). Learning and forgetting during and after post traumatic amnesia in head injured patients. *Society for Neuroscience Abstracts, 13*, 205.

Levin, H. S., High, W. M., Meyers, C. A., Von Laufen, A., Hayden, M. E., & Eisenberg, H. M. (1985). Impairment of remote memory after closed head injury. *Journal of Neurology, Neurosurgery and Psychiatry, 48*, 556–563.

Liddle, P. F., & Crow, T. J. (1984). Age disorientation in chronic schizophrenia is associated with global intellectual impairment. *British Journal of Psychiatry, 144*, 193–199.

Lloyd, P., Mayes, A., Manstead, A. S. R., Meudell, P. R., & Wagner, H. L. (1984). *Introduction to psychology: An integrated approach*. London: Fontana.

Luria, A. R. (1973). *The working brain*. Harmondsworth: Penguin.

Lynch, G., & Baudry, M. (1984). The biochemistry of memory: A new and specific hypothesis. *Science, 224*, 1057–1063.

Mackintosh, N. J. (1985). Varieties of conditioning. In N. M. Weinberger, J. L. McGaugh, & G. Lynch (Eds.), *Memory systems of the brain*. New York: Guilford Press.

Mair, W. G. P., Warrington, E. K., & Weiskrantz, L. (1979). Memory disorders in Korsakoff's psychosis: A neuropathological and neuropsychological investigation of two cases. *Brain, 102*, 749–783.

Mandler, G. (1980). Recognizing: The judgement of previous occurrence. *Psychological Review, 87*, 252–271.

Maragos, W. F., Greenamyre, J. T., Penney, J. B., & Young, A. B. (1987). Glutamate dysfunction in Alzheimer's disease: An hypothesis. *Trends in Neuroscience, 10*, 65–68.

Marcel, A. J. (1983). Conscious and unconscious perception: Experience and perceptual processes. *Cognitive Psychology, 15*, 238–300.

Maring, W., Deelman, B. G., & Brouwer, W. (1984, April). Retrieval from (very) long term memory after closed head injury. *INS Bulletin*, p. 14.

Markowitsch, H. J. (1985). Hypotheses on mnemonic information processing by the brain. *International Journal of Neuroscience, 27*, 191–227.

Markowitsch, H. J., & Pritzel, M. (1985). The neuropathology of amnesia. *Progress in Neurobiology, 25*, 189–287.

Marslen-Wilson, W. D., & Teuber, H. L. (1975). Memory for remote events in anterograde amnesia: Recognition of public figures from newsphotographs. *Neuropsychologia, 13*, 353–364.

Martone, M., Butters, N., Payne, M., Becker, J. T., & Sax, D. S. (1984). Dissociations between skill learning and verbal recognition in amnesia and dementia. *Archives of Neurology, 41*, 965–970.

Mayes, A. R. (1986). Learning and memory disorders and their assessment. *Neuropsychologia, 24*, 25–39.

Mayes, A. R. (1987). Varieties of human organic memory disorder. In H. Beloff & A. M. Colman (Eds.), *Psychology survey 6*. Leicester: BPS Press.

Mayes, A., & Meudell, P. (1983). Amnesia in humans and other animals. In A. Mayes (Ed.), *Memory in animals and humans*. Wokingham: Van Nostrand Reinhold.

Mayes, A. R., Meudell, P. R., & Pickering, A. (1985). Is organic amnesia caused by a selective deficit in remembering contextual information? *Cortex, 21*, 167–202.

Mayes, A. R., Meudell, P. R., & Som, S. (1981). Further similarities between amnesia and normal attenuated memory: Effects with paired-associate learning and context-shifts. *Neuropsychologia, 19*, 655–664.

Mayes, A. R., Pickering, A., & Fairbairn, A. (1987). Amnesic sensitivity to proactive interference: Its relationship to priming and the causes of amnesia. *Neuropsychologia, 25*, 211–220.

McCarthy, R., & Warrington, E. K. (1985a). A two-route model of speech production: Evidence from aphasia. *Brain, 107*, 463–485.

McCarthy, R., & Warrington, E. K. (1985b). Category specificity in an agrammatic patient: The relative impairment of verb retrieval and comprehension. *Neuropsychologia, 23*, 709–727.

McCarthy, R. A., & Warrington, E. K. (1987). Understanding: A function of short-term memory? *Brain, 110*, 1565–1578.

McCleod, P., & Posner, M. (1984). Privileged loops from percept to act, in D. G. Bouma & H. Bouwhuis (Eds.), *Attention and performance, X*. Hillsdale, N.J.: Erlbaum.

McDowall, J. (1979). Effects of encoding instructions and retrieval cueing on recall in Korsakoff patients. *Memory and Cognition, 7*, 232–239.

McEntee, W. J., & Mair, R. G. (1978). Memory impairment in Korsakoff's psychosis: A correlation with brain noradrenergic activity. *Science, 202*, 905–907.

McEntee, W. J., & Mair, R. G. (1984). Some behavioral consequences of neurochemical deficits in Korsakoff psychosis. In L. R. Squire & N. Butters (Eds.), *Neuropsychology of memory*. New York: Guilford Press.

McKenna, P., & Warrington, E. K. (1980). Testing for nominal dysphasia. *Journal of Neurology, Neurosurgery and Psychiatry, 43*, 781–788.

McNaughton, B. L., & Barnes, C. A. (1985). The hippocampus, synaptic enhancement and intermediate-term memory. *Behavioral and Brain Sciences, 8*, 507–508.

Meudell, P. (1983). The development and dissolution of memory. In A. R. Mayes (Ed.), *Memory in animals and humans*. Wokingham: Van Nostrand Reinhold.

Meudell, P., & Mayes, A. (1981). The Claparède phenomenon: A further example in amnesics, a demonstration of a similar effect in controls and a reinterpretation. *Current Psychological Research, 1*, 75–88.

Meudell, P. R., Mayes, A. R., Ostergaard, A., & Pickering, A. (1985). Recency and frequency judgements in alcoholic amnesics and normal people with poor memory. *Cortex, 21*, 487–511.

Milner, B. (1971). Interhemispheric differences in the localization of psychological processes in man. *British Medical Bulletin, 27*, 272–277.

Milner, B., Petrides, M., & Smith, M. L. (1985). Frontal lobes and the temporal organization of memory. *Human Neurobiology, 4*, 137–142.

Mishkin, M. (1978). Memory in monkeys severely impaired by combined but not separate removal of amygdala and hippocampus. *Nature, 273*, 297–298.

Mishkin, M. (1982). A memory system in the monkey. *Philosophical Transactions of the Royal Society of London B, 298*, 85–95.

Mishkin, M., & Bachevalier, J. (1983). Object recognition impaired by ventromedial but not dorsolateral prefrontal cortical lesions in monkeys. *Society for Neuroscience Abstracts, 9*, 29.

Mishkin, M., Malamut, B., & Bachevalier, J. (1984). Memories and habits: Two neural systems. In G. Lynch, J. L. McGaugh, & N. M. Weinberger (Eds.), *Neurobiology of learning and memory*. New York: Guilford Press.

Morris, R. G. M., Anderson, E., Lynch, G. S., & Baudry, M. (1986). Selective impairment of learning and blockade of long-term potentiation by an N-methyl-D-aspartate receptor antagonist, AP5. *Nature, 319*, 774–776.

Morton, J., Hammersley, R. H., & Bekerian, D. A. (1985). Headed records: A model for memory and its failures. *Cognition, 20*, 1–23.

Moscovitch, M. (1982). Multiple dissociations of function in amnesia. In L. S. Cermak (Ed.), *Human memory and amnesia*. Hillsdale, N.J.: Erlbaum.

Moscovitch, M. (1985). Memory from infancy to old age: Implications for theories of normal and pathological memory. *Annals of the New York Academy of Sciences, 444*, 78–96.

Murray, E. A., & Mishkin, M. (1985a). Amygdalectomy impairs crossmodal association in monkeys. *Science, 228*, 604–606.

Murray, E. A., & Mishkin, M. (1985b). Severe tactual as well as visual memory deficits follow combined removal of the amygdala and hippocampus in monkeys. *Journal of Neuroscience, 4*, 2565–2580.

Nelson, T. O., & Vining, S. K. (1978). Effects of semantic versus structural processing on long-term retention. *Journal of Experimental Psychology: Human Learning and Memory, 4*, 198–209.

Newcombe, F. (1985). Neuropsychology qua interface. *Journal of Clinical and Experimental Neuropsychology, 7*, 663–681.

Nielsen, J. M. (1958). *Memory and amnesia*. Los Angeles: San Lucas Press.

Nissen, M. J., & Bullemer, P. (1987). Attentional requirements of learning: Evidence from performance measures. *Cognitive Psychology*, *19*, 1–32.

Oakley, D. A. (1983). The varieties of memory: A phylogenetic approach. In A. R. Mayes (Ed.), *Memory in humans and animals*. Wokingham: Van Nostrand Reinhold.

Ogden, J. A. (1985). Autotopagnosia: Occurrence in a patient without nominal aphasia and with an intact ability to point to parts of animals and objects. *Brain*, *108*, 1009–1022.

Ojemann, G. A. (1983). The intrahemispheric organization of human language, derived with electrical stimulation techniques. *Trends in Neurosciences*, *6*, 184–189.

O'Keefe, J., & Nadel, L. (1978). *The hippocampus as a cognitive map*. Oxford: Clarendon Press.

Owen, M. J., & Butler, S. R. (1981). Amnesia after transection of the fornix in monkeys. Long-term memory impaired, short-term memory intact. *Behavioural Brain Research*, *3*, 115–123.

Parkin, A. (1986). *Human memory and its pathology*. Oxford: Blackwell.

Parkin, A. J., & Leng, N. R. C. (1987). Comparative studies of human amnesia. In H. Markowitsch (Ed.), *Information processing and the brain*. Toronto: Huber.

Parkinson, J. K., & Mishkin, M. (1982). A selective mnemonic role for the hippocampus in monkeys: Memory for the location of objects. *Society for Neuroscience Abstracts*, *8*, 23.

Passingham, R. E. (1985). Memory of monkeys (*Macaca mulatta*) with lesions in prefrontal cortex. *Behavioral Neuroscience*, *99*, 3–21.

Penfield, W., & Mathieson, G. (1974). Memory: Autopsy findings and comments on the role of the hippocampus in experiential recall. *Archives of Neurology*, *31*, 145–154.

Phillips, C. G., Zeki, S., & Barlow, H. B. (1984). Localization of function in the cerebral cortex: past, present and future. *Brain*, *107*, 328–361.

Pickering, A. (1987). *Does amnesia arise from a specific deficit in memory for contextual information?* Unpublished doctoral dissertation, Manchester University.

Rawlins, J. N. P. (1985). Associations across time: The hippocampus as a temporary memory store. *Behavioral and Brain Sciences*, *8*, 479–496.

Regard, M., & Landis, T. (1984). Transient global amnesia: Neuropsychological dysfunction during attack and recovery of two 'pure' cases. *Journal of Neurology, Neurosurgery and Psychiatry*, *47*, 668–672.

Rocchetta, A. I. della (1986). Classification and recall of pictures after unilateral frontal or temporal lobectomy. *Cortex*, *22*, 189–211.

Roland, P. E. (1984) Metabolic measurements of the working frontal cortex in man. *Trends in Neurosciences*, *7*, 430–435.

Rolls, E. T. (1984). Neurophysiological investigations of different types of memory in the primate. In L. R. Squire & N. Butters (Eds.), *Neuropsychology of memory*. New York: Guilford Press.

Rolls, E. T. (1986). Information representation processing, and storage in the brain: Analysis at the single neuron level. In J.-P. Changeux & M. Konishi (Eds.), *Neural and molecular mechanisms of learning*. Berlin: Springer-Verlag.

Ross, E. D. (1982). Disorders of recent memory in humans. *Trends in Neurosciences*, *5*, 170–172.

Roth, M., & Iversen, L. L. (Eds.). (1986). Alzheimer's disease. *British Medical Bulletin*, *42*.

Routtenberg, A. (1984). The CA3 pyramidal cell in the hippocampus: Site of intrinsic expression and extrinsic control of memory formation. In L. R. Squire & N. Butters (Eds.), *Neuropsychology of memory*. New York: Guilford Press.

Roy-Byrne, P. P., Weingartner, H., Bierer, L. M., Thompson, K., & Post, R. M. (1986). Effortful and automatic cognitive processes in depression. *Archives of General Psychiatry*, *43*, 265–267.

Russell, W. R. (1971). *The traumatic amnesias*. Oxford: Oxford University Press.

Sabol, K. E., Neill, D. B., Wages, S. A., Church, W. H., & Justice, J. B. (1985). Dopamine depletion in a striatal subregion disrupts performance on a skilled motor task in the rat. *Brain Research*, *335*, 33–43.

Sagar, H. J., Sullivan, E. V., Cohen, N. J., Gabrieli, S., Corking, S., & Growdon, J. (1985). Specific cognitive deficit in Parkinson's disease. *Journal of Clinical and Experimental Neuropsychology*, *7*, 158.

Saint-Cyr, J. A., Taylor, A. E., & Lang, A. E. (1987). Procedural learning impairment in basal ganglia disease. *Journal of Clinical and Experimental Neuropsychology*, *9*, 280.

Salmon, D. P., Zola-Morgan, S., & Squire, L. R. (1987). Retrograde amnesia following combined hippocampus-amygdala lesions. *Psychobiology*, *15*, 37–47.

Samuels, I., Butters, N., & Fedio, P. (1972). Short-term memory disorders following temporal lobe removals in humans. *Cortex*, *9*, 283–298.

Sanders, H. I., & Warrington, E. K. (1971). Memory for remote events in amnesic patients. *Brain*, *94*. 661–668.

Sarter, M., & Markowitsch, H. J. (1985). The amygdala's role in human mnemonic processing. *Cortex*, *21*, 7–24.

Sass, K. J., Novelly, R. A., & Spencer, D. D. (1987). Memory and callosotomy: Series I. *Journal of Clinical and Experimental Neuropsychology*, *9*, 63.

Saunders, R. C., & Mishkin, M. (1987). The effects of separate and combined lesions of the bed nucleus of the stria terminalis and the fornix on recognition memory. *Society for Neuroscience Abstracts*, *13*, 207.

Saunders, R. C., Murray, E. A., & Mishkin, M. (1984). Further evidence that amygdala and hippo-campus contribute equally to recognition memory. *Neuropsychologia*, *22*, 785–796.

Schacter, D. L. (1985). Priming of old and new knowledge in amnesic patients and normal subjects. *Annals of the New York Academy of Sciences*, *444*, 41–53.

Schacter, D. L. (1986). Amnesia and crime: How much do we really know? *American Psychologist*, *41*, 286–295.

Schacter, D. L. (1987a). Memory, amnesia and frontal lobe dysfunction. *Psychobiology*, *15*, 21–36.

Schacter, D. L. (1987b). Implicit memory: History and current status. *Journal of Experimental Psychology: Learning, Memory, and Cognition*, *13*, 501–518.

Schacter, D. L., Harbluk, J. L., & McLachlan, D. R. (1984). Retrieval without recollection: An experimental analysis of source amnesia. *Journal of Verbal Learning and Verbal Behavior*, *23*, 593–611.

Schacter, D. L., Wang, P. L., Tulving, E., & Freedman, M. (1982). Functional retrograde amnesia: A quantitative case study. *Neuropsychologia*, *20*, 523–532.

Shallice, T. (1982). Several impairments of planning. *Philosophical Transactions of the Royal Society of London B*, *298*, 199–209.

Shallice, T. (1986). Impairments of semantic processing: Multiple dissociations. In M. Colt-heart, M. Job, & G. Sartori (Eds.), *The cognitive psychology of language*. Hillsdale, N.J.: Erlbaum.

Shallice, T., & Warrington, E. K. (1979). Auditory–verbal short-term memory impairment and conduction aphasia. *Brain and Language*, *4*, 479–491.

Sheremata, W. (1984). Decreased cortical activation with random word recall in multiple sclerosis. *INS Bulletin*, 58–59.

Shimamura, A. P. (1986). Priming effects in amnesia: Evidence for a dissociable memory function. *Quarterly Journal of Experimental Psychology*, *38A*, 619–644.

Shimamura, A. P., Salmon, D. P., Squire, L. R., & Butters, N. (1987). Memory dysfunction unique to Alzheimer's disease: Impairment in word priming. *Journal of Clinical and Experimental Neuropsychology*, *9*, 20.

Shimamura, A. P., & Squire, L. R. (1986a). Korsakoff's syndrome: A study of the relation between anterograde amnesia and remote memory impairment. *Behavioral Neuroscience*, *100*, 165–170.

Shimamura, A. P., & Squire, L. R. (1986b). Memory and metamemory: A study of the feeling of knowing phenomenon in amnesic patients. *Journal of Experimental Psychology: Learning, Memory, and Cognition*, *12*, 452–460.

Shimamura, A. P., & Squire, L. R. (1987). A neuropsychological study of fact memory and source amnesia. *Journal of Experimental Psychology: Learning, Memory, and Cognition*, *13*, 464–473.

Shoqeirat, M. (1986). *Is schizophrenia caused by frontal and temporal lobe lesions?* Unpublished master's thesis, University of Manchester.

Signoret, J. L., & Lhemitte, F. (1976). *The amnesic syndromes and the encoding process*. Cambridge, Mass.: MIT Press.

Sperry, R. W. (1974). Lateral specialization in the surgically separated hemispheres. In F. O. Schmitt & F. G. Worden (Eds.), *The neurosciences: Third study program*. Cambridge, Mass.: MIT Press.

Squire, L. R. (1981). Two forms of amnesia: An analysis of forgetting. *Journal of Neuroscience, 1*, 633–640.

Squire, L. R. (1982). Comparisons between forms of amnesia: Some deficits are unique to Korsakoff's syndrome. *Journal of Experimental Psychology: Learning, Memory, and Cognition, 8*, 560–571.

Squire, L. R. (1986). Mechanisms of memory. *Science, 232*, 1612–1619.

Squire, L. R. (1987). *Memory and brain*. Oxford: Oxford University Press.

Squire, L. R., Amaral, D. G., Zola-Morgan, S., Kritchersky, M., & Press, G. (1987). New evidence of brain injury in the amnesic patient N.A. based on magnetic resonance imaging. *Society for Neuroscience Abstracts, 13*, 1454.

Squire, L. R., & Cohen, N. J. (1982). Remote memory, retrograde amnesia, and the neuropsychology of memory. In L. S. Cermak (Eds.), *Human memory and amnesia*. Hillsdale, N.J.: Erlbaum.

Squire, L. R., & Cohen, N. J. (1984). Human memory and amnesia. In G. Lynch, J. L. McGaugh, & N. M. Weinberger (Eds.), *Psychobiology of learning and memory*. New York: Guilford Press.

Squire, L. R., Cohen, N. J., & Nadel, L. (1984). The medial temporal region and memory consolidation: A new hypothesis. In H. Weingartner & E. S. Parker (Eds.), *Memory consolidation*. Hillsdale, N.J.: Erlbaum.

Squire, L. R., & Moore, R. Y. (1979). Dorsal thalamic lesion in a noted case of human memory dysfunction. *Annals of Neurology, 6*, 503–506.

Squire, L. R., & Zola-Morgan, S. (1985). The neuropsychology of memory: New links between humans and experimental animals. *Annals of the New York Academy of Sciences, 444*, 137–149.

Staubli, U., Fraser, D., Kessler, M., & Lynch, G. (1986). Studies on retrograde and anterograde amnesia of olfactory memory after denervation of the hippocampus by entorhinal cortex lesions. *Behavioral and Neural Biology, 46*, 432–444.

Strub, R. L., & Gardner, H. (1974). The repetition deficit in conduction aphasia: Mnestic or linguistic? *Brain and Language, 1*, 241–255.

Stuss, D. T., & Benson, D. F. (1984). Neuropsychological studies of the frontal lobes. *Psychological Bulletin, 95*, 3–28.

Stuss, D., Kaplan, E. F., Benson, D. F., Weir, W. S., Chulli, S., & Sarazin, F. F. (1982). Evidence for the involvement of orbitofrontal cortex in memory functions: An interference effect. *Journal of Comparative and Physiological Psychology, 96*, 913–925.

Summers, W. K., Majovski, L. V., Marsh, G. M., Tachiki, K., & Kling, A. (1986). Oral tetrahydroaminoacridine in long term treatment of senile dementia, Alzheimer type. *New England Journal of Medicine, 315*, 1241–1245.

Temple, C. M. (1986). Anomia for animals in a child. *Brain, 109*, 1225–1242.

Teyler, T. J., & DiScenna, P. (1986). The hippocampal memory indexing theory. *Behavioral Neuroscience, 100*, 147–154.

Thompson, R. E. (1986). The neurobiology of learning and memory. *Science, 233*, 941–947.

Timsit-Berthier, M., Mantanus, H., Jacques, M. C., & Legros, J. J. (1980). Utilité de la lysine vasopressine dans la traitement de l'amnesie post-traumatique. *Acta Psychiatrica Belgica, 80*, 728–747.

Tranel, D., & Damasio, A. R. (1985). Knowledge without awareness: An autonomic index of facial recognition. *Science, 228*, 1453–1454.

Troster, A. I., Staton, R. D., Rorabaugh, A. G., & Beatty, W. W. (1987). Effects of scopolamine on remote and anterograde memory. A test of the cholinergic hypothesis of Alzheimer's disease. *Journal of Clinical and Experimental Neuropsychology, 9*, 17.

Tulving, E. (1984). Précis of Elements of Episodic Memory. *Behavioral and Brain Sciences, 7*, 223–268.

Tyler, S. W., Hertel, P. T., McCallum, M. C., & Ellis, H. C. (1979). Cognitive effort and memory. *Journal of Experimental Psychology: Human Learning and Memory, 5*, 607–617.

Vallar, G., & Baddeley, A. D. (1984). Fractionation of working memory: Neuropsychological evidence for a phonological short-term store. *Journal of Verbal Learning and Verbal Behavior, 23*, 151–161.

Vallar, G., & Papagno, C. (1985). *Phonological short-term store and the nature of recency effect. Evidence from neuropsychology.* Paper presented at the International Meeting on Cognitive Neuropsychology, Venice, Italy.

Van Hoesen, G. W. (1985). Neural systems of the non-human primate forebrain implicated in memory. *Annals of the New York Academy of Sciences, 444*, 97–112.

Victor, M., Adams, R. D., & Collins, G. H. (1971). *The Wernicke-Korsakoff syndrome. A clinical and pathological study of 245 patients, 82 with post-mortem examinations.* Oxford: Blackwell.

Volpe, B. T., Holtzman, J. D., & Hirst, W. (1986). Further characterization of patients with amnesia after cardiac arrest: Preserved recognition memory. *Neurology, 36*, 408–411.

Volpe, B. T., Pulsineli, W. A., Tribuna, J., & Davis, H. P. (1984). Behavioural performance of rats following transient forebrain ischemia. *Stroke, 15*, 558–562.

Von Cramon, D. Y., Hebel, N., & Schuri, U. (1985). A contribution to the anatomical basis of thalamic amnesia. *Brain, 108*, 993–1008.

Warrington, E. K. (1975). The selective impairment of semantic memory. *Quarterly Journal of Experimental Psychology, 24*, 30–40.

Warrington, E. K. (1982). The fractionation of arithmetical knowledge skills: A single case study. *Quarterly Journal of Experimental Psychology, 34A*, 31–52.

Warrington, E. K. (1984). *Recognition memory test.* Windsor: NFER-Nelson.

Warrington, E. K., Galton, M., & Maciejewski, C. (1985). The WAIS as a lateralising and localising diagnostic instrument: A study of 656 patients with unilateral cerebral lesions. *Neuropsychologia, 24*, 223–240.

Warrington, E. K., & McCarthy, R. A. (1986). Neurological disorders of memory. In A. K. Asbury, G. N. McKhann, & W. J. McDonald (Eds.), *Diseases of the nervous system.* London: Ardmore Medical Books.

Warrington, E. K., & McCarthy, R. A. (1987). Categories of knowledge: Further fractionation and an attempted integration. *Brain, 110*, 1273–1296.

Warrington, E. K., & Rabin, P. (1971). Visual span of apprehension in patients with unilateral cerebral lesions. *Quarterly Journal of Experimental Psychology, 23*, 423–431.

Warrington, E. K., & Shallice, T. (1984). Category specific semantic impairments. *Brain, 107*, 829–855.

Warrington, E. K., & Taylor, A. M. (1973). Immediate memory for faces: Long- or short-term memory? *Quarterly Journal of Experimental Psychology, 25*, 316–322.

Warrington, E. K., & Weiskrantz, L. (1974). The effect of prior learning on subsequent retention in amnesic patients. *Neuropsychologia, 12*, 419–428.

Warrington, E. K., & Weiskrantz, L. (1982). A disconnection syndrome? *Neuropsychologia, 20*, 233–248.

Weinberger, D. R., Berman, K. F., & Zec, R. F. (1986). Physiologic dysfunction of dorsolateral prefrontal cortex in schizophrenia. *Archives of General Psychiatry, 43*, 114–124.

Weingartner, H., Gold, T., Ballenger, J. C., Mallberg, S. A., Summers, R., Rubinow, D. R., Post, R. M., & Goodwin, F. K. (1981). Effect of vasopressin on human memory function. *Science, 211*, 602–604.

Weingartner, H., Grafman, J., Boutelle, W., & Martin, P. (1983). Forms of cognitive failures. *Science, 221*, 380–382.

Weiskrantz, L. (1985). On issues and theories of the human amnesic syndrome. In N. M. Weinberger, J. L. McGaugh, & G. Lynch (Eds.), *Memory systems of the brain.* New York: Guilford Press.

Weiskrantz, L., & Warrington, E. K. (1979). Conditioning in amnesic patients. *Neuropsychologia*, *17*, 187–194.

Wickelgren, W. A. (1974). Single trace fragility theory of memory dynamics. *Memory and Cognition*, *2*, 775–780.

Wickelgren, W. A. (1979). Chunking and consolidation: A theoretical synthesis of semantic networks, configuring in conditioning, S-R versus cognitive learning, normal forgetting, the amnesic syndrome, and the hippocampal arousal system. *Psychological Review*, *86*, 44–60.

Wilkins, A. J., Shallice, T., & McCarthy, R. (1987). Frontal lesions and sustained attention. *Neuropsychologia*, *25*, 359–366.

Wilson, B. A., & Cockburn, J. (1988). The prices test: A simple test of retrograde amnesia. In M. M. Gruneberg, R. N. Sykes, & P. Morris (Eds.), *Practical aspects of memory—two*. New York: Wiley.

Winocur, G. (1985). The hippocampus and time. *Behavioral and Brain Sciences*, *8*, 512–513.

Winocur, G., & Kinsbourne, M. (1978). Contextual cueing as an aid to Korsakoff amnesics. *Neuropsychologia*, *16*, 671–682.

Winocur, G., Oxbury, S., Roberts, R., Agnetti, V., & Davis, C. (1984). Amnesia in a patient with bilateral lesions to the thalamus. *Neuropsychologia*, *22*, 123–143.

Yarnell, P. R., & Lynch, S. (1973). The ding: Amnestic states in football trauma. *Neurology*, *23*, 196–197.

Zola-Morgan, S., Cohen, N. J., & Squire, L. R. (1983). Recall of remote episodic memory in amnesia. *Neuropsychologia*, *21*, 487–500.

Zola-Morgan, S., Dabrowska, J., Moss, M., & Mahut, M. (1983). Enhanced preference for perceptual novelty in the monkey after section of the fornix but not after ablation of the hippocampus. *Neuropsychologia*, *21*, 433–454.

Zola-Morgan, S., & Squire, L. R. (1982). Two forms of amnesia in monkeys: Rapid forgetting after medial temporal lesions but not diencephalic lesions. *Society for Neuroscience Abstracts*, *8*, 24.

Zola-Morgan, S., Squire, L. R., & Mishkin, M. (1982). The neuroanatomy of amnesia: Amygdala–hippocampus versus temporal stem. *Science*, *218*, 1337–1339.

Zornetzer, S. F. (1985). Catecholamine system involvement in age-related memory dysfunction. *Annals of the New York Academy of Sciences*, *444*, 242–254.

Index